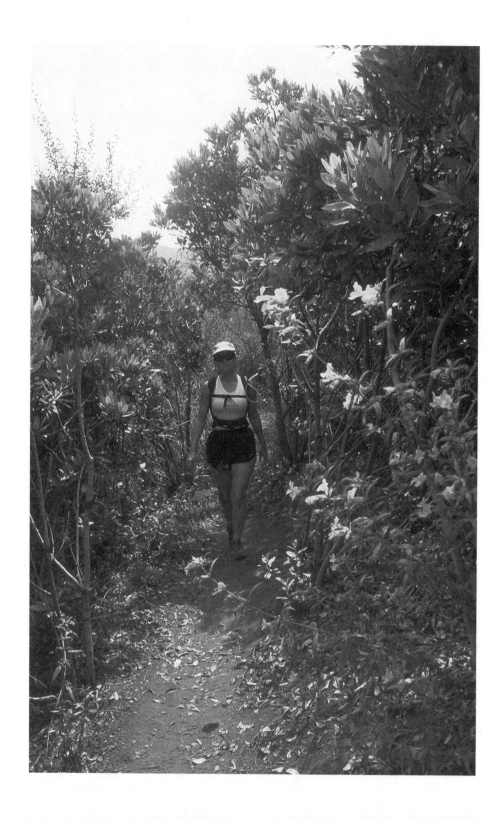

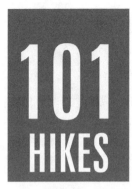

101 HIKES

in Southern California

Exploring Mountains, Seashore, and Desert

Jerry Schad

 WILDERNESS PRESS · BERKELEY, CA

101 Hikes in Southern California

1st EDITION July 1996
2nd EDITION February 2005
  2nd Printing November 2005

Copyright © 1996, 2005 by Jerry Schad

Front cover photos copyright © 2005 by Jerry Schad
Interior photos: Jerry Schad
Maps: Jerry Schad
Cover and book design: Larry B. Van Dyke
Book editor: Roslyn Bullas

ISBN 0-89997-351-5
UPC 7-19609-97351-5

Manufactured in the United States of America

Published by: **Wilderness Press**
                1200 5th Street
                Berkeley, CA 94710
                (800) 443-7227; FAX (510) 558-1696
                info@wildernesspress.com
                www.wildernesspress.com

Visit our website for a complete listing of our books and for ordering information.

Cover photos:	California poppies and Englemann oak *(background);*
	West shoulder of Whale Peak, Anza-Borrego Desert State Park *(top inset);*
	Holy Jim Falls, Cleveland National Forest *(bottom inset)*
Frontispiece:	Hiking through chaparrel,
	Santa Monica Mountains National Recreation Area

SAFETY NOTICE: Although Wilderness Press and the author have made every attempt to ensure that the information in this book is accurate at press time, they are not responsible for any loss, damage, injury, or inconvenience that may occur to anyone while using this book. You are responsible for your own safety and health. The fact that a trail is described in this book does not mean that it will be safe for you. Be aware that trail conditions can change from day to day. Always check local conditions and know your own limitations.

Preface

Just beyond the limits of Southern California's ever-spreading urban sprawl lies a world apart. In snippets of open space here, and in sprawling wilderness areas there, California's primeval landscape survives more or less untarnished. In hundreds of hidden places just over the urban horizon (and sometimes within the cities themselves), you can still find Nature's radiant beauty unfettered—or at least not too seriously compromised—by human intervention.

My purpose in writing this book is to entice you to explore some of these hidden places. In the pages ahead you will find updated versions of trips previously published in my *Afoot & Afield* series of guidebooks on Los Angeles, Orange, and San Diego counties, plus additional trips from eastern Ventura County, western San Bernardino County, and western Riverside County—a total of 101 hikes described in detail. The 101 Hikes Key Map on pages x and xi reveals how the majority of hikes chosen for this book cluster around the major urban areas of Los Angeles, Orange County, and San Diego. As a result, no matter where you live within Southern California, it is likely that 50 or more of these hikes are accessible to you in less than a two-hour drive.

Users of the *Afoot & Afield* books will already be familiar with the format and layout of this book. Each hike description includes a capsulized summary with icons allowing you to determine at a glance the nature and difficulty of the trip. Each trip is plotted on an easy-to-read sketch map. Photos of scenery and interesting features on or near the trails are sprinkled throughout the book.

All hikes described in this book were hiked at least once by me at one time or another, and every effort has been made to ensure that the information contained herein is up-to-date. Roads, trailheads, and trails can and do change every year, however. You can keep me apprised of recent developments and/or changes by writing me in care of Wilderness Press, or e-mailing me at schadj@worldnet.att.net. Your comments will be appreciated.

Jerry Schad
La Mesa, California
December 2004

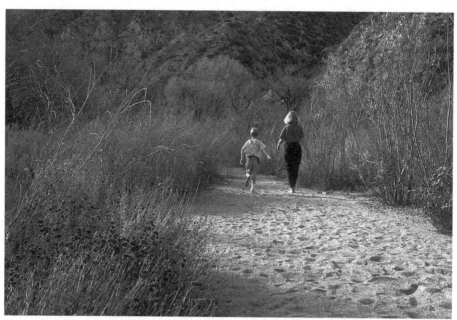

Lower Big Morongo Canyon (Hike 41)

Contents

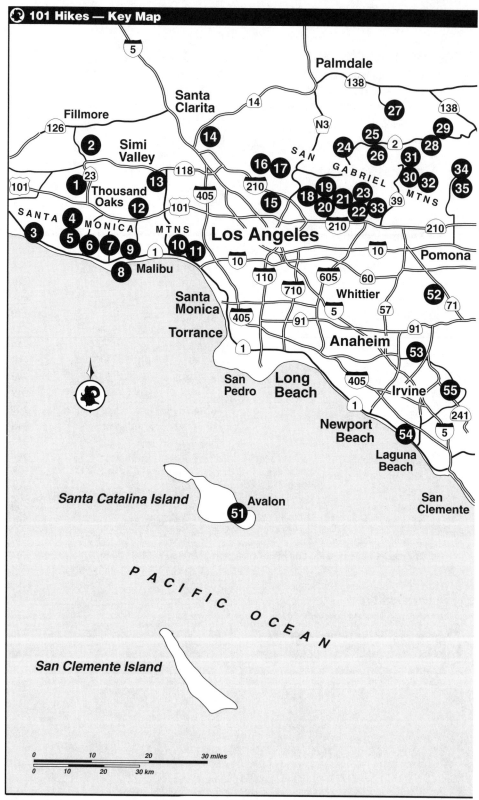

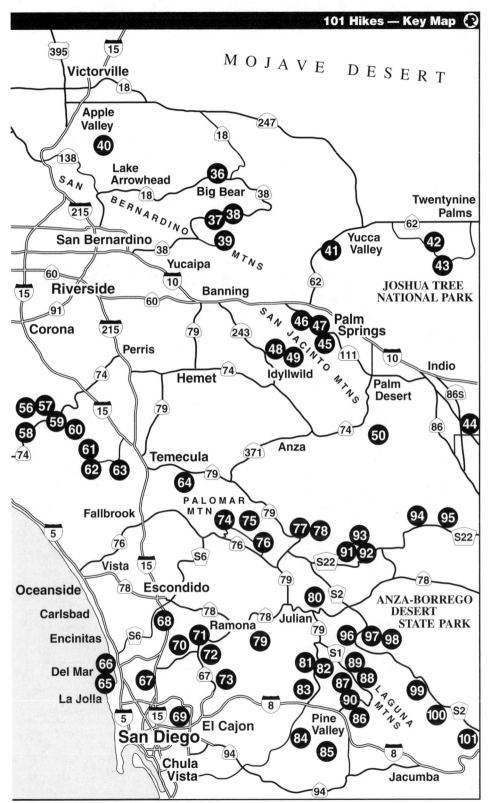

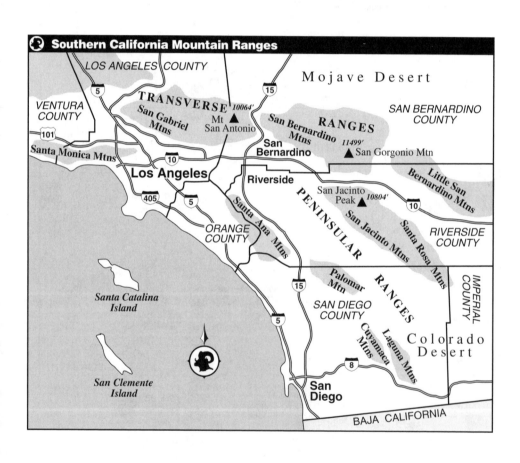

Southern California Mountain Ranges

LOS ANGELES COUNTY

Mojave Desert

VENTURA COUNTY

SAN BERNARDINO COUNTY

TRANSVERSE

San Gabriel Mtns

10064'
Mt San Antonio

RANGES

San Bernardino Mtns

101

Santa Monica Mtns

5

15

San Bernardino

11499'
San Gorgonio Mtn

10

Los Angeles

405

5

Riverside

Little San Bernardino Mtns

San Jacinto Peak

10804'

10

PENINSULAR

ORANGE COUNTY

Santa Ana Mtns

San Jacinto Mtns

Santa Rosa Mtns

RIVERSIDE COUNTY

Santa Catalina Island

15

Palomar Mtn

RANGES

IMPERIAL COUNTY

SAN DIEGO COUNTY

Colorado Desert

San Clemente Island

Cuyamaca Mtns

Laguna Mtns

8

San Diego

BAJA CALIFORNIA

Southern California's Wilderness Rim

Southern California sits astride one of the earth's most significant structural features—the San Andreas Fault. For more than 10 million years, earth movements along the San Andreas and neighboring faults have shaped the dramatic topography evident throughout the region today. The very complexity of the shape of the land has spawned a variety of localized climates. In turn, the varied climates, along with the diverse topography and geology, have resulted in a remarkably plentiful and diverse array of plant and animal life.

Living on the "active" edge of a continent has advantages and disadvantages that cannot be untangled. Like the proverbial silver lining in a dark cloud, the rumpled beauty of our youthful, ever-changing coastline, mountains, and desert redresses the ever-present threat of earthquakes, fires, and floods. Because much of South-

ern California is physically rugged, not all of it has succumbed to the plow or the bulldozer. When you've had the pleasure of hiking beside a crystal-clear mountain stream minutes from downtown L.A., or cooling off in the spray of a cottonwood-fringed waterfall just beyond suburban San Diego, you'll realize that not many regions in the world offer so great a variety of natural pleasures to a population of many millions.

Let us, in the next couple of pages, briefly explore the principal wild and semiwild natural areas bordering Southern California's coastal plain. When linked together, these natural areas form a broad, curving crescent around Southern California's urban population—now more than 20 million strong. About 90 percent of the hikes found in this book fall into this unpopulated or sparsely populated crescent.

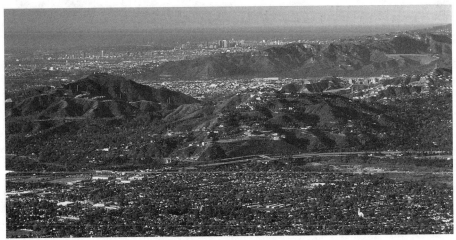

Los Angeles on a clear day from the Sam Merrill Trail (Hike 21)

1

The Santa Monica Mountains

We start with the Santa Monica Mountains, which rise abruptly from the Pacific shoreline west of (or "up the coast" from) Los Angeles. They, along with the San Gabriel and San Bernardino mountains, are part of the Transverse Ranges, so named because they trend east-west and stand crosswise to the usual northwest-southeast grain of nearly every other major mountain range in California. This anomaly, it is thought, is largely due to compression along the San Andreas Fault. There is a kink in the San Andreas Fault north of Los Angeles where the fault, running southeast from the San Francisco Bay Area, jogs east for a while before resuming its course toward the southeast. Compression against this kink has caused the land south of it to crumple and wrinkle upward. The devastating January 1994 Northridge earthquake was just one small episode in the slow but fitful uplift of the Transverse Ranges.

Compared to other Southern California ranges, the Santa Monicas are modest in size—barely more than 3000 feet high— but their rise from the sea is dramatic.

They are a shaggy looking range, clothed in tough, drought-resistant vegetation that falls into two principal categories: coastal sage scrub and chaparral. The *coastal sage scrub* plant "community" lies mostly below 2000 feet elevation, on primarily south-facing slopes in the Santa Monica Mountains and elsewhere in the coastal ranges of Southern California. Characterized by various aromatic sages (California sagebrush, black sage, white sage) along with buckwheat, laurel sumac, and lemonade berry shrubs and prickly pear cactus, sage scrub is fast disappearing in the Santa Monicas and elsewhere as urbanization encroaches on it. Much of the sage-scrub vegetation is dormant and dead-looking during the warmer half of the year, but green and aromatic during the cool, wet half.

The *chaparral* plant community is commonly found between 1000 and 5000 feet elevation—almost anywhere there's a slope that hasn't burned recently. Chaparral needs more moisture than sage scrub, so in the Santa Monicas it's often found on the shadier, north-facing slopes and other spots protected from the full

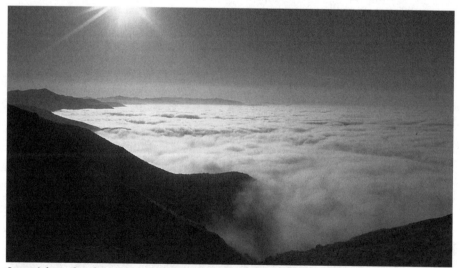

Late-night and early-morning low clouds (the "marine layer") typically cover Southern California's coastline during spring and summer.

glare of the sun. The dominant chaparral plants include chamise, scrub oak, manzanita, toyon, mountain mahogany, and various forms of ceanothus ("wild lilac"). Yuccas, known for their spectacular candle-shaped blooms, often frequent the chaparral zones. The chaparral plants are tough and intricately branched evergreen shrubs with deep root systems that help the plants survive during the long, hot summers. Chaparral is sometimes called "elfin forest"—a good description of a mature stand. Without benefit of a trail, travel through mature chaparral, which is often 15 feet high and incredibly dense from the ground up, is almost impossible.

A touch of the *southern oak woodland* and *riparian woodland* communities is present in the Santa Monicas and sparsely distributed nearly everywhere else in coastal Southern California. The Santa Monica Mountains include the southernmost stands of the valley oak, a massive, spreading tree that is as much a symbol of the Golden State as are the redwoods farther north. The southern oak woodland is very "parklike" in appearance, especially in the spring when attended by new growths of grass and wildflowers. Riparian (streamside) vegetation includes trees such as willows, sycamores, and alders that thrive wherever water flows year round—typically along the bottoms of the larger canyons. Strolling through the riot of growth in riparian zones is the nearest thing to a jungle experience you can have in arid Southern California. Both types of habitat have declined all over California as a result of urbanization and agricultural development, and the attendant exploitation of water resources.

Wildfire plays a dominant role in the ecology of the Santa Monica Mountains, and indeed almost everywhere else in coastal Southern California. Sage scrub and chaparral vegetation readily renews itself after fire. Before modern times wildfires would incinerate most hillsides every 5 to 15 years, and thick stands of chapar-

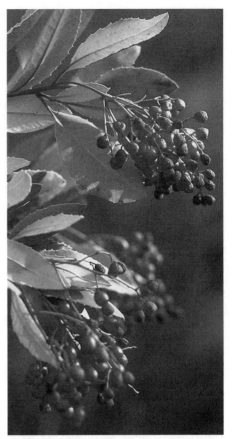

Toyon (California holly, the "holly" of Hollywood) is a common chaparral plant

ral seldom developed. Over the past century, however, the active prevention and suppression of fires has led to longer growth cycles and abnormally large accumulations of dead fuelwood. Once started, today's wildfires in chaparral zones are often difficult or impossible to control.

From Malibu east into L.A.'s west side, the Santa Monicas are steadily filling up with custom houses and subdivisions, all of which are in jeopardy from firestorms during the dry summer and fall seasons. Large and small wildfires will forever torment those who seek to establish permanent residence here.

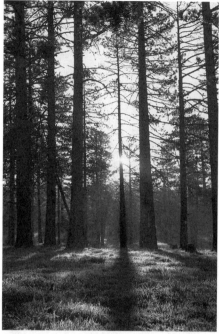

Jeffrey pines in the Laguna Mountains

Today the Santa Monicas are a patch-work quilt of private lands (many already built upon or slated for future development) and public lands, protected from urban development by inclusion within Santa Monica Mountains National Recreation Area, a unit of the National Park system.

The San Gabriel Mountains

Turning our attention farther north and east, we find the San Gabriel Mountains, another segment of the east-west trending Transverse Ranges. Behind the south ramparts of the San Gabriels, whose chaparraled slopes rise sheer from the Los Angeles Basin and the San Gabriel Valley, stands a series of high peaks, the tallest of which—Old Baldy, or Mt. San Antonio—exceeds 10,000 feet in elevation. Yawning gorges slash into the range, in one place offering more than a mile of vertical relief between canyon bottom and adjacent ridge.

Geologists figure that the San Gabriels are being squeezed horizontally about a tenth of an inch each year, and being thrust upward much more rapidly than that. Caught in this tectonic frenzy, the San Gabriel Mountains are surging upward as fast as any mountain range on the planet. They are also disintegrating at a spectacular rate. Although the San Gabriels consist mainly of durable granitic rocks, much like those in the sturdy Sierra Nevada, the San Gabriel rocks have been through a tectonic meat grinder. The tops of the San Gabriels are fairly rounded, but the slopes are often appallingly steep and unstable. An average of 7 tons of material disappears from each acre of the front face each year, most of it coming to rest behind debris barriers and dams in the L.A. Basin below.

The San Gabriel Mountains themselves are relatively young as upthrust units—only a few million years old. This is not true of the ages of most of the rocks that compose them. Some rocks exposed here are representative of the oldest found on the Pacific coast—over 600 million years of age.

Botanically, parts of the San Gabriel Mountains are extremely attractive, especially in zones above 4000 feet that receive enough precipitation. There the *coniferous forest* thrives. This has two phases in Southern California. The "yellow pine" phase includes conifers such as bigcone Douglas-fir, ponderosa pine, Jeffrey pine, sugar pine, incense-cedar, and white fir, and forms tall, open forest. These species are often intermixed with live oaks, California bay (bay laurel), and scattered chaparral shrubs such as manzanita and mountain mahogany. Higher than about 8000 feet, in the "lodgepole pine" phase, lodgepole pine, white fir, and limber pine are the prevailing trees. These trees, somewhat shorter and more weather-beaten than those below, exist in small, sometimes dense stands, interspersed with such shrubs as chinquapin, snowbrush, and manzanita.

Excluding relatively small parcels of private land, the bulk of the higher San Gabriel Mountains lies within Angeles National Forest. Hundreds of square miles of wilderness or near wilderness in the San Gabriels are available within easy reach of millions of Los Angeles residents.

The San Bernardino Mountains

Farther east, across the low gap of Cajon Pass, the Transverse Ranges soar again as the San Bernardino Mountains. With Lake Arrowhead, Big Bear Lake, and winter ski areas, the mid elevations of the San Bernardinos (5000–8000 feet elevation) draw millions of day trippers and vacationers yearly. Hikers and backpackers can explore the 10,000-foot-plus peaks of the San Gorgonio Wilderness, including 11,500-foot San Gorgonio Mountain itself—Southern California's high point. There it is possible to ascend through the yellow-pine and lodgepole belts to treeline and above.

As in the San Gabriel Mountains, islands of private land in the San Bernardinos are surrounded by large sections of national forest. San Bernardino National Forest encompasses much of the San Bernardino Mountains, as well as the San Jacinto and Santa Rosa mountains to the south.

The most dramatic change taking place in the high mountains of Southern California—especially the San Bernardinos—is a massive die-off of coniferous trees, which continues unabated as of this writing. The high-elevation areas in Southern California have been receiving less precipitation in recent decades. A string of very dry years beginning in 1998–99 triggered an acute infestation of bark beetles, which eventually resulted in sudden death for millions of drought-stressed pine, fir, and cedar trees. Wild-

fires in October 2003 destroyed some of these dead and dying trees, and many others are being removed by logging operations in an overall effort to thin the forest to attain a more healthy level of tree density. Heavy rains during the 2004-05 rainfall season renewed hopes for a healthier forest in the years to come.

The Mojave Desert

North and east of the San Gabriel and San Bernardino mountains lies the vast, arid sweep of the Mojave Desert, a zone only partly included in this book. The Mojave, sometimes known as the "high" desert for its generally high average elevation, becomes far less populated and more diverse in its natural features as we move toward eastern California. A few of the hikes in this book explore the transitional region between high mountain and

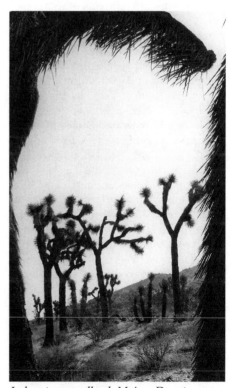

Joshua tree woodland, Mojave Desert

high desert. There, at elevations of 3000–5000 feet, thrives the *pinyon-juniper woodland*, largely characterized by the rather stunted looking one-leaf pinyon pine and the California juniper. Large sections of the Mojave, again in the elevation range of about 3000–5000 feet, are dominated by *Joshua tree woodland*. Here the indicator plant is an outsized member of the yucca family—the Joshua tree. Joshua Tree National Park preserves some, but hardly all, of the finest stands of these odd, tree-sized plants.

The San Jacinto Mountains

Moving south from the San Bernardino Mountains and Joshua Tree National Park, we find the northwest-southeast trending San Jacinto Mountains and their southerly extension, the Santa Rosa Mountains. These lofty ranges comprise the northern ramparts of what geologists call the Peninsular Ranges—so named because they extend, more or less continuously, south across the Mexican border and comprise the spine of the long, thin peninsula of Baja California.

As the highest peak in the entire Peninsular Ranges province, 10,800-foot San Jacinto Peak would outrank all other Southern California peaks were it not for the slightly higher San Gorgonio massif looming just 20 miles north. For sheer dramatic impact, however, San Jacinto wins hands down. Viewed from I-10 outside Palm Springs, the north and east escarpments of San Jacinto appear to rise nearly straight up from the desert floor—10,000 feet in 10 miles or less. Every plant community we have mentioned so far except Joshua tree woodland thrives at one level or another on the mountain.

San Jacinto's pine clad western slopes shelter several resort communities (such as Idyllwild); otherwise nearly all of the mountain's upper elevations lie within national-forest wilderness or state wilderness areas.

The Colorado Desert

East of the northernmost Peninsular Ranges lie Palm Springs, the Coachella Valley, and the Salton Trough (Salton Sea). They are within the domain known as the Colorado Desert—California's "low" desert—so called because it stretches west from the lower Colorado River, which divides California from Arizona. A 1000-square-mile chunk of the Colorado Desert lies within Anza-Borrego Desert State Park, by far the largest state park in California. Especially close and convenient for San Diegans, Anza-Borrego's vast acreage ranges from intricately dissected, desiccated terrain known as "badlands" to the pinyon-juniper and yellow-pine forests of the Peninsular Ranges.

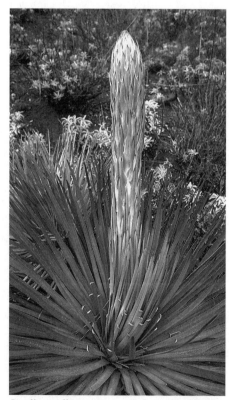

Lord's candle yucca ranges from the coast to the desert rim

The Laguna, Cuyamaca, Palomar, and Santa Ana Mountains

East and north of San Diego the Peninsular Ranges consist of a number of parallel ranges—primarily the Laguna, Cuyamaca, and Palomar ranges—each attaining heights of just over 6000 feet. Chaparral blankets the slopes of these mountains, while the higher elevations are dominated by the typical yellow-pine assemblage of oak, pine, cedar, and fir. Farther north and east, bordering the rapidly expanding urban zones of southwestern Riverside and southern Orange County, lie the Santa Ana Mountains. They are the northernmost coastal expressions of the Peninsular Ranges.

Suburban sprawl has crept into the foothills of these far-southern ranges, and in some cases threatens to degrade the

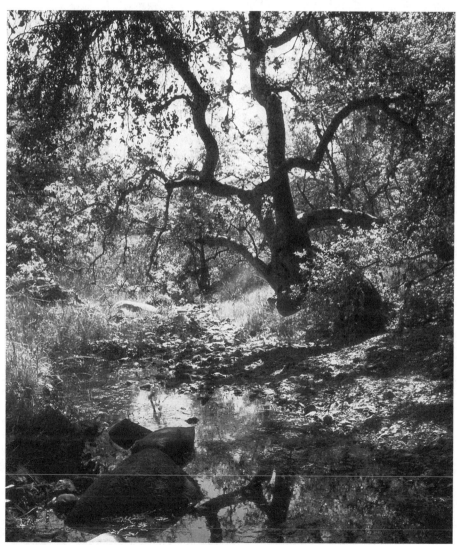

Oak woodland shelters Cole Creek, Santa Rosa Plateau Ecological Reserve (Hike 63)

higher elevations as well. Fortunately, large parts of this mountainous region lie within the jurisdiction of Cleveland National Forest and various state parks.

All the mountain ranges rimming San Diego have been hard-hit recently by both drought and catastrophic wildfire. The 300,000-acre Cedar Fire, which blazed an elongated path across central San Diego County in October 2003, burned through primarily chaparral and oak woodland, and secondarily through prime oak/coniferous forest, mostly in the Cuyamaca Mountains. The chaparral and oak woodlands of lower elevation, adapted to periodic fires, will likely fully recover in a decade or so. The formerly lush Cuyamaca Mountains may never look quite the same, however, unless the climate shifts back to a wetter regime.

Health, Safety and Courtesy

Good preparation is always important for any kind of recreational pursuit. Hiking the Southern California backcountry is no exception. Although most of the Southland's natural environments are seldom hostile or dangerous to life and limb, there are some pitfalls to be aware of.

Preparation and Equipment

An obvious safety requirement is being in good health. Some degree of physical conditioning is always desirable, even for the trips in this book designated as easy or moderate (rated ★ and ★★ in difficulty). The more challenging trips (rated ★★★, ★★★★ or ★★★★★) require increasing amounts of stamina and technical expertise. Running, bicycling, swimming, aerobics, or any similar exercise that develops both the leg muscles and the aerobic capacity of the whole body are recommended as preparatory exercise.

For the longest hikes in this book, there is no really adequate way to prepare other than hiking itself. Start with easy- or moderate-length trips, and then work gradually toward extending both distance and time.

Several of the hiking trips in this book reach elevations of 7000 feet or more—altitudes at which sea-level folks may notice a big difference in their rate of breathing and stamina. A few hours or a day spent at altitude before exercising will help almost anyone acclimate, but that's often impractical for short daytrips. Still, you might consider spending a night or two at a campground with some altitude before

tackling the likes of 11,500-foot San Gorgonio Mountain. Altitude sickness strikes some victims at elevations as low as 8000 feet. If you become dizzy or nauseous, or suffer from congested lungs or a severe headache, the antidote may be as simple as descending one or two thousand feet.

Your choice of equipment and supplies on the longer hikes in this book can be critically important. The essentials you should carry with you at all times in the remote backcountry are the things that would allow you to survive, in a reasonably comfortable manner, one or two unscheduled nights out. It's important to note that no one ever plans these nights! No one plans to get lost, injured, stuck, or pinned down by the weather. Always do a "what if" analysis for a worst-case scenario, and plan accordingly. These essential items are your safety net; keep them with you on dayhikes, and take them with you in a small day pack if you leave your backpack and camping equipment behind at a campsite.

Chief among the essential items is *warm clothing*. Inland Southern California is characterized by wide swings in day and night temperatures. In mountain valleys susceptible to cold-air drainage, for example, a midday temperature in the 70s or 80s is often followed by a subfreezing night. Carry light, inner layers of clothing consisting of polypropylene or wool (best for cool or cold weather), or cotton (adequate for warm or hot weather, but very poor for cold and damp weather). Include a thicker insulating layer of synthetic fill, wool, or down to put on whenever needed, especially when you are not moving around and generating heat. Add to this a cap, gloves, and a waterproof or water-resistant shell (a large trash bag will do in a pinch)—and you'll be quite prepared for all but the most severe weather.

In hot, sunny weather, sun-shielding clothing may be another "essential." This would normally include a sun hat and a light-colored, long-sleeve top.

Water and *food* are next in importance. Most streams and even some springs in the mountains have been shown to contain unacceptably high levels of bacteria or other contaminants. Even though most of the remote watersheds are probably pristine, it's wise to treat by filtering or chemical methods any water obtained outside of developed camp or picnic sites. Unless the day is very warm or your trip is a long one, it's usually easiest to carry (preferably in sturdy plastic bottles, or a "camelback") all the water you'll need. Don't underestimate your water needs: During a full day's hike in 80° temperatures you may require as much as a gallon of water. Know, too, that many springs and watercourses—even some shown as being "permanent" on topographic maps—may run dry at some point during the summer. Food is necessary to stave off the feeling of hunger and keep energy stores up, but it is not nearly as critical as water is in emergency situations in which water is needed to prevent dehydration.

Down the list further, but still "essential," are a *map* and *compass* (or a GPS unit and the knowledge of its use), *flashlight, fire-starting devices* (examples: waterproof matches or lighter, and candle), and *first-aid kit.*

Items not always essential, but potentially very useful and convenient, are sunglasses, pocket knife, whistle (or other signaling device), sunscreen, and toilet paper. [NOTE: Sunglasses are an essential item for travel over snow.]

The essential items mentioned above should be carried by every member of a hiking party, because individuals or splinter groups may end up separating from the party for one reason or another. If you plan to hike solo in the backcountry, being well-equipped is very important. If you hike alone, be sure to check in with a park ranger or leave your itinerary with a responsible person. In that way, if you do get stuck, help will probably come to the right place—eventually.

Special Hazards

Other than getting lost or pinned down by a rare sudden storm, the most common hazards found in the Southland are steep, unstable terrain; icy terrain; spiny plants; rattlesnakes; mountain lions, ticks; and poison oak.

Falls

Exploring some trails—especially those of the San Gabriel Mountains—may involve traveling over structurally weak rock on steep slopes. The erosive effects of flowing water, of wedging by roots and by ice, and of brush fires tend to pulverize such rock even further. Slips on such terrain usually lead to sliding down a hillside some distance. If you explore cross-country, always be on the lookout for dangerous run-outs, such as cliffs, below you. The sidewalls of many canyons in the San Gabriels may look like nice places to practice rock-climbing moves, but this misconception has been the cause of many deaths over the years.

Snow and Ice

Statistically, mishaps associated with snow and ice have caused the greatest number of fatalities in the San Gabriel and San Bernardino mountain ranges. This is not because our local mountains are inherently more dangerous than the Sierra Nevada, the Cascades, or other ranges. Rather, it is because inexperienced lowlanders, never picturing their backyard

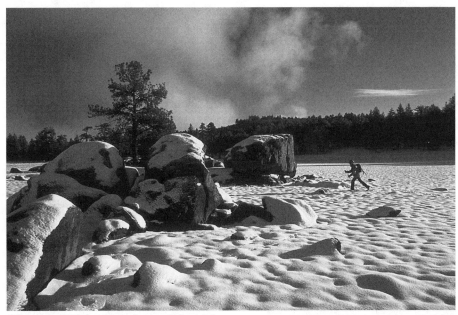

Winter at 6000 feet in the Laguna Mountains

mountains as true wilderness areas, are attracted here by the novelty of snow and the easy access by way of snow-plowed highways. Icy chutes and slopes capable of avalanching can easily trap such visitors unaware. Winter travel in the more gentle areas of the high country can be accomplished on snowshoes or skis; but the steeper slopes require technical skills and equipment such as ice ax and crampons, just as in other snow-covered mountain ranges.

Puncturing Plants

Most desert hikers will sooner or later suffer punctures by thorns or spines. This is most likely to happen during close encounters with the cholla ("jumping") cactus, whose spine clusters readily break off and attach firmly to your skin, clothes or boots. A comb can be used to gently pull away the spine clusters, and tweezers or lightweight pliers can be used to remove any individual embedded spines. Another problematic spiny plant is the agave, or century plant. It consists of a rosette of fleshy leaves, each tipped with a rigid

thorn containing a mild toxin. A headlong fall into either an agave or one of the more vicious kinds of cacti could easily make you swear off desert travel permanently. It's best to give these devilish plants as wide a berth as possible.

Rattlesnakes

Rattlesnakes are common everywhere in Southern California below an elevation of about 7000 feet. Seldom seen in either cold or very hot weather, they favor temperatures in the 75–90° range—spring and fall in the desert and coastal areas, and summer in the mountains. Most rattlesnakes are as interested in avoiding contact with you as you are with them. Watch carefully where you put your feet, and especially your hands, during the warmer months. In brushy or rocky areas where sight distance is short, try to make your presence known from afar. Tread with heavy footfalls, or use a stick to bang against rocks or bushes. Rattlesnakes will pick up the vibrations through their skin and will usually buzz (unmistakably) before you get too close for comfort. Most

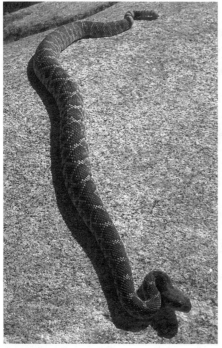

Red diamond rattlesnake

bad encounters between rattlesnakes and hikers occur in April and May, when snakes are irritable and hungry after a long hibernation period.

Mountain Lions

Mountain-lion attacks, although statistically rare, have been increasing all over California in the last two decades. This trend may continue as the natural habitat for these carnivorous cats becomes more and more fragmented by suburban and rural development. Several attacks and many more incidents of threatening behavior by mountain lions toward humans have taken place in urban-edge park and national-forest lands, such as those covered in this book. Here are some basic tips for dealing with this potential hazard:

- Hike with one or more companions.
- Keep children close at hand.
- Never run from a mountain lion. This may trigger an instinct to attack.

- Make yourself "large," face the animal, maintain eye contact with it, shout, blow a whistle, and do not act fearful. Do anything to convince the animal that you are not its prey.

Ticks

Ticks can sometimes be the scourge of overgrown trails in the coastal foothills and lower mountain slopes, particularly during the first warm spells of the year, when they climb to the tips of shrub branches and lie in wait for warm-blooded hosts. If you can't avoid brushing against vegetation along the trail, be sure to check yourself for ticks frequently. Upon finding a host, a tick will usually crawl upward in search of a protected spot, where it will try to attach itself. If you can be aware of the slightest irritation on your body, you'll usually intercept ticks long before they attempt to bite. Ticks would be of relatively minor concern here, except that tick-borne Lyme disease, which can have serious health effects, has been reported within Southern California.

Poison Oak

Poison oak grows profusely along many of the coastal and mountain canyons below 5000 feet elevation. It is often found on the banks of streamcourses in the form of a bush or vine, where it prefers semi-shady habitats. Quite often, it's seen beside or encroaching on well-used trails. Learn to recognize its distinctive three-leafed structure, and avoid touching it with skin or clothing. Since poison oak loses its leaves during the winter months (and sometimes during summer and fall drought), but still retains some of the toxic oil in its stems, it can be extra hazardous at that time because it is harder to identify and avoid. Mid-weight pants, like blue jeans, and a long-sleeve shirt will serve as a fair barrier against the toxic oil of the poison oak plant. Do, of course, remove these clothes as soon as

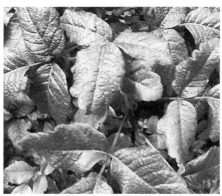

Poison-oak leaves

the hike is over, and make sure they are washed carefully afterward.

Other Safety Concerns

Deer-hunting season in Southern California usually runs through the middle part of the autumn. Although conflicts between hunters and hikers are rare, you may want to confine your autumn explorations to state and county parks, and wilderness areas where hunting is not permitted.

There is always some risk in leaving a vehicle unattended at a trailhead. It may be worthwhile to disable your car's ignition or attach an anti-theft device to your steering wheel. Never leave valuable property in an automobile, so as to be an invitation for a break-in. Report all theft and vandalism of personal or public property to the county sheriff or the appropriate park or forest agency.

Permits and Camping

All trails on national-forest lands (Angeles, San Bernardino, and Cleveland national forests) are at present subject to a "National Forest Adventure Pass" program. This applies only to vehicles parked on national forest land, and not to users who arrive on foot or by bicycle. Adventure passes are available at all national-forest offices, ranger stations, and fire stations. They are also sold though hun-

dreds of vendors—typically sport shops throughout the region, gas stations and markets near the principal national-forest entry roads, and small businesses within national-forest borders. Adventure passes cost $5 per day or $30 for a year. The adventure pass must be prominently displayed on your parked car—otherwise your car will likely be ticketed and fined.

If you plan to visit national-forest territory more than two or three times a year, it is time-efficient at the very least to purchase the $30 yearly pass instead of worrying about obtaining one each day you come up for a visit. Rules for the adventure pass program have a tendency to change rapidly; in fact, there remains the possibility the program will be rescinded in the future.

If you are planning an overnight trip of some type into the Southern California backcountry, be aware that camping in roadside campgrounds is not always a restful experience. Off-season camping (late fall through early spring) offers relief from crowds, but not from chilly nighttime weather. Most national forest campgrounds are less well supervised than those in state and county parks, and therefore sometimes attract a noisy crowd. In my experience, facilities with a "campground host" promise a better clientele, and a better night's sleep.

The nice advantage of a developed campground is that you can always have a campfire there—unless the facility itself is closed. On trails where backpacking is allowed, fire regulations vary. Most jurisdictions prohibit campfires all or part of the year. Others permit fires, as long as you have the necessary free permit.

Some of the national forest areas allow "remote," primitive-style camping: You are not always restricted to staying at a developed campground or designated trail camp. For sanitation reasons, you are required to locate your camp well away from the nearest source of water. And, of course, you must observe the fire regulations stated earlier. Always check with the Forest Service to confirm these rules if you intend to do any remote camping.

Most federally managed wilderness areas around the state require special wilderness permits for entry. Many in Southern California have self-registering permits at trailheads; others require permits only for overnight visits. The San Gorgonio and San Jacinto wilderness areas are so popular that trailhead quotas are sometimes implemented.

Trail Courtesy

Whenever you travel the backcountry, you take on a burden of responsibility—keeping the wilderness as you found it. Aside from common-sense prohibitions against littering, vandalism, and inappropriate campfires, there are some less obvious guidelines every hiker should be aware of. We'll mention a few:

Never cut trail switchbacks. This practice breaks down the trail tread and hastens erosion. Try to improve designated trails by removing branches, rocks, or other debris. Springtime growth can quite rapidly obscure pathways in the chaparral country, and funding for trail maintenance is often scarce—so try to do your part by joining a volunteer trail crew or by performing your own small maintenance

tasks while walking the trails. Report any damage to trails or other facilities to the appropriate ranger office.

When backpacking, be a "no trace" camper. Leave your campsite as you found it—or leave it in an even more natural condition.

Collecting specimens of minerals, plants, animals, and historical objects without a special permit is generally prohibited in most jurisdictions. This means common things, too, such as pine cones, wildflowers, and lizards. These should be left for all visitors to enjoy. Some limited collecting of items like pine cones may be allowed on the national forest lands—check first.

We've covered most of the general regulations associated with Southern California's public lands. But you, as a visitor, are responsible for knowing any additional rules as well. The capsulized summary for each hike described in this book includes a reference to the agency responsible for the area you'll be visiting. Phone numbers for those agencies appear in the back of this book. Internet research is often helpful, too. Using a search engine, just enter key words for the park or area in question to find an abundance of information. The quality of this information, however, varies, and it is important to note the date of its posting, if given.

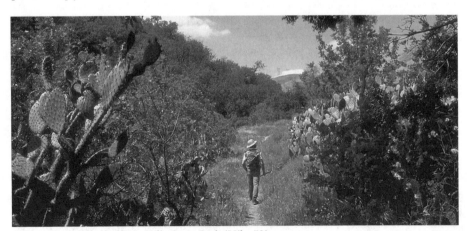

Water Canyon Trail, Chino Hills State Park (Hike 52)

Using This Book

There are three principal ways to find hiking trips in this book suitable for you. First, you can check the key map for all 101 hikes in this book, pages *x* and *xi*, and restrict your search to a specific geographic area. Second, you can leaf through the book, browsing hike summaries, descriptions, and photos. Third, you can scan the "Summary of Hikes" matrix in the back of this book.

Please take the time to carefully read, below, about the meaning of the special symbols and other bits of capsulized information that appear before each hike description in this book.

Sketch maps are provided for each hike in this book. The boxed "T" (trailhead) symbol on each map denotes the start point of the hike depicted on that map. Point-to-point hikes have two "T" symbols—one for the beginning of the hike and one for end of the hike. For nearly all hikes described in this book, the sketch map we provide is adequate for basic navigation. For a few hikes, a detailed topographic map is recommended in the capsulized summary.

The following is an explanation of the small symbols and capsulized information appearing at the beginning of each hike description. If you're simply browsing through this book, these summaries alone can be used as a tool to eliminate from consideration hikes that are either too difficult, or perhaps too trivial, for your abilities.

Symbols

 Easy Terrain. Roads, trails and easy cross-country hiking

 Moderate Terrain. Cross-country boulder hopping and easy scrambling

 Difficult Terrain. Nontechnical climbing required

Only *one* of these three symbols appears for a given hike, indicating the general character of the terrain encountered. A hike almost entirely on roads and trails, but including a short section of boulder-hopping, for example, will be rated as easy terrain, and the difficulties will be duly noted in the text. As the symbols suggest, light footwear (running shoes) is appropriate for easy terrain, while sturdy hiking boots are recommended for more difficult terrain.

Nontechnical climbing includes everything up to and including Class 3 on the rock-climber's scale. While ropes and climbing hardware are not normally required, a hiker should have a good sense of balance, and enough experience to recognize dangerous moves and situations. In difficult terrain, these hikes should be attempted only by suitably equipped, experienced hikers adept at traveling over steep or rocky terrain requiring the use of the hands as well as the feet.

Bushwhacking

Cross-country travel through dense brush. This symbol is included for hikes requiring a substantial amount of off-trail "bushwhacking." Wear long pants and be especially alert for ticks and rattlesnakes.

Only *one* of these two symbols appears:

 Marked Trails/Obvious Routes

 Navigation by Map and Compass Required

Unambiguous cross-country routes—up a canyon, for example—are included in the first category. The hiker, of course, should never be without a map, even if there are marked trails or the route seems obvious. Other cross-country trips should be attempted only by hikers skilled in navigation techniques.

 Point-to-Point Route

Out-and-Back Route

 Loop Route

Only *one* of these three symbols appears, reflecting the hike as described. There is some flexibility, of course, in the way in which a hiker can actually follow the hike.

 Suitable for Backpacking

A few trips in this book are suitable for overnight camping. Sometimes, overnight camping is permitted at some spot off the route but nearby. This icon indicates when backpacking is an attractive option for a particular hike.

 Suitable for Mountain Biking

The route, as described, is open to mountain biking, and is reasonably safe for that activity. Since regulations governing the use of mountain bikes on trails may change, it is a good idea to check with the agency having jurisdiction over the area.

 Dogs Allowed

This icon indicates that dogs are allowed on the trail, generally on a leash no longer than 6 feet.

 Good for Kids

These trips are especially recommended for inquisitive children. They were chosen on the basis of their safety and ease of travel, and their potential for entertaining the whole family.

Capsulized Summaries

Location. The general location of the hike is stated: a well-known park, mountain range, or nearby city or town.

Highlights. One or two engaging features of the hike are mentioned.

Distance. An estimate of total distance is given. Out-and-back trips show the sum of the distances of the out and back segments.

Total Elevation Gain/Loss. These are estimates of the sum of all the vertical gain segments and the sum of all the vertical loss segments along the total length of the route (both ways for out-and-back trips). This is often considerably more than the net difference in elevation between the high and low points of the hike.

Hiking Time. This figure is for the average hiker, and includes only the time spent in motion. It *does not* include time spent for rest stops, lunch, etc. Fast walkers can complete the routes in perhaps 30% less time, and slower hikers may take 50% longer. We assume the hiker is traveling with a light day pack. [IMPORTANT NOTE: "Hiking time" stated in this book is for *time-in-motion* only. Also, hikers carrying heavy packs could easily take nearly twice as long, especially if they are traveling under adverse weather conditions. Remember, too, that the progress made by a group as a whole is limited by pace of the slowest member or members.]

Optional/Recommended Map(s). The topographic maps listed are nearly all U.S. Geological Survey 7.5-minute series topographic maps. Usually, these are the most complete and accurate maps of the physical features (if not always the cultural features and trails) of the area you'll be traveling in. These maps are typically stocked by backpacking, outdoor sports, and map shops around the Southland. Topographic maps on CD format and topographic-map images downloadable from the internet are becoming popular alternatives to purchasing hard-copy topographic maps.

Best Times. Because of the extreme heat, the longer desert trips in this book should generally be avoided during any period except the one recommended here. Trips elsewhere in Southern California are usually safe enough at other than "best" times, but usually less rewarding.

Agency. These code letters refer to the agency, or office, that has jurisdiction or management over the area being hiked management of the area being hiked (for example, CNF/TD means Cleveland National Forest, Trabuco District). You can contact the agency for more information. Full names, phone numbers, and some addresses (of larger agencies) are listed in Agencies & Information Sources in the back of this book.

Difficulty. The author's subjective, overall rating takes into account the length of the hike and the nature of the terrain. The following are general definitions of the five categories:

★ *Easy.* Suitable for every member of the family.

★★ *Moderate.* Suitable for all physically fit people.

★★★ *Moderately Strenuous.* Long length, substantial elevation gain, and/or difficult terrain. Recommended for experienced hikers only.

★★★★ *Strenuous.* Full day's hike (or a backpack trip) over a long and/or challenging route. Suitable only for experienced hikers in excellent physical condition.

★★★★★ *Very Strenuous.* Long and rugged route in extremely remote area. Suitable only for experienced hikers/climbers in top physical condition. (Only two hikes in this book, 32, Down the East Fork, and 47, San Jacinto Peak, Hard Way, get this rating.)

Each higher level represents more or less a doubling of the difficulty. On average, ★★ trips are twice as hard as ★ trips, ★★★ trips are twice as hard as ★★ trips, and so on.

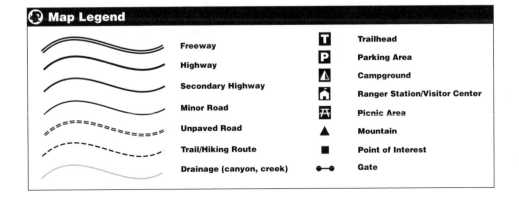

Map Legend	
～～～ Freeway	**T** Trailhead
～～～ Highway	**P** Parking Area
～～～ Secondary Highway	**⚠** Campground
～～～ Minor Road	**⌂** Ranger Station/Visitor Center
==== Unpaved Road	**⊞** Picnic Area
- - - - Trail/Hiking Route	▲ Mountain
～～～ Drainage (canyon, creek)	■ Point of Interest
	●—● Gate

101 Hikes...

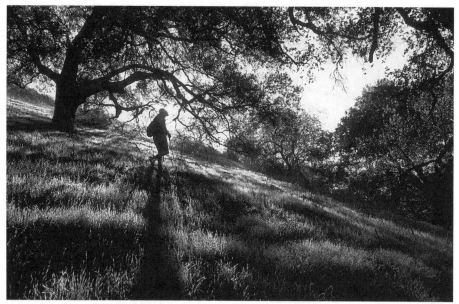

Late-afternoon sunlight in Water Canyon (Hike 52)

HIKE 1

Paradise Falls

Location	Wildwood Park, City of Thousand Oaks
Highlights	Gem of a waterfall in a steep gorge
Distance	3.0 miles
Total Elevation Gain/Loss	400'/400'
Hiking Time	2 hours
Optional Map	USGS 7.5-min *Newbury Park*
Best Times	All year
Agency	CRPD
Difficulty	★★

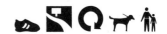

Wildwood Park in Thousand Oaks is Ventura County's most scenic suburban park. The scenery here has been imprinted in the minds of many in the over-50 age group: The area was once an outdoor set for old Hollywood movies, as well as for television's "The Rifleman," "Gunsmoke," and "Wagon Train." The short but steep hike—down and then up—described here takes you to Wildwood Park's scenic gem: the Arroyo Conejo gorge and Paradise Falls.

To Reach the Trailhead: Exit Highway 101 at Lynn Road in Thousand Oaks and follow Lynn Road north 2.5 miles to Avenida de los Arboles. Turn left and follow Avenida de los Arboles 1 mile west. At this point traffic goes sharply right on Big Sky Drive; you make a U-turn and park on the right at Wildwood Park's principal trailhead, open 8 A.M. to 5 P.M. Nearby curbside parking is also available.

Description: Three trails radiate from the Avenida de los Arboles trailhead. Two are wide and relatively unscenic dirt roads. The third (the one you want), the narrow and scenic Moonridge Trail, descends sharply from the east side of the parking area. This is the left side of the parking area as you drive in. Right away you come to a T-intersection amid oak woods. Turn right, remaining on the Moonridge Trail. The trail descends a

sunny slope covered with aromatic sage-scrub vegetation and dappled with succulent live-forever plants that sprout white, comical-looking flower stalks. There's a brief passage across a shady ravine using wooden steps and a plank bridge. At 0.5 mile, you cross over a dirt road and continue on the narrow Moonridge Trail.

Ahead, the trail curls around a deep ravine without gaining or losing a lot of elevation, edging into the crumbly sedimentary rock. This passage is exciting enough for hikers, and could be worrisome for parents with small kids. At 0.9 mile you join another dirt road and use it

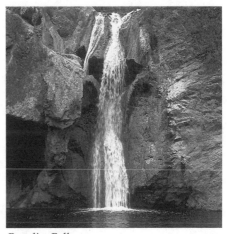

Paradise Falls

to descend toward a large wooden teepee structure on a knoll just below. Make a right at the tepee, further descending into the Arroyo Conejo gorge. As you descend, watch for the narrow side trail on the left that will take you straight down to Paradise Falls—a beautiful, 30-foot-high cascade that makes its presence known by sound before sight. The high water table in the canyon bottom ensures a nearly year-round flow of water.

After you've admired the falls, continue by climbing back up the slope in the direction you came, and by taking the fenced, cliff-hanging trail around the left (east) side of the falls. Beyond that fenced stretch, the narrow trail descends a little and sidles up alongside the creek, where large coast live oaks spread their shade. Soon, you'll find yourself continuing on a path of dirt-road width. Stay with that path until you reach a major crossroads. The small Wildwood Nature Center is just around the bend to the right, a short spur path to the walk-through Indian Cave lies on the left, and your return route up along Indian Creek is straight ahead.

On the Indian Creek Trail, you pay your debt to gravity by ascending nearly 300 feet in about 0.7 mile. The beautifully tangled array of live oak and sycamore limbs along this trail keeps your mind off the climb. At one point, you can look down into a deep ravine where an inaccessible mini-waterfall and pool lie practically hidden. When you finally reach Avenida de los Arboles, turn left and then return a short distance to the trailhead parking lot.

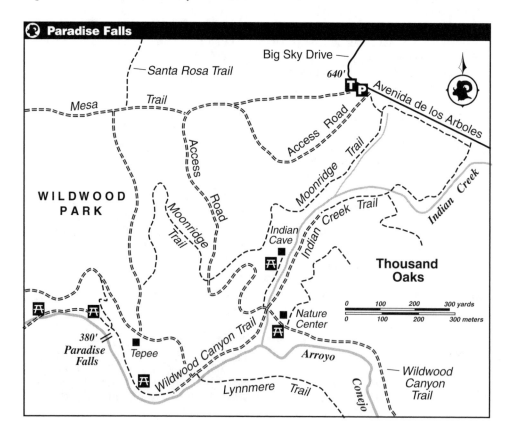

HIKE 2

Happy Camp Canyon

Location	Near Moorpark and Simi Valley
Highlights	Prime oak woodland; strange rock formations
Distance	9.4 miles
Total Elevation Gain/Loss	700'/700'
Hiking Time	5 hours
Optional Map	USGS 7.5-min *Simi*
Best Times	October through June
Agency	SMMC
Difficulty	★★★

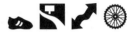

Happy Camp Canyon nuzzles in a crease between the long, rounded ridge called Big Mountain, just north of Simi Valley, and Oak Ridge, a taller parallel ridge to the north. These ridges and plenty more, like the Santa Monica Mountains, are caterpillar-like, parallel segments of the Transverse Ranges, which stretch from Santa Barbara County in the west to San Bernardino County to the east.

Oil-bearing shales predominate in this region, evidenced by various oil wells and dirt roads built to access them scattered across the surrounding hillsides. On your ramble through the lower and middle parts of the canyon, keep an eye out for bright red stones, sometimes exhibiting a glassy texture, some right under you feet and others visible in outcrops. These rocks were formed by the slow combustion of

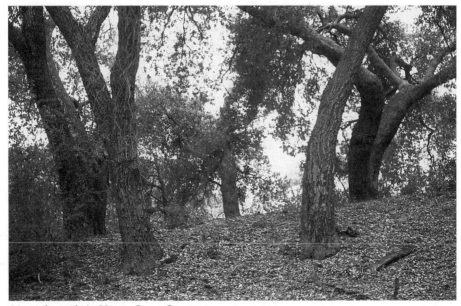

Live-oak woods in Happy Camp Canyon

organic material trapped in layers of
shale.

Happy Camp Canyon itself remains
quite pristine. Several groups of Chumash
Indians called this place home in past cen-
turies; later it became a part of an immense cattle ranch founded by a pioneer
Simi Valley family. Purchased as a future
state park in the late 1960s, it was later
traded to Ventura County for use as a regional park. Today, save for a few dirt
roads and a smattering of artifacts from
the days of cattle ranching, the 3000-acre
canyon park serves as prime natural habitat for native plants and animals, and a
restful retreat for hikers seeking to escape
from the sights and sounds of city and
suburban life. The October 2003 Simi Fire
consumed most of the canyon's hillside
sage-scrub and chaparral vegetation, and
it is likely that the next few years will feature impressive displays of fire-following
wildflowers during the late winter and
spring seasons.

To Reach the Trailhead: To get to the
Happy Camp Canyon's principal trailhead, follow the 118 Freeway west from
Simi Valley or the 23 Freeway north from
Thousand Oaks to the New Los Angeles
Avenue exit. Go west 1 mile to Moorpark
Avenue (signed Highway 23), turn right,
and proceed 2.6 miles to where Highway
23 makes a sharp bend to the left. Keep
going straight here, but then make an immediate right turn on Broadway. Proceed
a short way to the east end of Broadway,
which is where you will find a spacious
dirt parking lot and trailhead.

Description: On foot, follow the trail
which winds north and east along gentle,
grassy slopes down onto the wide floor
of Happy Camp Canyon. As you look

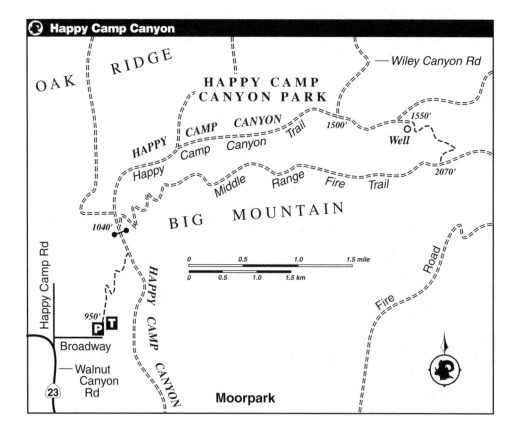

down on a golf course at the canyon's mouth, note the terraced aspect of the landscape on both sides. These are fluvial (streamside) terraces—sedimentary deposits from earlier flows of Happy Camp Canyon's Creek.

At 1.0 mile you join a dirt road in the bottom of the canyon, and 0.2 mile later you pass through a gate marking the start of the "wilderness" section of Happy Camp Canyon Park. Ignoring dirt roads on the right and left, keep straight (north) into the main canyon.

By 2.0 miles, the canyon floor has become narrow, you've turned decidedly east, and are strolling through beautiful coast live-oak woods (plus native sycamore and walnut trees), which continue intermittently up the canyon in the next 3 miles. A little stream flows in the bottom of the canyon during and for some weeks or months after the winter rains. You're climbing at a gentle rate of about 200 feet of elevation gain per mile. You pass the ascending Wiley Canyon Road

on the left at 4.1 miles, and at 4.7 miles you reach the site of an old well and pump. Large oak trees nearby provide enough shade for a convenient lunch stop. Savor the splendid isolation of this secluded retreat before you head back the same way.

An alternative to the out-and-back trip described above is available if you are interested and energetic, especially if the air is clear enough to enjoy distant views: Continue following the graded dirt road about 300 yards past the well. The road ends, but a bulldozed track, eroded and very steep at first, curls 0.7 mile up the south slope of Happy Camp Canyon then joins Middle Range Fire Trail on the crest of Big Mountain. Use that ridge-running fire trail to return to lower Happy Camp Canyon at a point just above the gate marking the wilderness area boundary. This looping alternative route (beginning and ending at the trailhead) measures 10.5 miles, with elevation gains and losses of 1300 feet.

HIKE 3

La Jolla Valley Loop

Location	Point Mugu State Park
Highlights	Spectacular ocean views; rare native vegetation
Distance	10.8 miles
Total Elevation Gain/Loss	1950'/1950'
Hiking Time	6 hours
Optional Map	USGS 7.5-min *Point Mugu*
Best Times	October through June
Agency	PMSP
Difficulty	★★★

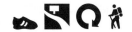

Lazily curving up the rumpled slopes of the western Santa Monica Mountains, the Ray Miller Trail takes in sweeping views of the Point Mugu coastline and the distant Channel Islands. This is the westernmost link in the nearly completed Backbone Trail, which skims along the crest of the Santa Monicas for some 65 miles. The Ray Miller Trail offers a well-graded and scenic approach to the rounded ridge that divides the two largest canyons in Point Mugu State Park: La Jolla and Big Sycamore canyons.

The Ray Miller Trail is just the start of the big loop we're suggesting here: a comprehensive trek through the western quadrant of Point Mugu State Park. If this is too big a chunk to bite off for a single day, there are short cuts, as our map suggests. You could also extend your trip by staying overnight at La Jolla Valley (walk-in) Camp. For that, you must register with a park ranger first.

To Reach the Trailhead: Point Mugu State Park lies some 32 miles west of Santa Monica via Pacific Coast Highway. Park at the Ray Miller Trailhead, off the coast highway and just west of Thornhill Broome Beach Campground.

Description: Two trails diverge from the parking lot. The wide one going up along the dry canyon bottom ahead is the La Jolla Canyon Trail—your return route.

To begin, take the narrower Ray Miller Trail to your right. It doggedly climbs 2.4 miles to a junction with the Overlook Trail, a wide fire road. This is the major ascent along the loop—better to get it over with at the beginning. Ever-widening views of the ocean and fine, springtime wildflower displays keep your mind off the effort.

Turn left when you reach the Overlook Trail, and wend your way around several bumps on the undulating ridge. You arrive at a saddle (4.5 miles from the start), where five wide trails diverge. Take the trail to the left (west) that descends into the green- or flaxen-colored (depending on the season) La Jolla Valley.

The valley is managed by the state park as a natural preserve to protect the native bunchgrasses that flourish there. Because so much of California's coast ranges have been biologically disturbed by grazing for more than a century, opportunistic, non-native grasses have taken over just about everywhere. The authentic California "tall-grass prairie" in parts of La Jolla Valley is a notable exception.

The La Jolla Valley Walk-in Camp ahead has piped water, restrooms, and oak-shaded picnic tables. Just south of there, beside a trail leading directly back to the Ray Miller Trailhead, you'll find a tule-fringed pond, seasonally dry in some years. Look for chocolate lilies on the slopes around it.

From the camp, continue west in the direction of a military radar installation on Laguna Peak. Stay right where marked trails diverge to the left, circling the perimeter of the La Jolla Valley grassland, and rising sharply on the Chumash Trail to a saddle (6.7 miles) on the northwest shoulder of the Mugu Peak ridge. At that saddle you'll have a great view of the Pacific Ocean. The popping noises you may hear below are from a military shooting range, near Pacific Coast Highway. Up the coast lies the Point Mugu Naval Air Station.

From the saddle, Chumash Trail descends sharply to Pacific Coast Highway. You veer left on the Mugu Peak Trail, and contour south and east around the south flank of Mugu Peak. You arrive (7.7 miles) at another saddle just east of Mugu's 1266-foot summit. Five minutes of climbing on a steep path puts you on top, where there's a dizzying view of the east-west-oriented coastline. You can look down upon The Great Sand Dune (coastal dunes) and Pacific Coast Highway where it barely squeezes past some coastal bluffs. On warm days there's a desertlike feel to this rocky and sparsely vegetated mountain, oddly juxtaposed with the sights and sounds of the surf below.

Return to the saddle east of the peak and continue descending to a junction in a wooded recess of La Jolla Canyon. Turn right, proceed east along a hillside, and then hook up with the La Jolla Canyon Trail (9.7 miles), where you turn right.

There's an exciting stretch down through a rock-walled section of La Jolla Canyon, where you'll see magnificent springtime displays of giant coreopsis. This plant is quite common in the Channel Islands, but found only in scattered coastal locales from far western Los Angeles County to San Luis Obispo County. Some coreopsis plants have forked stems towering as high as 10 feet, head and shoulders above the surrounding scrub.

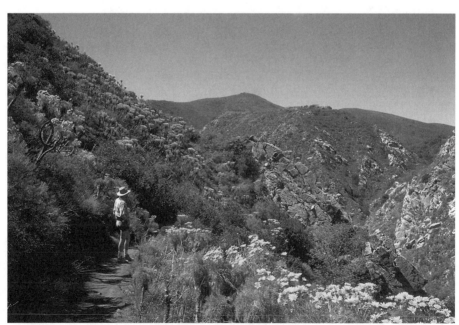

La Jolla Canyon Trail, with giant coreopsis in bloom

The massed, yellow, daisylike flowers are an unforgettable sight in March and April.

Descending toward the canyon's mouth, you'll pass a little grove of native walnut trees and a small, seasonal waterfall. After a final descent, you'll join a dirt road built to haul stone out of the area for the construction of the coast highway, and arrive a few minutes later at the Ray Miller Trailhead.

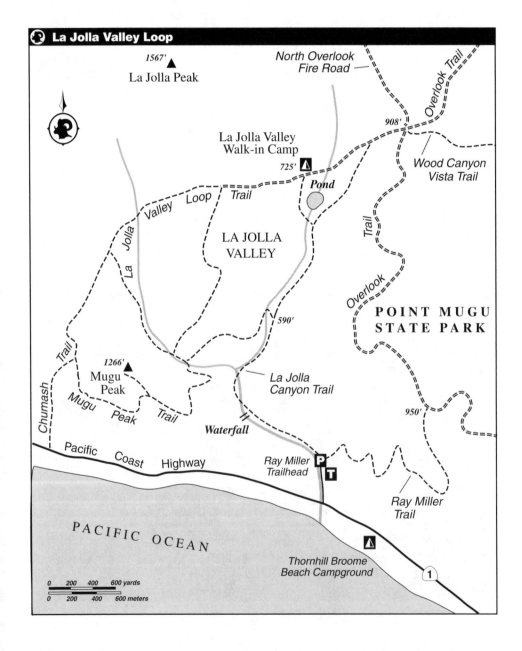

La Jolla Valley Loop

HIKE 4

Sandstone Peak

Location	Circle X Ranch
	(Santa Monica Mountains National Recreation Area)
Highlights	Most inclusive view in the Santa Monicas;
	volcanic rock formations
Distance	5.8 miles
Total Elevation Gain/Loss	1400'/1400'
Hiking Time	3 ½ hours
Optional Maps	USGS 7.5-min *Triunfo Pass, Newbury Park*
Best Times	October through June
Agency	SMMNRA
Difficulty	★★★

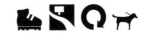

Sandstone Peak is the quintessential destination for peak baggers in the Santa Monica Mountains. The 3111-foot summit can be efficiently climbed from the east via the Backbone Trail in a mere 1.5 miles, but the far more scenic way to go is the looping route outlined below. Take a picnic lunch and plan to make a half day of it. Try to come on a crystalline day in late fall or winter to take best advantage of the skyline views. Or, if it's wildflowers you most enjoy, come in April or May, when the native vegetation blooms best at these middle elevations. In addition to blue-flowering stands of ceanothus, the early-to-mid-spring floral bloom includes monkeyflower, nightshade, Chinese houses, wild peony, wild hyacinth, morning glory, and phacelia. Delicate, orangish Humboldt lilies unfold by June.

Sandstone Peak lies within Circle X Ranch—formerly owned by the Boy Scouts of America, and now a federally managed unit of the Santa Monica Mountains National Recreation Area.

To Reach the Trailhead: The trailhead is located near the western end of the Santa Monica Mountains, a few miles (by crow's flight) south of Thousand Oaks. You can get there by following Yerba Buena Road 6.4 miles north from Pacific Coast Highway, or by following Little Sycamore Canyon and Yerba Buena roads 4.5 miles west from Mulholland Highway. On either approach, you face a white-knuckle drive on paved, but very narrow and curvy roads.

Description: Start hiking at the large parking lot on the north side of Yerba Buena Road, 1 mile east of the Circle X Ranch park office. Proceed on foot past a gate and up a fire road 0.3 mile to where the marked Mishe Mokwa Trail branches right. On it, right away you plunge into tough, scratchy chaparral vegetation. The hand-tooled route is delightfully primitive, but requires frequent maintenance so as to keep the chaparral from knitting together across the path. Both your hands and your feet will come into play over the next 40 or 50 minutes as you're forced to scramble a bit over rough-textured outcrops of volcanic rock. You'll make intimate acquaintance with mosses and ferns and several of the more attractive chaparral shrubs: toyon, holly-leaf cherry, manzanita, and red shanks (a.k.a. ribbonwood), which is identified by its wispy foliage and perpetually peeling, rust-colored bark. You'll also pass several small bay trees. After about a half hour on the Mishe Mokwa Trail, keep an eye out for an amazing balanced rock that rests precariously on the opposite wall of the canyon that lies just below you.

By 1.7 miles from the start you will have worked your way around to the north flank of Sandstone Peak, where you suddenly come upon a couple of picnic tables and "Split Rock," a fractured volcanic boulder with a gap wide enough to walk through (please do so to maintain the Scouts' tradition). From then on, you continue on an old dirt road that crosses the aforementioned canyon and turns west (upstream). You pass beneath some hefty volcanic outcrops and at 2.8 miles come to a junction with the Backbone Trail. That leg of the Backbone Trail, a narrow path, goes west into Point Mugu State Park. Keep straight (south) on the graded fire road ahead, signed BACKBONE TRAIL, and gradually circle east.

A few minutes beyond some water tanks on the right, look for a side path going right. This takes you about 50 yards to the top of a rock outcrop—Inspiration Point. The direction-finder there indicates local features as well as very distant points such as Mt. San Antonio (Old Baldy), Santa Catalina Island, and San Clemente Island.

Press on with your ascent. At a point just past two closely spaced hairpin turns

in the wide Backbone Trail, make your way up a slippery path to Sandstone Peak's windswept top. The plaque on the summit block honors W. Herbert Allen, a long-time benefactor of the Scouts and Circle X Ranch. To the Scouts this mountain is "Mt. Allen," although that name has not, so far, been accepted by cartographers. In any event, the peak's real name is misleading. It, along with Boney Mountain and most of the western crest of the Santa Monicas, consists of beige- and rust-colored volcanic rock, not unlike sandstone when seen from a distance.

On a clear day the view is truly amazing from here, with distant mountain ranges, the hazy L.A. Basin, and the island-dimpled surface of the ocean occupying all 360° of the horizon. To complete the loop, return to the Backbone Trail and resume your travel eastward. One and a half miles of twisting descent will take you back to the trailhead.

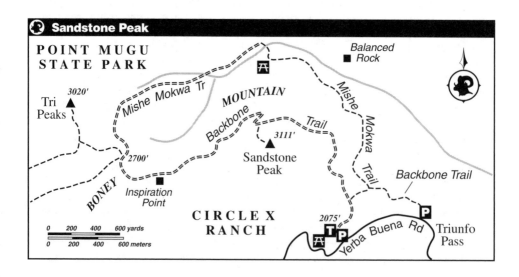

HIKE 5

The Grotto

Location	Circle X Ranch
	(Santa Monica Mountains National Recreation Area)
Highlights	Spooky rock formations; live oak groves
Distance	2.8 miles round trip
Total Elevation Gain/Loss	650'/650'
Hiking Time	2 hours (round trip)
Optional Map	USGS 7.5-min *Triunfo Pass*
Best Times	All year
Agency	SMMNRA
Difficulty	★★

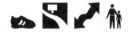

The 1655-acre Circle X Ranch, formerly run by the Boy Scouts of America but now administered by the National Park Service, is positively riddled with Tom Sawyer-esque hiking paths. Chief among those is the Grotto Trail, perfect for young, or young-in-thought, adventurers. Note that this hike is almost entirely downhill on the way in, and uphill on the way back. Plan accordingly and bring enough drinking water along.

To Reach the Trailhead: The trailhead is located near the western end of the Santa Monica Mountains, a few miles (by crow's flight) south of Thousand Oaks. You can get there by following Yerba Buena Road 5.4 miles north from Pacific Coast Highway, or by following Little Sycamore Canyon and Yerba Buena roads 5.5 miles west from Mulholland Highway. On either approach, you face a white-knuckle drive on paved, but very narrow and curvy roads.

Description: Start hiking at the Circle X Ranch park office. Walk down to the group campground, where you can find

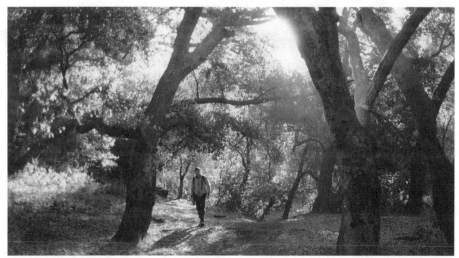

Live-oak woodland, West Fork Arroyo Sequit

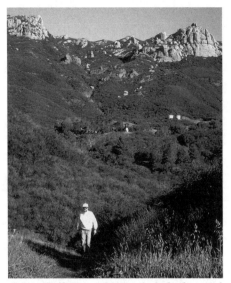

Grotto Trail, Boney Mountain in background

and follow the Grotto Trail heading south down along a shady, seasonal creek. Keep going downhill as you pass the Canyon View Trail intersecting on the left. Shortly afterward, you cross the creek at a point immediately above a 30-foot ledge, which becomes a trickling waterfall in winter and spring. You then go uphill, gaining about 50 feet of elevation, and cross an open meadow offering fine views of both Boney Mountain above and a deep-cut

gorge (the west fork of Arroyo Sequit) below. Maintain your descent, which becomes sharper as you get closer to the bottom of the gorge.

When you come upon an old roadbed at the bottom, stay left, cross the creek, and continue downstream on a narrowing trail along the shaded east bank. Curve left when you reach a grove of fantastically twisted live oaks at the confluence of two stream forks. On the edge of this grove, an overflow pipe coming out of a tank discharges tepid spring water. Continue another 200 yards down along the now-lively brook to The Grotto, a narrow, spooky constriction flanked by sheer volcanic-rock walls. If your sense of balance is good, you can clamber over gray-colored rock ledges and massive boulders fallen from the canyon walls—just as thousands of Boy Scouts have done in the past. At one spot you can peer cautiously into a gloomy cavern, where the subterranean stream is more easily heard than seen. Water marks on the boulders above are evidence that this part of the gorge probably supports a two-tier stream in times of flood.

When you've had your fill of adventuring, return by the same route, uphill almost the whole way.

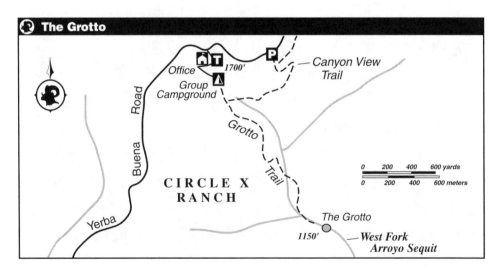

HIKE 6

Charmlee Wilderness Park

Location	Santa Monica Mountains
Highlights	Spring wildflowers; ocean views
Distance	2.8 miles
Total Elevation Gain/Loss	500'/500'
Hiking Time	1 ½ hours
Optional Map	USGS 7.5-min *Triunfo Pass*
Best Times	All year
Agency	CW
Difficulty	★★

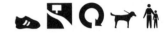

Charmlee Wilderness Park (a.k.a. Charmlee Natural Area), 590 acres of meadow, oak woodland, sage scrub, and chaparral, was first opened to the public in 1981 as a unit of the Los Angeles County park system. Today the City of Malibu administers the park, which lies on that coastal city's western extremity. Never designed to accommodate a large number of visitors, Charmlee's parking lot is often full on the weekends. A spider web of trails totaling 8 miles covers the park, making it a great place to ramble with family and friends for the purpose of wildflower spotting in spring, and ocean watching on any clear day. Out of the maze of footpaths and old ranch roads in the park, I've pieced together the perimeter route described here.

To Reach the Trailhead: To reach Charmlee Wilderness Park from Santa Monica, drive 25 miles west on Pacific Coast Highway (Highway 1), turn north on Encinal Canyon Road, and proceed north 4 miles to the park's well-marked entrance. Gates are open 8 A.M. to sunset daily.

Description: From the parking lot, walk on pavement to the nature center (inside, pick up a guide for the Fire Ecology Trail and other interpretive materials). Bear right on a paved road, soon dirt, that bends north up a slope. Make an acute left turn at the top, follow a ridge road past a hilltop water tank (detour and walk around the tank for a good overview of the park and the ocean), and then curve down to a T-intersection. Jog right, then go left on the Fire Ecology Trail. After a few minutes you will be passing under some fire-singed coast live oaks, which are well known for their ability to survive fast-moving wildfires.

At post 10 on the Fire Ecology Trail, go right on a road that winds along the west edge of Charmlee's large, central meadow.

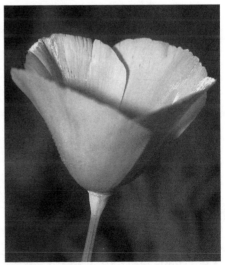

California poppy

Continue all the way to a dry ridge topped by some old eucalyptus trees and a concrete-lined cistern, both relics of cattle-ranching days. From there descend south (stay right at the next junction) to the "Ocean Vista," which really delivers in a big way what its name suggests, especially on clear days. In addition to miles of surf and sand seemingly at your feet, your eyes drink in perhaps a thousand square miles of wind-ruffled ocean.

Circle north from Ocean Vista around the hill with the cistern and then along the east side of the meadow. When you come to the northeast part of the meadow and the dirt road curves west, pick up the hard-to-spot Botany Trail on the right. It winds through mostly chaparral vegetation and takes you to the picnic area just above your starting point.

If it's a spring day and you've kept a tally of wildflowers spotted on the hike, you may be surprised to find your list includes as many as two dozen or more.

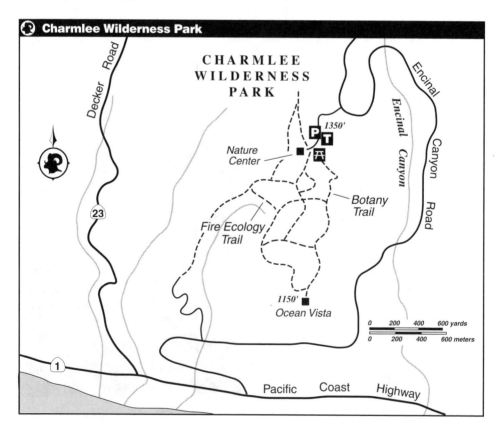

HIKE 7

Zuma Canyon

Location	Santa Monica Mountains
Highlights	Spectacular, wild canyon trek; ocean views on the return
Distance	8.0 miles
Total Elevation Gain/Loss	1700'/1700'
Hiking Time	6 hours
Optional Map	USGS 7.5-min *Point Dume*
Best Times	October through June
Agency	SMMNRA
Difficulty	★★★★

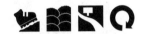

Although it slices only 6 miles inland from the Pacific shoreline, Zuma Canyon harbors one of the deepest gorges in the Santa Monica Mountains. Easily on a par with nearby Malibu and Topanga canyons in scenic wealth but much less known, Zuma Canyon holds a further distinction of never having suffered the invasion of a major road. Under cover of junglelike growths of willow, sycamore, oak and bay, the canyon's small stream cascades over sculpted sandstone boulders and gathers in limpid pools adorned with ferns. These natural treasures yield their secrets begrudgingly, as they should, only to those willing to scramble over boulders, plow through sucking mud and cattails, and thrash through scratchy undergrowth.

On this challenging trek, you'll proceed straight up the canyon's scenic midsection, climb out of the canyon depths via a powerline service road, and loop back to your starting point on the ridge-running Zuma Ridge Trail (a fire road). The roads are shadeless, yet they offer great vistas of the canyon, the ocean, and the seemingly interminable east-west sweep of the Santa Monica Mountains.

Hiking the canyon bottom is least problematical in the fall season before the heavy rains set in. The stream may have shrunk to isolated pools by then, and you'll step mostly on dry rocks with good

traction. Winter flooding can render the canyon impassable, but such episodes are rare and short-lived. During spring, the stream flows heartily and there's plenty of greenery and wildflowers; at the same time there's an increased threat of exposure to poison oak (which is found in fair abundance along the banks) and you're likely to surprise a rattlesnake. Summer days are usually too oppressively warm and humid for such a difficult hike. Whatever the season, take along plenty of water; the water in the canyon is not potable.

To Reach the Trailhead: A good starting place is the north end of Bonsall Drive, in the Point Dume area of Malibu. From the intersection of Kanan Dume Road and Pacific Coast Highway, drive 0.9 mile west on PCH to Bonsall Drive, turn right, and continue 1 mile to where Bonsall Drive ends at a trailhead for the Zuma Canyon trail system.

Description: From the end of Bonsall Drive, walk north on the main path following Zuma Canyon's winter-wet, summer-dry creek. You'll pass statuesque sycamores, tall laurel sumac bushes, and scattered wildflowers in season. This is a promising area for spotting wildlife anytime—squirrels, rabbits, and coyotes are commonly seen, deer and bobcats less so.

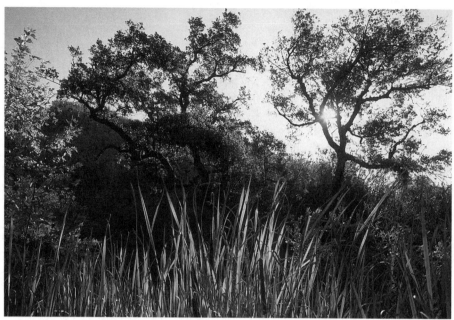

The wilds of Zuma Canyon

After about a mile's walk along the creek or dry canyon bottom, the canyon walls close in tighter, oaks appear in greater numbers, and you'll notice a small grove of eucalyptus trees on a little terrace. Not long afterward, the path abruptly ends at a pile of sandstone boulders. During the dry months, surface water may get only this far down the canyon. Often, however, the water trickles or tumbles past here, disappearing at some point downstream into the porous substrate of the canyon floor. Now you begin a nearly 2-mile stretch of boulder-hopping (and possibly wading), 2 or 3 hours worth depending on the conditions. Other than a few rusting pieces of pipeline from an old dam and irrigation system, you may find that the canyon is completely litter-free; please keep it that way.

The great variety of rocks that have been washed down the stream or have fallen from the canyon walls says a lot about the geologic complexity of the Santa Monicas. You'll scramble over fine-grained siltstones and sandstones, con-

glomerates that look like poorly mixed aggregate concrete, and volcanic rocks of the sort that make up Saddle Rock (a local landmark near the head of Zuma Canyon) and the Goat Buttes of nearby Malibu Creek State Park. Some of the larger boulders attain the dimensions of mid-sized trucks, presenting an obstacle course that must be negotiated by moderate hand-and-foot climbing.

About 0.5 mile shy of the Edison service road crossing, you'll pass directly under a set of high-voltage transmission lines—so high they're hard to spot. These lines, plus the graded road built to give access to the towers, represent the major incursion of civilization into Zuma Canyon. If you can ignore them, however, it's easy to imagine what all the large canyons in the Santa Monicas were like only a century ago.

When you finally reach the Edison Road, turn left and follow it to the top of the west ridge. From there, turn left on the Zuma Ridge Trail (another dirt road) and follow its lazily curving, downhill course toward the coastal plain, enjoying clear-air vistas of the vast Pacific Ocean much of the way. This and many other utility service roads in the Santa Monicas are closed to unauthorized motorized vehicles, and are popular among hikers and mountain bikers. When you reach the bottom of the Zuma Ridge Trail, where Busch Drive and Cuthbert Road meet, take the path across the hillside to your left (east). You lose about 300 feet of elevation as you zigzag down to the bottom of the Zuma Canyon flood plain. Turn right when you reach the main Zuma Canyon trail and walk a short distance over to where you began your hike.

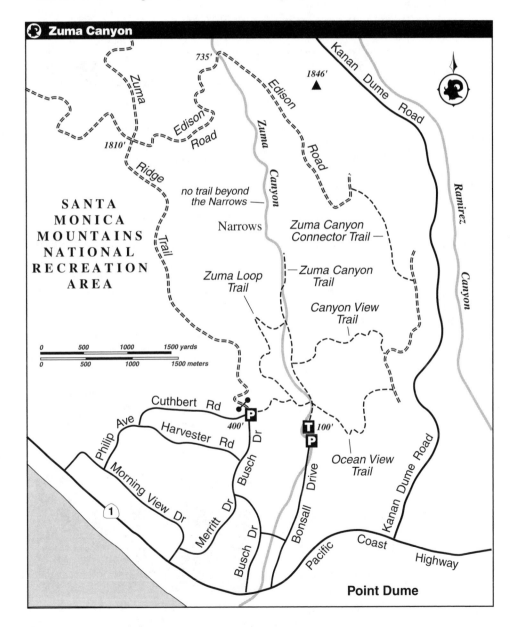

HIKE 8

Point Dume to Paradise Cove

Location	Malibu coast
Highlights	Panoramic ocean vistas; superb intertidal exploration
Distance	2.1 miles one way
Total Elevation Gain/Loss	(Nearly flat)
Hiking Time	1 ½ hours
Optional Map	USGS 7.5-min *Point Dume*
Best Times	All year (passable during low tides)
Agency	SMMNRA
Difficulty	★★

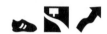

Like the armored bow of an ice-breaker, flat-topped Point Dume juts into the Pacific about 20 miles west of Santa Monica. Just east of the point itself, an unbroken cliff wall shelters a secluded beach from the sights and sounds of the civilized world. Below the sometimes-narrow stretch of sand east of Point Dume, a strip of rocky coastline harbors tidal pools and a mind-boggling array of plant and animal life.

A pleasant walk anytime the tide is low, this trip is doubly rewarding when the tide dips as low as -2 feet. Here are some of the creatures we spotted one warm October afternoon during a -1.5 foot tide: limpets, periwinkles, chitons, tube snails, sandcastle worms, sculpins, mussels, shore and hermit crabs, green and aggregate anemones, three kinds of barnacles, and two kinds of sea stars. Extreme low tides occur during the afternoon two or three times each month from October through March. During the summer, negative tides are rarer, and you'll have to get up early to catch them. Consult tide tables to find out exactly when.

To Reach the Trailhead: From the intersection of Pacific Coast Highway and Kanan Dume Road on Malibu's west side, drive 1 mile west on PCH to the turnoff for Zuma and Westward county beaches. Drive down Westward Beach Road to the roadend at Westward Beach (open daylight hours—parking fee charged).

Description: Starting out at Westward Beach you have a choice between two routes: over the top of the point or around the end of the point at sea level. The shorter, much easier route (and the only practical alternative during all but extremely low tides) is the first one, the trail slanting left up the cliff. On top you'll come to an area popular for sighting gray whales during their southward migration in winter. You'll also discover a state historic monument. Point Dume, you'll learn, was christened by the British naval commander George Vancouver, who sailed by in 1793.

As you stand on Point Dume's apex, note the marked contrast between the lighter sedimentary rock exposed on the cliff faces both east and west, and the darker volcanic rock just below. This unusually tough mass of volcanic rock has

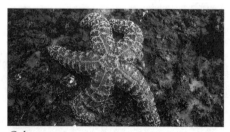

Ochre sea star

thus far resisted the onslaught of the ocean swells. After you descend from the apex, some metal stairs will take you down to crescent-shaped Dume Cove.

The alternate route is for expert climbers only. During the very lowest tides, you round the point itself, making your way by hand-and-toe climbing in a couple of spots over huge, angular shards of volcanic rock along the base of the cliffs. The tidepools here and to the east along Dume Cove's shoreline have some of the best displays of intertidal marine life in Southern California. This visual feast will remain for others to enjoy if you refrain from taking or disturbing in any way the organisms that live there. (WARNING: Exploring the lower intertidal zones can be hazardous. Be very cautious when traveling over slippery rocks, and always be aware of the incoming

swells. Don't let a rogue wave catch you by surprise.)

The going is easy once you're on Dume Cove's ribbon of sand. Signs posted here warn against nude bathing and sunning. This was once a popular nude beach, much to the chagrin of some of those living in the cliffside mansions overlooking the area.

When you reach the northeast end of Dume Cove, swing left around a lesser point and continue another mile over a somewhat wider beach to Paradise Cove, site of an elegant beach-side restaurant, private pier, and parking lot (public welcome, fee charged). If you've parked a second car here, then your hike ends here. Otherwise you can return the way you came or wend your way along the residential streets of Point Dume to return to Westward Beach.

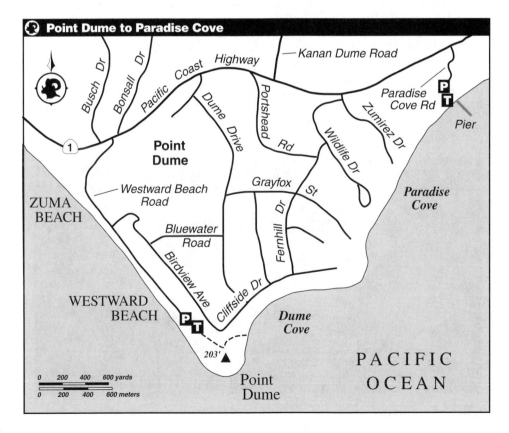

HIKE 9

Solstice Canyon Park

Location	Santa Monica Mountains (Malibu)
Highlights	Superb oak woodland; lessons in fire ecology
Distance	2.4 miles round trip (to Tropical Terrace)
Total Elevation Gain/Loss	350'/350'
Hiking Time	1 ½ hours (round trip)
Optional Maps	USGS 7.5-min *Malibu Beach, Point Dume*
Best Times	All year
Agency	SMMNRA
Difficulty	★

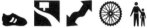

The easy-going but superbly scenic Solstice Canyon Trail takes you through the grounds of the former Robert's Ranch—now Solstice Canyon Park, a site administered by the National Park Service. The canyon once hosted a private zoo where giraffes, camels, deer, and exotic birds roamed. At trail's end you come to Tropical Terrace, the site of an architecturally noted grand home that burned in a 1982 wildfire.

To Reach the Trailhead: Solstice Canyon Park's gateway is located on Corral Canyon Road, 0.2 mile north of Pacific Coast Highway in Malibu. There's over-

flow parking space for several cars right at the entrance, and a more spacious lot 0.3 mile farther inside at the main trailhead. Parking is free. Carpooling is encouraged since parking space is limited. Posted park hours are 8 A.M. to sunset. We assume in this trail description that you start from the inside parking lot.

Description: Since the Solstice Canyon Trail is paved, it accommodates road bikes as well as mountain bikes, and all travel by foot and even wheelchairs. Starting at the main trailhead, pass through a gate and continue upstream alongside the canyon's melodious creek. You travel

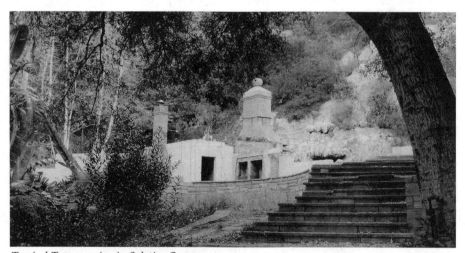

Tropical Terrace ruins in Solstice Canyon

through a fantastic woodland of alder, sycamore, bay, and live oak—the latter with trunks up to 18 feet in circumference. After 15 minutes or so, you pass an 1865 stone cottage on the right—thought to be the oldest existing stone building in Malibu.

At 1.2 miles, you arrive at the remains of Tropical Terrace. In a setting of palms and giant birds-of-paradise, curved flagstone steps sweep toward the roofless remains of what was for 26 years one of Malibu's grand homes. Beyond the house, crumbling stone steps and pathways lead to what used to be elaborately decorated rock grottoes, and a waterfall on Solstice Canyon's creek. Large chunks of sandstone have cleaved from the canyon walls, adding to the rubble. Hidden among the Tropical Terrace ruins are the remains of a concrete bomb shelter. For all its per-

fectly natural setting, Tropical Terrace's destiny was that of a temporary paradise, defenseless against both fire and flood.

Those on foot may want to try out the steep, rugged Sostomo or Rising Sun trails, which ascend the canyon walls and offer coastline views stretching from the Palos Verdes peninsula to Point Dume. Otherwise, you can turn around at Tropical Terrace and start an easy, gentle descent back to the trailhead.

Back at the trailhead parking lot you may want to check out the Dry Creek Trail, which goes northeast up an oak-shaded ravine for about 0.6 mile before entering private property. An outrageously cantilevered "Darth Vader" house overlooks the ravine as well as a 150-foot-high precipice that infrequently becomes a spectacular waterfall.

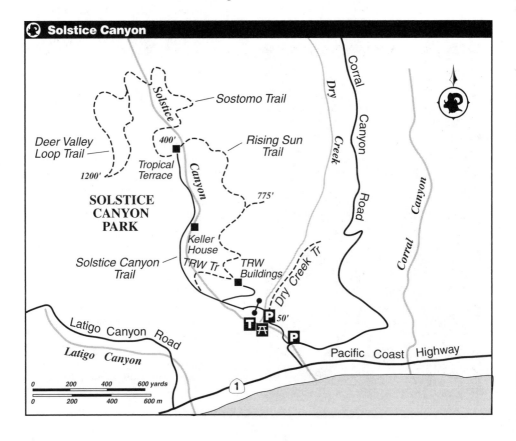

HIKE 10

Temescal Canyon

Location	Santa Monica Mountains (Pacific Palisades)
Highlights	Pseudo-aerial coastline views; shady riparian/oak woodland
Distance	2.8 miles
Total Elevation Gain/Loss	850'/850'
Hiking Time	1 ½ hours
Optional Map	USGS 7.5-min *Topanga*
Best Times	All year
Agency	SMMNRA
Difficulty	★★

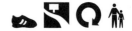

Spring lingers long on the coastal slopes of the Santa Monica Mountains, which are frequently bathed from May till July in the sopping-wet breath of the marine layer. This is quintessential coastal sage-scrub and chaparral country, a particular habitat that is fast succumbing to

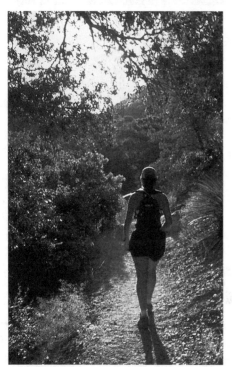

Slope above Temescal Canyon

urban development all over Southern California. All through spring and early summer, you can enjoy the scents of sage and wildflowers on the trails of Temescal Canyon, part of the Santa Monica Mountains National Recreation Area and Topanga State Park. With an early start on a foggy morn, you may find yourself punching right through the mist as you ascend into the bright, sunny world above.

To Reach the Trailhead: Begin at Temescal Gateway Park, just north of the intersection of Sunset Boulevard and Temescal Canyon Road in Pacific Palisades, 1 mile north of Pacific Coast Highway by way of Temescal Canyon Road. Park for a fee inside the gateway park, sunrise to sunset, or find a curbside space in the commercial district of Pacific Palisades across Sunset Boulevard. Pets are allowed on the short paths in the Gateway park itself, but not on the outlying trails ahead, which enter Topanga State Park.

Description: This hike traverses the Temescal loop clockwise, climbing the scrubby west wall of Temescal Canyon on the way up, and then making a nice, easy descent down through the canyon. To do this, head north toward several buildings that comprise the former Presbyterian conference grounds, and pick up the Temescal Ridge Trail. The narrow trail immediately starts a vigorous ascent up the scrubby canyon slope to the west. After several twists and turns, the trail gains a moderately ascending crest and sticks to it. Pause often so you can turn around and look at the ever-widening view of the coastline curving from Santa Monica Bay to Malibu. One winter afternoon on this ridge, I watched a leaden cumulus cloud drop its load over Temescal Canyon and then move on, leaving a vivid rainbow in its wake.

Ahead, two short trails (the Leacock and Bienveneda trails) strike off to the left toward the end of Bienveneda Avenue. Ignore those paths and continue a junction (1.3 miles from the start) with the former Temescal Ridge fire road, which is signed TEMESCAL RIDGE TRAIL to the north, and TEMESCAL CANYON TRAIL to the south. At this juncture you have the option of mak-

ing a side trip north 0.4 mile to a wind-carved, sandstone outcrop known as Skull Rock. To stay on the loop route, turn right and follow the Temescal Canyon Trail into the shady bottom of Temescal Canyon.

At the bottom you cross Temescal Canyon's creek on a footbridge. Above and below that bridge are small, trickling waterfalls and shallow, limpid pools. You can poke around the creek a bit for a look at its typical denizens—water striders and newts. When you've finished sightseeing, continue down the canyon trail back to the conference buildings, a mile away. That final stretch follows the canyon bottom, and then contours along a slope behind the buildings. Lots of live oak, sycamore, willow, and bay trees, their woodsy scents commingling on the ocean breeze, highlight your return.

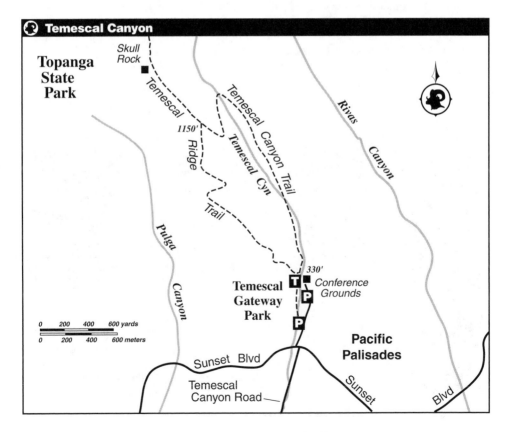

HIKE 11

Will Rogers Park

Location	Santa Monica Mountains (Pacific Palisades)
Highlights	City, ocean, and mountain views in a single stance
Distance	2.0 miles
Total Elevation Gain/Loss	350'/350'
Hiking Time	1 hour
Optional Map	USGS 7.5-min *Topanga*
Best Times	All year
Agency	WRSHP
Difficulty	★

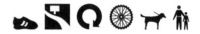

Drive up a short mile from the speedway known as Sunset Boulevard toward Will Rogers State Historic Park, and you'll instantly leave the rat race behind. Especially on weekdays or early on weekend mornings, this quiet spot is perfect for getting some exercise and taking advantage of multimillion-dollar views of Santa Monica, West L.A. and downtown L.A.

Newspaperman, radio commentator, movie star and pop-philosopher Will Rogers purchased this 182-acre property in 1922 and lived with his family here from 1928 until his death in 1935. Historic only by Southern California standards, his 31-room mansion is nevertheless interesting to tour. Our main goal, however, is to reach Inspiration Point, a flat-topped bump on a ridge overlooking the entire spread.

To Reach the Trailhead: Drive 1.5 miles east on Sunset Boulevard from the com-

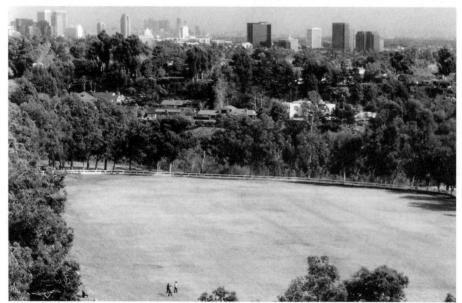

The polo field at Will Rogers Park

mercial district of Pacific Palisades (Sunset Boulevard and Temescal Canyon Road) to reach the Will Rogers Park entry road. Or take Sunset Boulevard 4 miles west from Interstate 405 to reach the same entry. The park is open daily, except certain holidays, from 8 A.M. to sunset. A parking fee is charged.

Description: You may want to obtain a copy of the detailed hikers' map, available at the gift shop in a wing of the home. Printed on the map is one of Will's memorable (if not apropos) aphorisms, "...if your time is worth anything, travel by air. If not, you might just as well walk." To reach Inspiration Point, follow the main, wide, riding and hiking trail that makes a 2-mile loop, starting at the north end of the big lawn adjoining the Rogers home. Or use any of several shorter, more direct paths (mountain bikes and leashed pets are only allowed on the main, looping trail, however).

Relaxing on the benches at the top on a clear day, you can admire true-as-advertised, inspiring vistas stretching east to the front range of the San Gabriel Mountains and southeast to the Santa Ana Mountains. South past the swelling Palos Verdes peninsula you can sometimes spot Santa Catalina Island, rising in ethereal majesty from the shining surface of the sea.

Will Rogers Park serves as the east terminus of the Backbone Trail, which skims some 65 miles along the crest of the Santa Monica Mountains. The west end of that same trail lies in Point Mugu State Park, and is described in Hike 3.

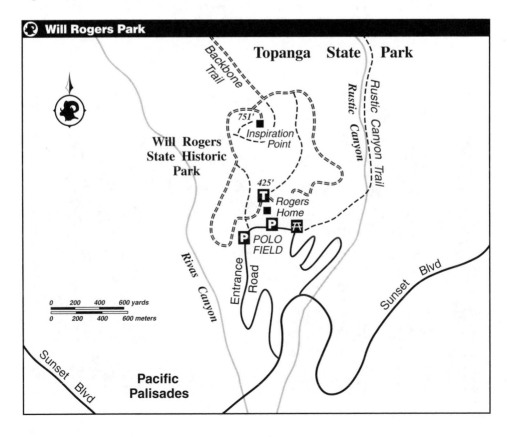

HIKE 12

Cheeseboro and Palo Comado Canyons

Location	Simi Hills (east of Thousand Oaks)
Highlights	Classic California green/golden grassland dotted with oaks
Distance	10.3 miles
Total Elevation Gain/Loss	1200'/1200'
Hiking Time	5 hours
Optional Map	USGS 7.5-min *Calabasas*
Best Times	October through June
Agency	SMMNRA
Difficulty	★★★

The Cheeseboro/Palo Comado Canyons park site, a unit of the Santa Monica Mountains National Recreation Area, serves as an important wildlife corridor between the interior Transverse Ranges in the north and the Santa Monica Mountains to the south. Self-propelled travelers by the thousands have discovered the place, but there's plenty of room for visitors to spread out. The long, leisurely loop route described here visits the two canyons, both surprisingly serene and pristine despite extensive suburban development in the surrounding region. Deer, bobcats, coyotes, rabbits, owls, and various birds of prey can be spotted in both canyons, especially in the early morning.

Without question, the period between the emergence of tender green grass (December or January) and the shift from green to gold (April or May) is the very best time to visit Cheeseboro and Palo Comado canyons. July through September brings midday temperatures in the 90s, making this area unpleasant for all but

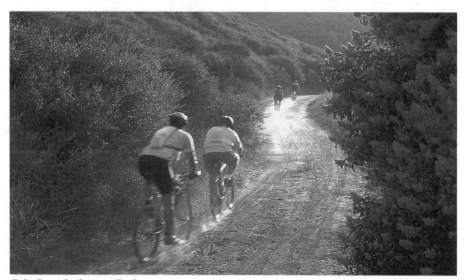

Palo Comado Canyon Trail

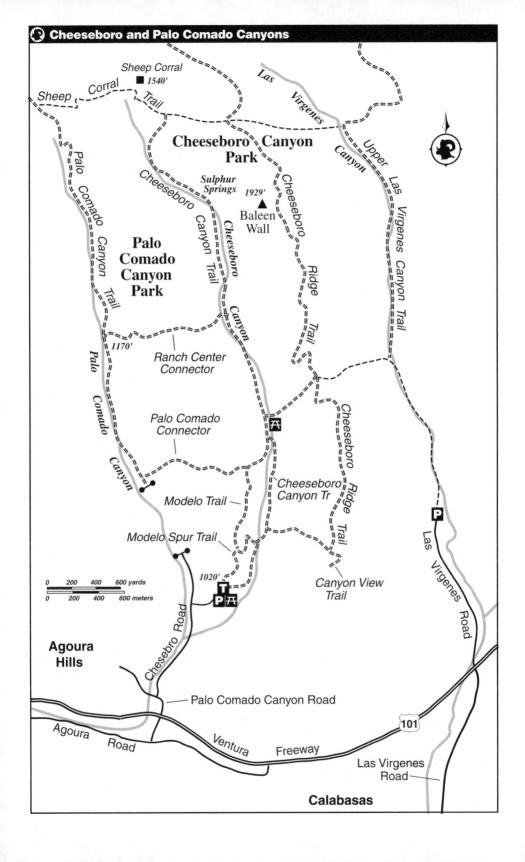

perhaps mountain bikers, who may enjoy the benefit of evaporative cooling if they move fast enough.

How to Reach the Trailhead: From Highway 101 in Agoura Hills, take the Chesebro (sic) Road exit, go north about 200 yards on what is signed Palo Comado Canyon Road, then turn right on Chesebro Road. Drive 0.7 mile north to the main entrance to the Cheeseboro/Palo Camado Canyons site, on the right. Gates to the trailhead parking lot swing open at 8 A.M.—but often earlier on weekends, when volunteers staff a National Park Service information booth here. A fenced trail into Cheeseboro Canyon bypasses the parking area, and hikers, bikers, and equestrians use it even when the gates are shut. Be aware that soggy trail conditions may close the park.

Description: From the trailhead parking lot, follow the wide Cheeseboro Canyon Trail, which goes briefly east and then bends north up along the wide, nearly flat canyon floor. Two kinds of oak trees dominate the Cheeseboro landscape: evergreen coast live oaks clustering along the canyon bottoms, and deciduous valley oaks, widely spaced, striking statuesque poses in the meadows and on the hillsides. This looks like typical California cattle-grazing land, and indeed it was for a period of about 150 years. Now that the cattle have been removed, oak seedlings are taking root in increasing numbers, and native spring wildflowers are returning to the hillsides, creating splashes of color across the grassy hillsides.

At 1.6 miles on Cheeseboro Canyon Trail, near the Palo Comado Connector trail joining from the west, you come upon a pleasant trailside picnic area. Stay on the main, wide trail going north through the canyon bottom. At 3.3 miles you pass Sulphur Springs. Let your nose be your guide for locating the springs. There's not much to see—the springs are mere seeps.

As you continue, the oaks clustering along the canyon bottom thin out, and you can gaze upward, to your right, at the whitish sedimentary outcrop known as the Baleen Wall. By 4.5 miles from the trailhead, in the corner of Shepherds Flat, you'll reach an old sheep corral made of wire. Pause here for a picnic, perhaps, before resuming your trip.

From the corral continue west on a narrow trail through the brush. You pass over a saddle and briefly descend to meet the graded-dirt Palo Comado Canyon Trail (5.2 miles). Turn left now, and commence a short mile of crooked descent on the wide dirt road. You look down on a lovely tapestry of canyon-bottom woods and slopes adorned with dense patches of chaparral and sandstone outcrops. Soon you are amid those woods, which are mostly live oaks and sycamores. The going is easy for another 2 miles as you proceed almost imperceptibly downhill along the canyon bottom.

At 8.2 miles, there's a forced left turn out of the canyon (off-limits private land lies ahead) and onto the Palo Comado Connector Trail. You meander uphill for a mile to a rounded ridge, where you meet the Modelo Trail on the right. Use it, and later the Modelo Spur, to return to the trailhead by the most expeditious route.

Beginning with the opening of Cheeseboro Canyon in the late 1980s, public agencies have been busy buying and trading properties to assemble a huge chunk of open-space centered on Cheesboro Canyon. Contiguous, protected open spaces in this part of the Simi Hills now cover about 30 square miles. The most recently purchased parcels of open-space land include upper Las Virgenes Canyon, and the former Ahmanson Ranch to the east, which links with existing parkland on the west rim of the San Fernando Valley. The National Park volunteers staffing the information center at the trailhead can give you the latest maps and information about these new areas.

HIKE 13

Old Stagecoach Road

Location	Santa Susana Pass
Highlights	Valley views, historical interest
Distance	2.6 miles round trip
Total Elevation Gain/Loss	650'/650'
Hiking Time	1 ½ hours (round trip)
Optional Maps	USGS 7.5-min *Oat Mountain, Santa Susana*
Best Times	October through June
Agency	SSPSHP
Difficulty	★★

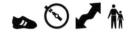

Clear-air vistas of the San Fernando Valley and surrounding mountain ranges are as spectacular as they come when seen from the Old Stagecoach Road above Chatsworth. The boulder-stacked hillsides rising from the valley seem strongly reminiscent of the golden backdrops seen in old Western movies and television shows, because they really did play a background role in many of those productions.

The area traversed by the Old Stagecoach Road has recently been incorporated into the new, 670-acre Santa Susana Pass State Historic Park. The pass has been (and continues to be) a key link in a major coastal transportation corridor connecting northern and southern California. The Spanish Army Captain Gaspar de Portola passed this way in 1769, blazing a trail from San Diego to Monterey Bay. The route later became a part of the El Camino Real (King's Highway) which linked together the Spanish system of presidios, pueblos, and missions along California's coast and coastal-inland valleys. Today, railroad tracks and the Simi Valley Freeway traverse the Santa Susana Pass slightly north of where an earlier, devilishly steep road, called the Devil's Slide, was built to accommodate stagecoaches. Surprisingly, this long-abandoned stage route can be traced today on foot.

Because the state historic park is new and a plan for development of marked trails is in the works, the directions here may differ slightly from what you will find there.

To Reach the Trailhead: You'll begin at Chatsworth Park South, at the west end of Devonshire Street, 0.5 mile west of Topanga Canyon Boulevard in Chatsworth. The park is open from 8 A.M. to sunset daily.

Description: As you walk into Chatworth Park South, look for the path signed OLD STAGECOACH ROAD on the left. You soon cross into Santa Susana Pass State Historic Park and start climbing into the bouldered hills, where a maze of roads and old vehicle tracks may complicate route-finding. Head generally southwest and uphill to a low ridge distinguished by a row of bushy olive trees (0.6 mile). From there, turn right (northwest) up the ridge and aim toward a large, white, rectangular plaque embedded in sandstone on the hillside about 0.4 mile away. You're now on a well-preserved section of the Devil's Slide, a key link in the 1860–90 coastal stage road linking Los Angeles and San Francisco. As you walk up the hard sandstone bed, notice the carefully hewn drainage chutes on both sides. With a little detective work you may also find a couple of old cisterns, used to capture rainwater for relay teams of horses that pulled wagons up the formidable grade.

The tiled historical plaque, installed in 1939, remains in good shape. Beyond the plaque, you can follow the stagecoach road bed another 0.3 mile to the Devil's Slide summit (1630'), where you cross the L.A.-Ventura county line and reach a trailhead sign on Lilac Lane in an area of scattered residences. North, behind a hill, is today's Santa Susana Pass, threaded by the Simi Valley Freeway and the older Santa Susana Pass Road. Some 600 feet below you is the 1.4-mile-long Santa Susana railroad tunnel, whose east entrance can be seen back near Chatsworth Park South.

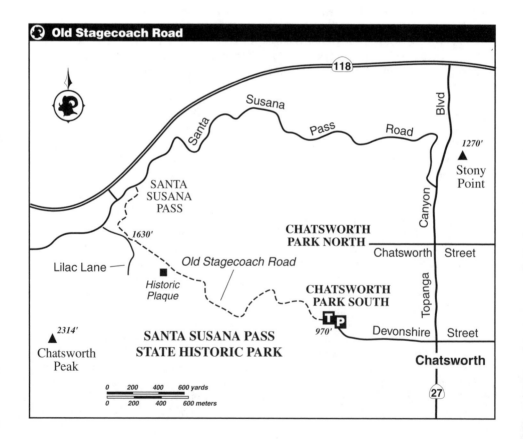

HIKE 14

Placerita Canyon

Location	Santa Clarita
Highlights	Wooded ravines; waterfall; historical interest
Distance	5.0 miles round trip (to waterfall)
Total Elevation Gain/Loss	700'/700'
Hiking Time	2 ½ hours (round trip)
Optional Maps	USGS 7.5-min *Mint Canyon, San Fernando*
Best Times	October through June
Agency	PCP
Difficulty	★★

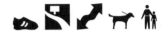

Barely 10 minutes drive from northern San Fernando Valley and the sprawling suburban city of Santa Clarita, Placerita Canyon Park nestles comfortably at the foot of one of the more verdant slopes of the San Gabriel Mountains. The park's wild backcountry sector (the subject of this hike, as described) is complemented by a very civilized nature center—the envy of many a national park—housing exhibits on local history, pre-history, geology, plants, and wildlife.

Placerita Canyon's fascinating history is highlighted by the discovery of gold there in 1842. That event, which touched off California's first (and relatively trivial) gold rush, predated by six years John Marshall's famous discovery of gold at Sutter's Mill in Northern California. By the 1950s, Placerita Canyon had become one of the more popular generic Western site locations used by Hollywood's movie makers and early television producers. The canyon was eventually acquired as parkland—first by the state, then by the county.

To Reach the Trailhead: Take the Placerita Canyon exit from Antelope Valley Freeway (Highway 14) at Newhall, and drive east 1.5 miles to reach the park's main gate, open 9 A.M. to 5 P.M. Nearby lie the nature center and a paved path leading under Placerita Canyon Road to the

"Oak of the Golden Dream," the exact site (according to legend) where gold was discovered in 1842 by a herdsman pulling up wild onions for his after-siesta meal.

Description: To start the somewhat ambitious hike described here, head east from the nature center on the Placerita Canyon Trail. The canyon's melodious creek flows decently about half the year (winter and spring), caressing the ears with white noise that echoes from the canyon walls. During the fall, when the creek may be bone-dry, you make your own noise instead by crunching through the crispy leaf litter of sycamore and live oak. Down by the grassy banks are wild

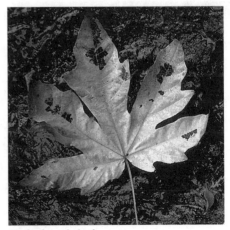

Bigleaf maple leaf

blackberry vines, lots of willows, and occasionally cottonwood and alder trees.

Soaring canyon walls ahead tell the story of thousands of years of natural erosion, as well as the destructive effects of hydraulic mining, which involved aiming high-pressure water hoses at hillsides to loosen and wash away ores. Used extensively in Northern California during the big Gold Rush, "hydraulicking" was finally banned in 1884 after catastrophic damages to waterways and farms downstream. At Placerita Canyon, several hundred thousand dollars worth of gold were ultimately recovered, but at considerable cost, effort, and general messiness.

After about 1 mile you reach a split. Go either way; the two paths join later. After the two paths converge, you reach the scant remains of some early-20th-Century cottages hand-built by settler Frank Walker, his wife, and some of his 12 children. The area is now used as a group campground; drinking water is available.

Our way lies ahead, along the Waterfall Trail, which leads into Los Pinetos Canyon. Don't confuse this trail with the better-traveled Los Pinetos Trail on the right. The Waterfall Trail momentarily slants upward along the canyon's steep west wall, and then drops onto the canyon's sunny flood plain. Presently you bear right into a narrow ravine (Los Pinetos Canyon), avoiding a wider tributary bending left (east).

Continue, now on an ill-defined path, past and sometimes over water-polished, metamorphic rock. Live oaks and bigcone Douglas-firs cling to the slopes above, and a few bigleaf maples grace the canyon bottom. About 0.2 mile after the first fork in the canyon, there's a second fork. Go right and continue 50 yards to a sublime little grotto, cool and dark except when the sun passes almost straight overhead, and a small waterfall. As you listen to water dashing or dribbling down the chute, enjoy the serenity of this private place and contemplate that it lies only 3 miles—but a world away—from the creeping boundary of the L.A. metropolis. Return the way you came.

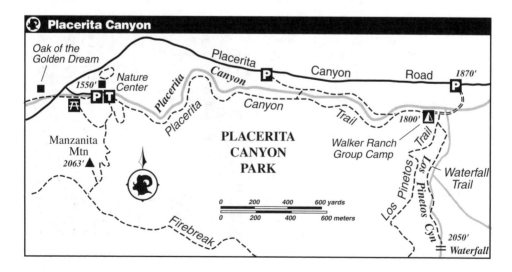

HIKE 15

Verdugo Mountains, South End Loop

Location	Glendale
Highlights	Incomparable city and regional views
Distance	5.5 miles
Total Elevation Gain/Loss	1500'/1500'
Hiking Time	3 ½ hours
Optional Maps	USGS 7.5-min *Pasadena, Burbank*
Best Times	November through May
Agency	SMMC
Difficulty	★★★

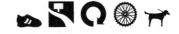

The Verdugo Mountains stand as a remarkable island of undeveloped land—a haven for wildlife such as deer and coyotes—completely encircled by an urbanized domain. Public access to the network of trails and fire roads on the mountain is by foot, horse, or mountain bike—great news if you're looking for a quick escape

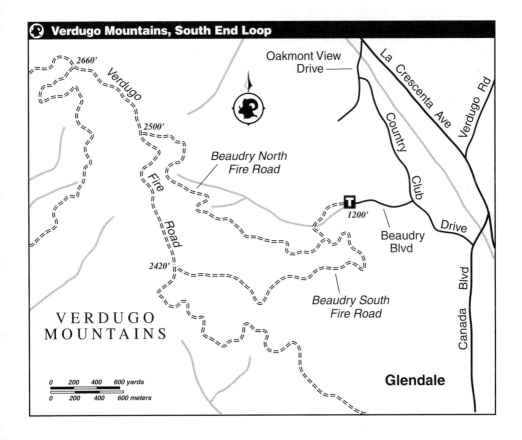

from the ubiquitous automobile and the pressures of city life.

Along the south crest of the Verdugos, your gaze takes in the San Gabriel Mountains, much of the L.A. megalopolis, and even the ocean on occasion. Do this trip late in the day if you want to enjoy both a spectacular sunset and a blaze of lights after twilight fades. At best, try this on any cloud-free, smog-free day that falls within two weeks on either side of the winter solstice (December 21). During that period, the sun sets on the flat ocean horizon behind Santa Monica Bay, at around 5 P.M. At other times of year, the sun's sinking path is likely to intersect the coastal mountains. The seemingly strange fact of the sun setting over land most of the year is a consequence of the east-west orientation of California's coastline in the first miles "up-coast" from Los Angeles.

To Reach the Trailhead: You'll find the starting point for this hike on Beaudry Boulevard, 0.4 mile west of Country Club Drive in the city of Glendale (not to be confused with Country Club Drive in nearby Burbank). Park on the street.

Description: From Beaudry Boulevard, walk up a paved segment of fire road, bypass a vehicle gate, and continue on dirt past a debris basin to where the fire road splits (0.3 mile). Choose for your way the shadier but less viewful right branch, Beaudry North Fire Road. You'll return to this junction by way of the left branch, the Beaudry South Fire Road. About halfway up the north road you'll come to a trickling spring and a water tank nestled in a shady ravine, a good place for a breather.

When you reach the summit ridge (2.3 miles), turn sharply left on Verdugo Fire Road and continue climbing another 0.4 mile toward a cluster of brightly painted radio towers atop a 2656-foot bump—the highest point along this hike. From the towers, continue south along the ridge 0.6 mile to a road junction at 2420 feet. The right branch descends to Sunshine Drive

in Glendale; you take the left branch and return along an east ridge to the split just above the debris basin.

HIKE 16

Trail Canyon Falls

Location	San Gabriel Mountains, near Sunland
Highlights	Lively stream and waterfall (in the wet season)
Distance	3.0 miles round trip
Total Elevation Gain/Loss	700'/700'
Hiking Time	1 ½ hours (round trip)
Optional Map	USGS 7.5-min *Sunland*
Best Times	December through May
Agency	ANF/LARD
Difficulty	★★

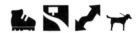

Rising starkly behind the San Fernando and La Crescenta valley communities of Sylmar, San Fernando, Sunland and Tujunga, the western ridges of the San Gabriel Mountains have a lean and hungry look. Yet there is a gentler, mostly hidden side, to these mountains, too. That's what you'll discover along Trail Canyon, where riparian glens and pocket forests of oak squeeze between canyon walls punctuated by eroding, angular rock outcrops and blanketed by tough chaparral.

When soaking rains come, Trail Canyon's normally indolent flow becomes a lively torrent. After tumbling through miles of rock-bound constrictions and sliding across many gently inclined declivities, the water comes to the lip of a real precipice. There the bubbly mixture momentarily attains weightlessness during a free-fall of about 30 feet. If you can manage to ignore the vastly smaller scale of this spectacle, you might easily imagine yourself in Yosemite Valley during spring runoff.

The falls in Trail Canyon are easy to approach, except during the most intense flooding, when the several fords you must cross on the way may be dangerously deep. Sturdy footwear (which is not needed during most of the year) may be helpful at some of the deeper crossings if the water is high.

To Reach the Trailhead: From the foothill community of Sunland, off I-210, take either Oro Vista Avenue or Mt. Gleason Avenue north to Big Tujunga Canyon Road, and turn right. Some 5 miles up Big Tujunga Canyon, on the left (mile 2.0 according to highway mile markers), look for a dirt-road turnoff and (perhaps) a sign reading TRAIL CANYON TRAIL. Turn left (north) there, drive 0.2 mile uphill to a fork, go right, and descend 0.2 mile to an oak-shaded parking area on the right, just

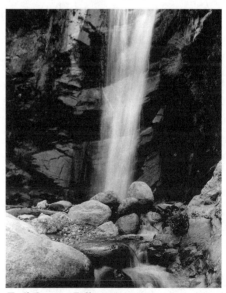

Trail Canyon Falls

above Trail Canyon's melodious creek. A National Forest Adventure Pass is needed for parking.

Description: From the parking lot, continue up the same road on foot, passing a few cabins and fording the creek for the first time. The now-very-deteriorated road goes on to follow an east tributary for a while, doubles back, contours around a ridge, and drops into Trail Canyon again (0.6 mile). The road ends there, and you continue up-canyon on a footpath. The path clings to the banks for 0.5 mile, crossing the stream several times, and then climbs the west wall to avoid a narrow, alder-choked section of the canyon. The falls come into view as you round a sharp bend about 1.5 miles from the parking area.

Although many people have obviously done so, it's difficult and dangerous to slide down from the trail to the base of the falls. The falls can also be reached by bushwhacking up the canyon from the point where the trail begins its ascent of the west wall; this might be fun scrambling for some during low water, but is hazardous during high water. Those sensitive to poison oak might think twice about stepping off the trail.

Past the falls, Trail Canyon Trail continues upstream to cozy Tom Lucas Trail Camp (4 miles from the start) and onward to a junction with the Condor Peak Trail. Ambitious hikers and backpackers can set their sights on a significant high point, Condor Peak, straightforwardly reached by means of a short, steep scramble from the Condor Peak Trail. One or more of the Channel Islands, floating above the coastal haze or smog, are frequently seen from Condor Peak's windswept summit.

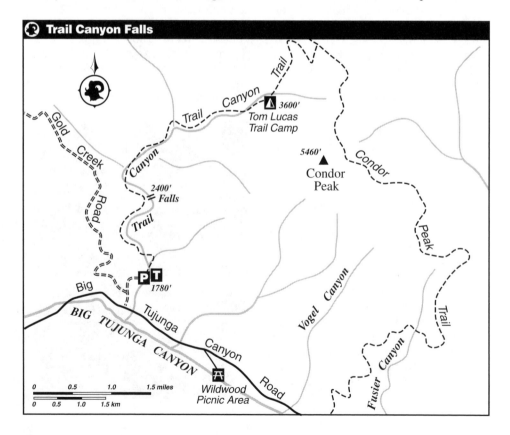

Trail Canyon Falls

HIKE 17

Mt. Lukens-Grizzly Flat Loop

Location	San Gabriel Mountains, near Sunland
Highlights	Urban, mountain, and ocean vistas
Distance	12.2 miles
Total Elevation Gain/Loss	3400'/3400'
Hiking Time	8 hours
Recommended Map	USGS 7.5-min *Condor Peak*
Best Times	October through May
Agency	ANF/LARD
Difficulty	★★★★

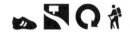

This all-day adventure lets you explore the massive flanks and the top of Mt. Lukens, the highest elevation in the city limits of Los Angeles. After a grueling climb up the Stone Canyon Trail, you circle back by way of a long, gradually descending route that passes through secluded Grizzly Flat. The hike feels best on a cool day, but beware of periods following heavy rain: The trip begins and ends with crossings of Big Tujunga creek, which can be hazardous in high water. Contact the Forest Service to check on flood conditions when appropriate and to get up-to-date information on the Grizzly Flat Trail, which is the last leg of your looping route. Despite the presence of a fancy trailhead interpretive panel at the bottom of the Grizzly Flat Trail, the trail itself has been infrequently maintained in

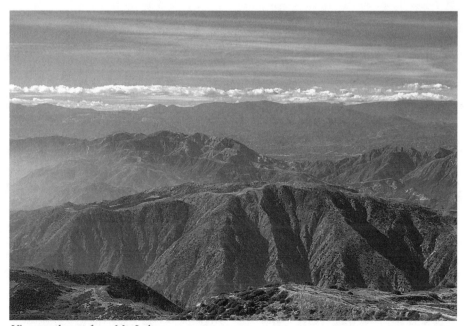
View northwest from Mt. Lukens

recent years and may be overgrown and difficult to follow.

Angeles National Forest generally permits "remote camping" in most seasons, but with strict restrictions on the use of open fires and sometimes restrictions on the use of camp stoves. This opens up the possibility of backpacking the route, perhaps with a layover night at Grizzly Flat. Again, contact the Forest Service to check on these rules if you are contemplating a two-day trek.

To Reach the Trailhead: From the foothill community of Sunland, off I-210, take either Oro Vista Avenue or Mt. Gleason Avenue north to Big Tujunga Canyon Road, and turn right. Some 7 miles up the canyon, on the right (south) side, is the well-marked turnoff to the Vogel Flat/Big Tujunga Station. Drive to the bottom of the hill, and either turn right to park at Vogel Flat Picnic Area (open 8 A.M. to 6 P.M.) or turn left to park at Stonyvale Picnic Area (open 6 A.M. to 10 P.M.). A National Forest Adventure Pass is required for parking at either place.

Description: On foot, head west from Vogel Flat along a narrow, paved road (private, but with public easement) through the cabin community of Stonyvale. When the pavement ends after 0.7 mile, continue on dirt for another ¼ mile or so. Choose a safe place to ford Big Tujunga creek, wade across, and find the Stone Canyon Trail on the far bank. From afar you can spot this trail going straight up the sloping terrace just left (east) of Stone Canyon's wide, boulder-filled mouth. Once you're on the terrace, settle into a pace that will allow you to persevere over the next 3 miles and 3200 feet of vertical ascent.

From the vantage point of the first switchback, you can look down on the thousands of storm-tossed granitic boulders filling Stone Canyon from wall to wall. Although the boulders are frozen in place, you can almost sense their movement over geologic time. Indeed, floods

continue to reshape this canyon and many others in the San Gabriels during every major deluge.

Ahead, you twist and turn along precipitous slopes covered by a thick blanket of chaparral. At or near ground level, a profusion of ferns, mosses, and herbaceous plants forms its own pygmy understory.

The dizzying view encompasses a long, obviously linear stretch of Big Tujunga Canyon. This segment of the canyon is underlain by the San Gabriel Fault and its offshoot, the Sierra Madre Fault. The latter fault splits from the former near Vogel Flat and continues southeast past Grizzly Flat, following a course roughly coincident with the final leg of our loop hike. According to current understanding, the San Gabriel Fault is presently inactive and not likely to be the cause of major movement or earthquakes in the foreseeable future. The impressive depth of Big Tujunga Canyon and the steepness of its walls are due primarily to stream cutting following uplift of the whole mountain range.

Between 1.8 and 2.6 miles (from Vogel Flat, as the assumed starting point), the trail hovers above an unnamed canyon to the east, nearly equal in drainage to Stone Canyon, but very steep and narrow. Down below you can often hear, and barely glimpse, an inaccessible waterfall. Long and short switchback segments take you rapidly higher to a steep, bulldozed track leading to the bald summit ridge of Mt. Lukens. Go 0.5 mile farther (connecting with Mt. Lukens Road along the way) to reach the highest point on the ridge (4.2 miles), which is occupied by several antenna structures. The summit lies within the city limit of Los Angeles, and is the highest point in any incorporated city in the county. Glendale almost claims this honor, as its corporate limit reaches within 300 yards of the summit. Both cities encompass parts of the Angeles National Forest. The views of the city below and the ocean in the distance can be fabulous—but only when strong winds evict the nearly ever-present smog from the L.A. basin and valleys below.

The remaining two-thirds of the hike is almost entirely downhill—a little monotonous at times, but not too jarring on the knees. Follow Mt. Lukens Road southeast down the main ridge, keeping left at the next two road junctions. At 7.2 miles you begin descending toward a saddle. At the four-way junction there (9.0 miles), choose the road to the far left and continue on a zigzag course past beautiful oaks and bay laurels to Grizzly Flat (10.0 miles), where planted pines fill most of a terrace sloping down to a ravine called Vasquez Creek. The leftmost of several diverging roads on the flat leads to a water tank. Behind that you may find a remnant of the old Dark Canyon Trail from Ange-

les Crest Highway to Big Tujunga Canyon—roughly the escape route used by the infamous outlaw Tibercio Vasquez and his unsuccessful pursuers during a hot chase over a century ago.

From the water tank, follow the Grizzly Flat Trail down to a creek bedecked with woodwardia fern and wild strawberry. You then descend moderately through oak forest, descend sharply down a ridge overlooking the pitlike gorge of Silver Creek, and finally reach a wildflower-dotted bench along Big Tujunga creek. Wild fruit trees and eucalyptus there silently speak of former homesteads. Head downstream, wading or stepping across the creek five times in the next mile, to reach Stonyvale Picnic Area, just shy of Vogel Flat.

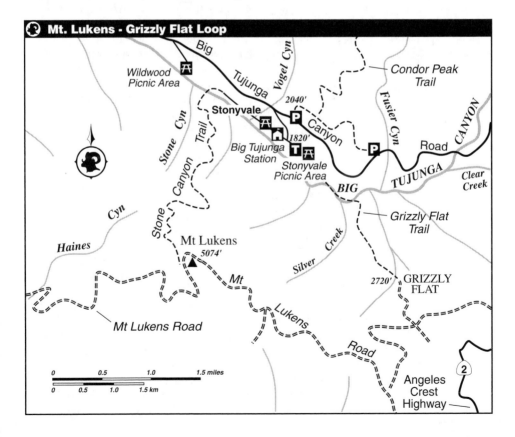

HIKE 18

Down the Arroyo Seco

Location	San Gabriel Mountains, above Pasadena
Highlights	Sylvan glens and a sparkling stream
Distance	9.6 miles
Total Elevation Gain/Loss	450'/2600'
Hiking Time	5 hours
Optional Maps	USGS 7.5-min *Condor Peak, Pasadena*
Best Times	October through June
Agency	ANF/LARD
Difficulty	★★★

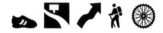

The Spanish colonists who christened Arroyo Seco ("dry creek") evidently observed only its lower end—a hot, boulder-strewn wash emptying into the Los Angeles River. Upstream, inside the confines of the San Gabriels, Arroyo Seco is a scenic treasure—all the more astounding when you consider that its exquisite sylvan glens and sparkling brook lie just 12–15 miles from L.A.'s city center. If you haven't yet been freed from the notion that Los Angeles is nothing but a seething megalopolis, walk down the canyon of the Arroyo Seco. You'll be convinced otherwise.

A botanist's and wildflower seeker's dream, the canyon features generous growths of canyon live oak, western sycamore, California bay, white alder, bigleaf maple, bigcone Douglas-fir, and arroyo willow. A quick census one spring day (in a dry year, no less) yielded for me the following blooming plants: golden yarrow, prickly phlox, western wall-flower, Indian pink, live-forever, wild pea, deerweed, bush lupine, Spanish broom, baby-blue-eyes, yerba santa, phacelia, chia, black sage, bush poppy, California buckwheat, shooting star, western clematis, Indian paintbrush, sticky mon-keyflower, scarlet bugler, and purple nightshade.

Some kind of car-shuttle or drop-off-and-pick-up transportation arrangement is obviously required for this long one-way trip.

To Reach the Trailhead (*Switzer Picnic Area*): Switzer Picnic Area is one of the most popular destinations in the San Gabriel Mountains. Plan to arrive early—gates normally swing open at 8 A.M. By 10 A.M. on weekends the picnic area's adjacent parking lot is usually filled to capacity. Overflow and off-hours parking is available at the well-marked entrance to the picnic area, at mile marker 34.2 on Angeles Crest Highway, 10 miles from I-210 at La Cañada. If you park at this entrance, you must hike down a narrow paved road to the picnic area, adding 0.4 mile and 250 feet of elevation loss to your one-way trip. A National Forest Adventure Pass is required for any car left at or near this upper trailhead.

To Reach the Trailhead (*Pasadena*): Exit I-210 at Arroyo Boulevard/Windsor Avenue, and drive north on Windsor Avenue for 0.8 mile to the intersection of Windsor Avenue and Ventura Street. Free trailhead parking is available here, at the trailhead for the Gabrielino Trail.

Description: You'll be traveling the westernmost leg of the Gabrielino Trail, one of four routes in Angeles National Forest specially designated as "National

Recreation Trails." The Arroyo Seco stretch of the Gabrielino Trail receives considerable use—and also a lot of much-needed maintenance—by mountain-bike club members. The upper and middle portions, which are in places narrow with steep drops to one side, are challenging even for expert riders, although not at all hard for hikers. The lower end consists of remnants of an old road built as far up the canyon as the Oak Wilde resort (now Oakwilde Campground) in the 1920s.

Several rest stops and picnic sites line the trail's lower half, making this a great route for a leisurely saunter. Most of these stops are located on the sites of early tourist camps or cabins erected in the early 1900s. Virtually all the structures were either destroyed by flooding in 1938 or removed through condemnation proceedings (based on water and flood-control needs) in the '20s, '30s, and '40s.

Carry along whatever drinking water you'll need for the duration of the trip; there may be piped water at one or another of the rest stops along the way, but don't count on it. Pleasantly shaded Oakwilde Campground near the midpoint is the best place to stay if you're backpacking the route.

For the easier, downhill direction we are suggesting here, you will start hiking from the west end of Switzer Picnic Area on the signed Gabrielino Trail. Make your way past outlying picnic tables, and then down along the alder-shaded stream. Soon nothing but the clear-flowing stream and rustling leaves disturb the silence. Remnants of an old paved road are occasionally underfoot. In a couple of spots you ford the stream by boulder-hopping—no problem except after heavy rain.

One mile down the canyon you come upon the foundation remnants of Switzer's Camp—now occupied by a trail campground. Established in 1884, the camp became the San Gabriels' premier wilderness resort in the early 1900s, patronized by Hollywood celebrities as well as anyone who had the gumption to hike or ride a burro up the tortuous Arroyo Seco trail from Pasadena. After the con-

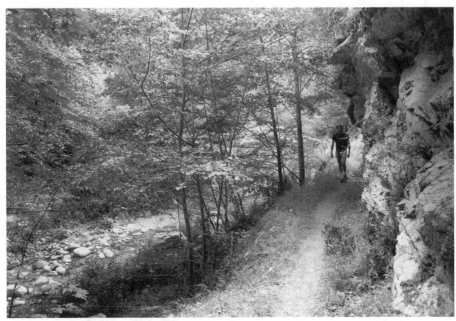

The Gabrielino Trail above Oakwilde

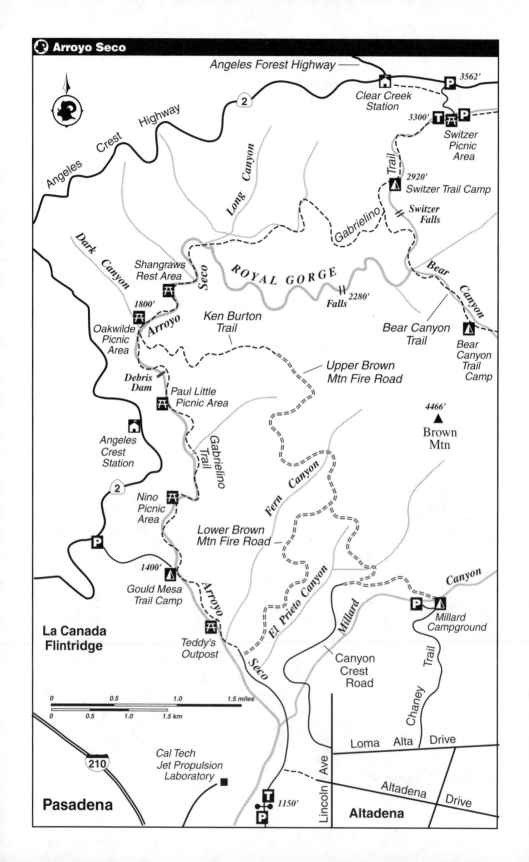

Angeles Forest Highway

2

Angeles Crest Highway

Long Canyon

Clear Creek Station

3562'

Switzer Picnic Area

3300'

Gabrielino Trail

2920'
Switzer Trail Camp

Switzer Falls

Dark Canyon

Shangraws Rest Area

Seco

ROYAL GORGE

Bear Canyon

1800'

Oakwilde Picnic Area

Arroyo

Ken Burton Trail

Falls 2280'

Bear Canyon Trail

Bear Canyon Trail Camp

Debris Dam

Paul Little Picnic Area

Upper Brown Mtn Fire Road

4466'
▲
Brown Mtn

Angeles Crest Station

Gabrielino Trail

2

Nino Picnic Area

Fern Canyon

Lower Brown Mtn Fire Road

Canyon

1400'

Gould Mesa Trail Camp

Arroyo

P

Millard Campground

La Canada Flintridge

Teddy's Outpost

El Prieto Canyon

Millard

Canyon Crest Road

Chaney Trail

Seco

0   0.5   1.0   1.5 miles
0   0.5   1.0   1.5 km

Loma   Alta   Drive

Lincoln Ave

Altadena   Drive

Cal Tech Jet Propulsion Laboratory ■

210

Pasadena

1150'

Altadena

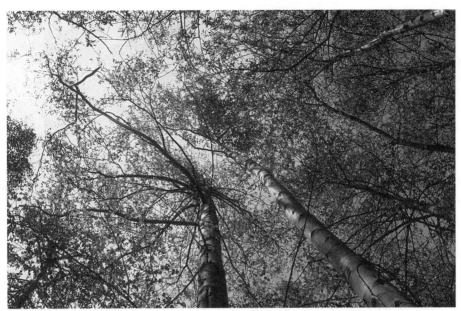

Alders in Arroyo Seco

struction of Angeles Crest Highway in the early '30s and a severe flood in the 1938, the resort lost its appeal. It was finally razed in the late '50s.

Walk down to a fork in the trail 0.2 mile beyond the trail camp. You will probably hear, if not clearly see, the 50-foot cascade known as Switzer Falls, to the east. Our way continues on the right fork (Gabrielino Trail), which now begins a mile-long traverse through chaparral. This less-than-perfectly-scenic stretch avoids a narrow, twisting trench called Royal Gorge, through which the Arroyo Seco stream tumbles and sometimes abruptly drops.

At 2.3 miles (from the start) the trail joins a shady tributary of Long Canyon, and later Long Canyon itself, replete with a trickling stream. Alongside the trail you'll discover at least five kinds of ferns, plus mosses, poison oak, and Humboldt lilies (in bloom during early summer).

At 3.4 miles, the waters of Long Canyon swish down through a sculpted grotto to join Arroyo Seco. The trail descends to Arroyo Seco canyon's narrow

floor and stays there, crossing and recrossing many times over the next few miles. The stretch from Long Canyon to Oakwilde Campground (4.5 miles) is perhaps the most gorgeous of all, flanked by soaring walls and dappled with shade cast by the ever-present alders. Bigleaf maples put on a great show here in November, their bright yellow leaves boldly contrasting with the earthy greens, grays, and browns of the canyon's dimly lit bottom.

Beyond Oakwilde Campground the canyon widens a bit and the trail assumes a more gentle gradient. There's a sharp climb at 5.3 miles—to bypass the large Brown Canyon Debris Dam—then a long trek out to the mouth of the canyon with no further significant climbing. Toward the end, the trail becomes a dirt road, and finally a paved service road, complete with bridged crossings of the Arroyo Seco (purists can follow a narrow, equestrian trail alongside). During the last couple of miles you're likely to run into lots of cyclists, joggers, parents pushing strollers, and even skateboarders.

HIKE 19

Mt. Lowe

Location	San Gabriel Mountains, above Pasadena
Highlights	Mountain, city, and ocean views
Distance	3.2 miles round trip
Total Elevation Gain/Loss	500'/500'
Hiking Time	1 ½ hours (round trip)
Optional Map	USGS 7.5-min *Mount Wilson*
Best Times	All year
Agency	ANF/LARD
Difficulty	★★

Late in the year, when the smog light-ens, but temperatures still hover within a moderate register, come up to Mt. Lowe to toast the setting sun. You can sit on an old bench, pour the champagne and watch Old Sol sink into Santa Monica Bay.

To Reach the Trailhead: To reach the starting point from I-210 at La Cañada, drive up Angeles Crest Highway for 14 miles to Red Box Divide and turn right

on Mt. Wilson Road. Proceed 2.4 miles to a large roadside parking area at un-marked Eaton Saddle.

Description: Walk past the gate on the west side and proceed up the dirt road (Mt. Lowe fire road) that carves its way under the precipitous south face of San Gabriel Peak. As you approach a short tunnel (0.3 mile) dating from 1942, look for the remnants of a former cliff-hanging

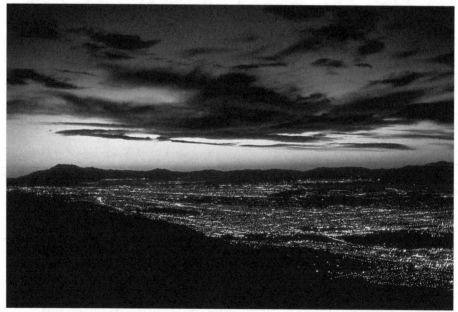

San Gabriel Valley at dawn from Mt. Lowe

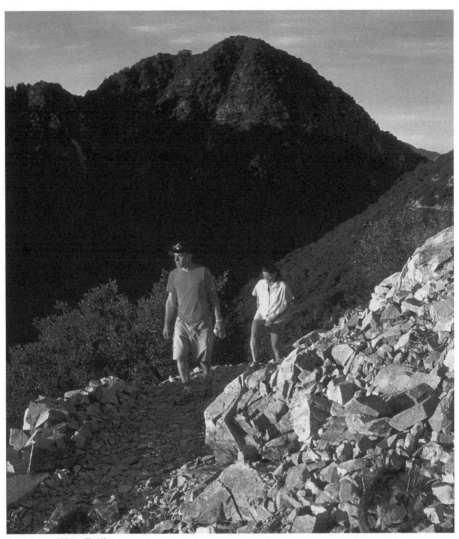

Mt. Lowe West Trail

trail to the left of the tunnel's east entrance. At Markham Saddle (0.5 mile) the fire road starts to descend slightly. Don't continue on the road. Instead, find the unmarked Mt. Lowe Trail on the left (south). On it, you contour southwest above the fire road for about 0.6 mile, and then start climbing across the east flank of Mt. Lowe without much change of direction.

At 1.3 miles, make a sharp right turn. Proceed 0.2 mile uphill, then go left on a short spur trail to Mt. Lowe's barren summit. Mt. Lowe was the proposed upper terminus for Professor Thaddeus Lowe's famed scenic railway (see Hike 21). Funding ran out, however, and tracks were never laid higher than Ye Alpine Tavern, 1200 feet below. During the railway's heyday in the early 1900s, thousands disembarked at the tavern and tramped Mt. Lowe's east- and west-side trails for world-class views of the basin and the

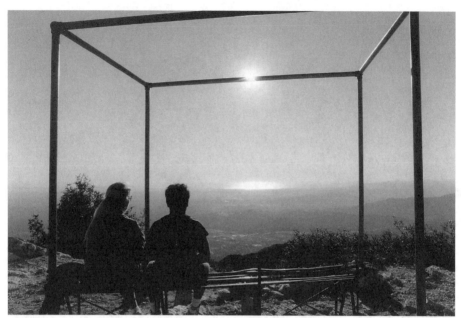

Summit of Mt. Lowe

surrounding mountains. Some reminders of that era remain on the summit of Mt. Lowe and along some of the trails: volunteers have repainted, relettered, and returned to their proper places some the many sighting tubes that helped the early tourists familiarize themselves with the surrounding geography.

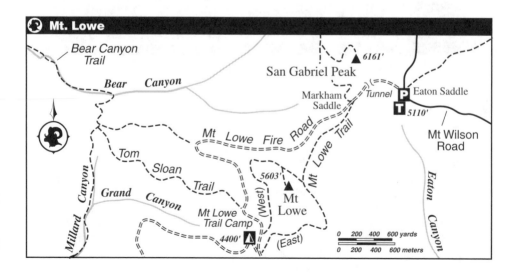

HIKE 20

Millard Canyon

Location	San Gabriel Mountains, above Pasadena
Highlights	Beautiful canyon stream; historical interest
Distance	5.6 miles
Total Elevation Gain/Loss	1600'/1600'
Hiking Time	3 ½ hours
Optional Map	USGS 7.5-min *Pasadena*
Best Times	October through June
Agency	ANF/LARD
Difficulty	★★★

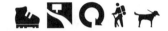

Millard Canyon's happily splashing stream, presided over by oaks, alders, maples, and bigcone Douglas-firs, is the main attraction on this hike. But you can also do a little snooping around the site of the Dawn Mine, one of the more promising gold prospects in the San Gabriels, worked intermittently from 1895 until the early 1950s.

An early start is emphatically recommended. That way you'll take advantage of shade during the climbing phase of the hike, and you'll be assured of finding a place to park your car at the trailhead (which is as popular with mountain bikers as with hikers).

To Reach the Trailhead: From Loma Alta Drive in Altadena, drive up the Chaney Trail (past a locked gate that swings open at 6 A.M. and clangs shut at 10 P.M.) to the top of Sunset Ridge, where there's parking by the roadside.

Description: Walk east on the gated, paved Sunset Ridge fire road. After about 100 yards, you pass a foot trail on the left leading down to Millard Campground. Continue another 300 yards to a second foot trail on the left (Sunset Ridge Trail). Take it. On it you contour north and east along Millard Canyon's south wall, passing above a sometimes-vociferous 50-foot waterfall. You begin climbing in earnest at about 0.7 mile and soon reach a trail fork.

The left branch (your return route) goes down 100 yards past a private cabin to the canyon bottom. You go right, uphill. Switchbacks long and short take you farther up along the pleasantly shaded canyon wall to an intersection with Sunset Ridge fire road (2.3 miles), just below a rocky knob called Cape of Good Hope.

Turn left on the fire road, and walk past Cape of Good Hope. The trail to Echo Mountain, intersecting on the right, and the fire road ahead are both part of the original Mt. Lowe Railway bed—now a self-guiding historical trail. Continue your

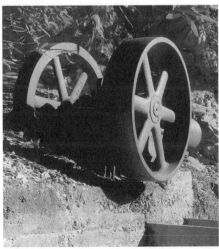

Mining machinery, Dawn Mine

ascent on the fire road/railway bed to post #4 on the left (2.8 miles). There you'll find a trail descending to Dawn Mine in Millard Canyon. This is a recently re-worked but primitive version of the mule path once used to haul ore from the mine to the railway above. On the way down you may encounter a dicey passage or two across loose talus.

After reaching the gloomy canyon bottom (3.4 miles), the trail goes upstream along the east bank for about 100 yards to the long-abandoned Dawn Mine, perched on the west-side slope. The gaping entrance to the lower shaft may seem inviting to explore, but it could collapse without warning.

From the mine, head down-canyon past crystalline mini-pools, the flotsam and jetsam of the mining days, and storm-tossed boulders. Much of the original trail

in the canyon has been washed away, but a new generation of hikers has beaten down a pretty good semblance of a path. About ½ mile below the mine a wider area of the canyon, with a high and dry terrace on the right, could be used as a wilderness campsite for backpackers.

After swinging around an abrupt bend to the right, the canyon becomes dark and gloomy once again. After another 0.5 mile you'll come to the aforementioned exit trail climbing up to the left. Pass the private cabin and hook up with the Sunset Ridge Trail, which will take you back to the Sunset Ridge fire road and your car.

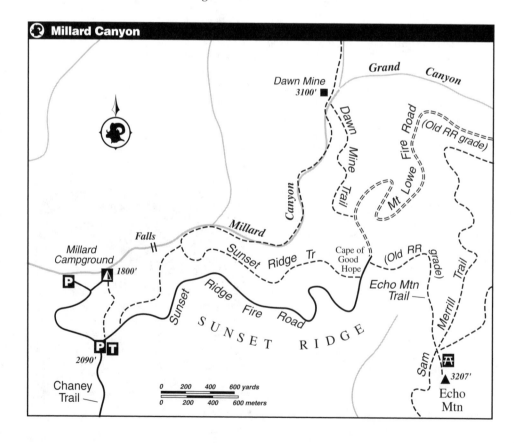

HIKE 21

Mt. Lowe Railway

Location	San Gabriel Mountains, above Pasadena
Highlights	Grand vistas; historical interest
Distance	11.4 miles
Total Elevation Gain/Loss	2800'/2800'
Hiking Time	6 hours
Optional Maps	USGS 7.5-min *Mount Wilson, Pasadena*
Best Times	October through May
Agency	ANF/LARD
Difficulty	★★★

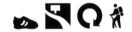

An engineering marvel when built in the 1890s, the Mt. Lowe Railway has lived a checkered past full of both glory and destruction. Before its final abandonment in the mid-1930s, the line carried over 3 million passengers—virtually all of them tourists. Unheard of by millions of Southland newcomers today, the railway was for many years the most popular outdoor attraction in Southern California.

Today hikers are taking a new interest in the old road bed; the Rails-to-Trails Conservancy (which promotes the conversion of abandoned rail corridors into recreation trails) ranked the Lowe Railway as one of the nation's 12 most scenic and historically significant recycled rail lines.

The line consisted of three stages, of which almost nothing remains today. Passengers rode a trolley from Altadena into lower Rubio Canyon, then boarded a steeply inclined cable railway that took them 1300 feet higher to Echo Mountain, where two hotels, a number of small tourist attractions, and an observatory stood. At Echo Mountain, non-acrophobic passengers hopped onto the third phase, a mountain trolley that climbed another 1200 vertical feet along airy slopes to the end of the line—Ye Alpine Tavern (later Mt. Lowe Tavern, on whose ruins stands today's Mt. Lowe Trail Camp).

The Forest Service and volunteers have put together a self-guiding trail, featuring ten markers fashioned from railroad rails, along the route of the mountain trolley. The middle portion of the old railway bed can be reached by hiking either the paved road or the trail coming up from the Chaney Trail above Millard Canyon. The more direct, easier, and more exciting way to reach Station 1 at Echo Mountain, however, is to go by way of the Sam Merrill Trail from Altadena, which is what we describe here.

To Reach the Trailhead: The Sam Merrill trailhead lies on the grounds of the long-demolished Cobb Estate, at the intersection of Lake Avenue and Loma Alta Drive in Altadena. Take the Lake Avenue exit from east- or west- bound I-210 in Pasadena, and drive about 3 miles north to where Lake Avenue turns left (west) and becomes Loma Alta Drive. Park on the street (no Adventure Pass needed).

Description: Walk east past the stone pillars at the Cobb Estate entrance and continue 150 yards on a narrow, blacktop driveway. The driveway bends left, but you keep walking straight (east). Soon you come to a water fountain on the rim of Las Flores Canyon and a sign indicating the start of the Sam Merrill Trail. This trail goes left over the top of a small debris dam and begins a switchback ascent of

Las Flores Canyon's precipitous east wall, while another trail (the Altadena Crest equestrian trail) veers to the right, down the canyon.

Inspired by the fabulous views (assuming you're doing this early on one of L.A.'s clear winter days), the 2.5 miles of steady ascent on the Sam Merrill Trail may seem to go rather quickly. Turn right at the top of the trail and walk south over to Echo Mountain, which is more like the shoulder of a ridge. There you'll find a historical plaque and some picnic tables near a grove of incense cedars and bigleaf maples. Poke around and you'll find many foundation ruins and piles of concrete rubble. An old "bullwheel" and cables for the incline railway were thoughtfully left behind after the Forest Service cleared away what remained of the buildings here in the 1950s and '60s. After visiting Echo Mountain, you'll go north on the signed Echo Mountain Trail, where you'll walk over railroad ties still imbedded in the ground.

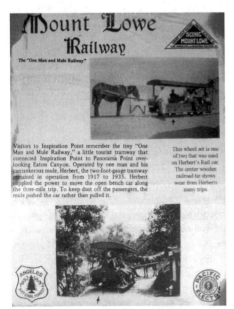

Interpretive display at Inspiration Point

Since the self-guiding brochure for the rail bed ahead is not always available from the Forest Service, I'll briefly summarize the stops. Numbers in parentheses refer to hiking mileage starting from Echo Mountain.

Station 1 (0.0) Echo Mountain. This was known as the White City during its brief heyday in the late 1890s, but most of its tourist facilities were destroyed by fire or windstorms in the first decade of the 1900s. The mountain remained a transfer point for passengers until the mid-'30s.

Station 2 (0.5) View of Circular Bridge. You can't see it from here, but passengers at this point first noticed the 400-foot-diameter circular bridge (Station 6) jutting from the slope above. As you walk on ahead, you'll notice the many concrete footings that supported trestles bridging the side ravines of Las Flores Canyon.

Station 3 (0.8) Cape of Good Hope. You're now at the junction of the Echo Mountain Trail and Sunset Ridge fire road. The tracks swung in a 200° arc around the rocky promontory just west— Cape of Good Hope. (Walk around the Cape, if you like, to get a feel for the experience.) North of this dizzying passage, riders were treated to the longest stretch of straight track—only 225 feet long. The entire original line from Echo Mountain to Ye Alpine Tavern had 127 curves and 114 straight sections. [NOTE: plenty of mountain bikers use this section of the old railroad grade. They mostly arrive by way of the Sunset Ridge fire road.]

Station 4 (1.0) Dawn Station/Devil's Slide. Dawn Mine lies below in Millard Canyon. Gold-bearing ore, packed up by mules from the canyon bottom, was loaded onto the train here. Ahead lay a treacherous stretch of crumbling granite, the Devil's Slide, which was eventually bridged by a trestle. (The current fire road has been shored up with much new concrete, and cement-lined spillways seem to do a good job of carrying away flood debris.)

Station 5 (1.2) Horseshoe Curve. Just beyond this station, Horseshoe Curve enabled the railway to gain elevation above Millard Canyon. The grade just beyond Horseshoe Curve was 7 percent—steepest on the mountain segment of the line.

Station 6 (1.6) Circular Bridge. An engineering accomplishment of worldwide fame, the Circular Bridge carried startled passengers into midair over the upper walls of Las Flores Canyon. Look for the concrete supports of this bridge down along the chaparral-covered slopes to the right.

Station 7 (2.0) Horseshoe Curve Overview. Passengers here looked down

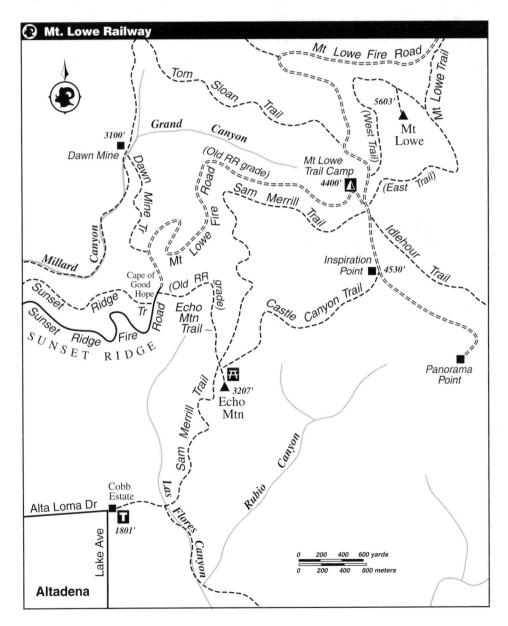

on Horseshoe Curve, and could also see all three levels of steep, twisting track climbing the east wall of Millard Canyon.

Station 8 (2.4) Granite Gate. A narrow slot carefully blasted out of solid granite on a sheer north-facing slope, Granite Gate took 8 months to cut. Look for the electric wire support dangling from the rock above.

Station 9 (3.4) Ye Alpine Tavern. The tavern, which later became a fancy hotel, was located at Crystal Springs, the source that still provides water (which now requires purification) for backpackers staying overnight at today's Mt.Lowe Trail Camp. The rails never got farther than here, although it was hoped they would one day reach the summit of Mt. Lowe, 1200 feet higher.

Station 10 (3.9) Inspiration Point. From Ye Alpine Tavern, tourists could saunter over to Inspiration Point along part of the never-finished rail extension to Mt. Lowe. Sighting tubes (still in place there) helped visitors locate places of interest below.

Inspiration Point is the last station on the self-guiding trail. The fastest and easiest way to return is by way of the Castle Canyon Trail, which descends directly below Inspiration Point. After 2 miles you'll arrive back on the old railway grade just north of Echo Mountain. Retrace your steps on the Sam Merrill Trail.

HIKE 22

Eaton Canyon

Location	Altadena/Pasadena
Highlights	Lessons in fire ecology; waterfall
Distance	3.4 miles round trip (to waterfall)
Total Elevation Gain/Loss	400'/400'
Hiking Time	1 ½ hours (round trip)
Optional Map	USGS 7.5-min *Mount Wilson*
Best Times	All year
Agency	ECNA
Difficulty	★★

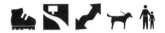

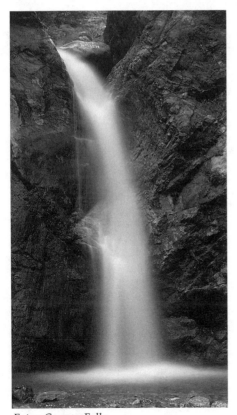

Eaton Canyon Falls

On October 27, 1993, the floor of lower Eaton Canyon (along with 118 homes in surrounding neighborhoods) was reduced to white ash and black cinders by the fast-moving Altadena Fire. By the following spring, which came on the heels of a wetter-than-average rainy season, visitors to the 184-acre Eaton Canyon Natural Area could only gasp in wonder as they beheld millions of wildflowers, swaying in the breeze, on the canyon floor. It is a California truism that from what seems the worst possible disaster, new life—and hope—can emerge triumphantly.

The brash, fire-following wildflowers have diminished with every passing season, and the oaks and chaparral shrubbery on the canyon rim have fully regenerated by now. A new Nature Center building, replacing the earlier one that burned, was dedicated in 1998. Perhaps a few decades hence, history will repeat itself when another Santa-Ana-wind-driven fire blows into town.

Upstream from the park, where the waters of Eaton Canyon have carved a raw groove in the San Gabriel Mountains, you'll discover Eaton Canyon Falls. Impressive only during the wetter half of the year, the falls possesses, as John Muir once put it, "a low sweet voice, singing like a bird." The falls are well worth visiting, especially in the aftermath of a larger winter storm, if only to witness the power of large (by Southern California standards) volumes of falling water.

To Reach the Trailhead: From the intersection of Altadena Drive and New York Drive in the eastern part of Pasadena, about 1.5 miles north of I-210, drive north on Altadena Drive for a block to the Eaton Canyon Nature Center/Natural Area entrance on the right. Drive down to the canyon floor, where you can park in a large lot near the nature center.

(If you prefer, you can shorten the walk to the falls by starting from the lower gate of Mt. Wilson Toll Road on Pinecrest Drive in Altadena. Be sure to observe any signs about parking restrictions in that neighborhood.)

Description: Three short, looping trails can be found near the nature center and parking lot: the Junior Nature Trail, Fire Ecology Trail, and Oak Terrace Trail. Our way, though, follows the Eaton Canyon Trail upstream along the canyon's cobbled

flood plain or stream. Beyond, the trail sticks to an elevated stream terrace, passing some beautiful live-oak woods. At 1.1 miles you rise to meet the Mt. Wilson Toll Road bridge over Eaton Canyon. Cross to the west end of the bridge, descend on the upstream side, and make your way up the trailless canyon (don't do this if the stream is too lively and dangerous to ford). You'll skip across rocks in the stream several times, or perhaps resort to wading. Except for a line of alders along part of the stream and some live oaks on benches just above the reach of floods, the canyon bottom and the precipitous walls are desolate and desertlike. After a half mile of canyon-bottom travel, you come to the falls, where the water slides and then free-falls a total of about 35 vertical feet down a narrow chute in the bedrock.

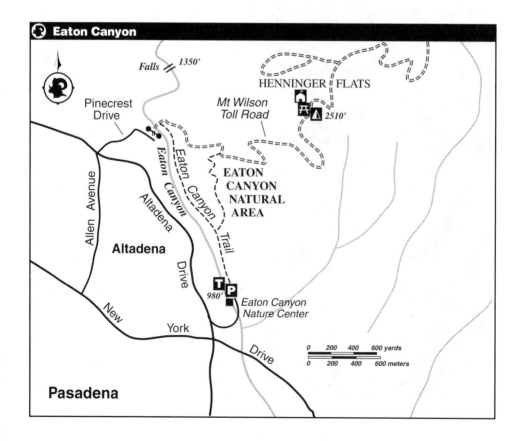

HIKE 23

Santa Anita Canyon Loop

Location	San Gabriel Mountains, above Arcadia
Highlights	Sparkling streams; botanical and historical interest
Distance	9.4 miles
Total Elevation Gain/Loss	2100'/2100'
Hiking Time	5 ½ hours
Optional Map	USGS 7.5-min *Mount Wilson*
Best Times	October through June
Agency	ANF/LARD
Difficulty	★★★

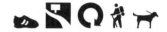

In the lush, shady recesses of Santa Anita Canyon and its tributary, Winter Creek, you can easily lose all sight and sense of the hundreds of square miles of dense metropolis, and the millions of people, that lie just over the ridge to the south. With easy access from the San Gabriel Valley by city street and mountain road, you can be strolling along a fern-lined path less than half an hour after leaving the freeway traffic behind.

To Reach the Trailhead: From I-210 in Arcadia, follow Santa Anita Avenue north. Continue to the edge of the city, pass a sturdy gate (open 6 A.M. to 10 P.M.), and ascend along a curling and precipitous ribbon of asphalt to your destination at the end of the road: Chantry Flat. Spacious, but often inadequate parking lots (National Forest Adventure Pass required), a ranger station, a picnic ground, and a mom-and-pop concession stand are here.

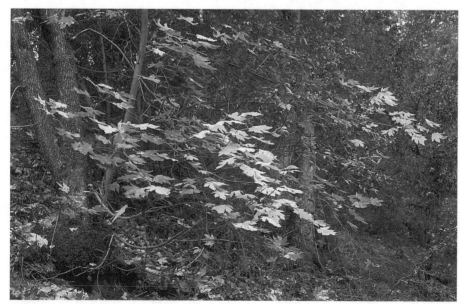

Bigleaf maples in Santa Anita Canyon

Chantry Flat also features an old-fashioned freight business—the last pack station operating year round in California. Most every day, horses, mules and burros carry supplies and building materials from the station down into canyon bottom, where an anachronistic cabin community has survived since the early 1900s.

Description: In this scenic loop trip from Chantry Flat, you'll climb by way of the Gabrielino Trail to historic Sturtevant Camp, and return by way of the Mt. Zion and Upper Winter Creek trails. Do it in a day, or take your time on an overnight backpacking trip, with a stay at Spruce Grove Trail Camp. The trail camp is a popular one, so plan to get there early to secure a spot on the weekend—or go on a weekday.

From the south edge of the lower parking lot at Chantry Flat, hike the first, paved segment of the Gabrielino Trail down to the confluence of Winter Creek and Santa Anita Canyon (0.6 mile). Pavement ends at a metal bridge spanning Winter Creek. Pass the restrooms and continue up alder-lined Santa Anita Canyon on a wide road bed following the left bank. Edging alongside a number of small cabins, the deteriorating road soon assumes the proportions of a foot trail.

At 1.4 miles, amidst a beautiful oak woodland, you come to a 4-way junction of trails. The right branch goes up-canyon to the base of 50-foot-high Sturtevant Falls, a worthy side trip during the wet season. The middle and left branches join again about a mile upstream. The left, upper trail is recommended for horses. Take the middle (lower) trail—the more scenic and exciting alternative—unless you fear heights. The lower trail slices across a sheer wall above the falls and continues through a veritable fairyland of miniature cascades and crystalline pools bedecked with giant chain ferns.

A half mile past the reconvergence of the upper and lower trails, you come upon Cascade Picnic Area (2.8 miles—

you'll find tables and restrooms here), named for a smooth chute in the stream bottom just below. Press on past a hulking crib dam (flood check dam) to reach Spruce Grove Trail Camp, 3.5 miles, named for the bigcone Douglas-fir (bigcone spruce) trees that attain truly inspiring proportions on the surrounding hillsides.

A little higher, at a fork, the Gabrielino Trail goes right. You go left on the signed Sturtevant Trail. After only 0.1 mile, Sturtevant Camp comes into view. This is both the oldest (1893) and the only remaining resort in the Santa Anita drainage. Run by the Methodist Church as a retreat (but available to other groups by reservation), the camp remains accessible only by foot trail. All supplies are packed in from Chantry Flat on the backs of pack animals, not unlike a century ago.

Next, you cross above a crib dam to the opposite side of the creek from the camp, continue another 0.1 mile, and look for stone steps rising on the left—the beginning of the Mt. Zion Trail (3.9 miles). This restored version of the original trail to Sturtevant Camp (reconstructed in the late 1970s and early '80s) winds delightfully upward across a ravine and then along timber-shaded, north-facing slopes.

When the trail crests at a notch just northwest of Mt. Zion, take the short side path up through manzanita and ceanothus to the summit, where a broad if somewhat unremarkable view can be had of surrounding ridges and a small slice of the San Gabriel Valley.

Return to the main trail and begin a long, switchback descent (1000 feet of elevation loss in about 1.5 miles) down the dry, north canyon wall of Winter Creek—a sweaty affair if the day is sunny and warm. At the foot of this stretch you reach the cool canyon bottom and a T-intersection with the Winter Creek Trail (6.7 miles), lying just above Hoegee's Trail Camp. Turn right, going upstream momentarily, follow the trail across the creek, and climb to the next trail junction. Bear left on the Upper Winter Creek Trail and complete the remaining 2.6 miles of easy, mostly level hiking, cool and semi-shaded nearly all the way.

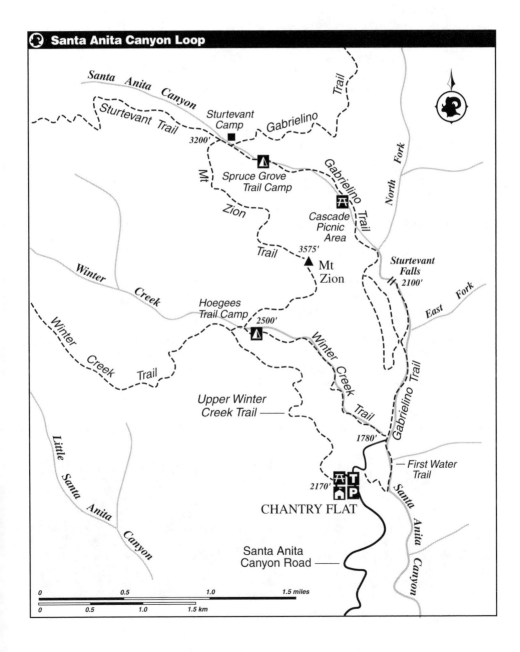

Santa Anita Canyon Loop

HIKE 24

Vetter Mountain

Location	Central San Gabriel Mountains
Highlight	Mountain vistas from an old fire lookout
Distance	3.3 miles
Total Elevation Gain/Loss	700'/700'
Hiking Time	1 ½ hours
Optional Map	USGS 7.5-min *Chilao Flat*
Best Times	All year
Agency	ANF/LARD
Difficulty	★★

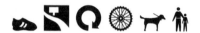

Vetter Mountain lies within Angeles National Forest's Charlton-Chilao Recreation Area—a gateway of sorts to the high country of the San Gabriel Mountains. Here, Angelenos heading up Angeles Crest Highway from the west first come upon what looks like true forest—stately pines, firs and cedars.

Vetter Mountain's pint-sized fire-lookout building, perched on a rounded summit nearly devoid of vegetation, takes advantage of a 360° view over the midsection of the San Gabriels. The lookout reopened for service in 1998 after an 18-year hiatus. The facility is staffed on weekends and on some weekdays during the fire season (summer and fall). The public is welcome to hike to the summit anytime.

The hike to Vetter's lookout can be as short as 1.4 miles round trip, via the Vetter Mountain service road. Or, you can incorporate a visit to the lookout into a longer, looping route of 3.3 miles (described here), which includes pleasant passages through Charlton Flats' heterogeneous forest of live oak, Coulter pine, Jeffrey pine, sugar pine, incense cedar, and bigcone Douglas-fir. With binoculars, a bird book, and a wildflower guide, you and your kids can take your sweet time, stopping as you please to admire a soaring hawk or raven, a noisy acorn woodpecker or Steller's jay, or an unfamiliar plant in bloom.

To Reach the Trailhead: To get to the starting point from I-210 in La Cañada, drive 24 miles east on Angeles Crest Highway to reach the Charlton Flats Picnic Area—at mile 47.5 according to the roadside mileage markers. During the off-season, part or all of the picnic area may be

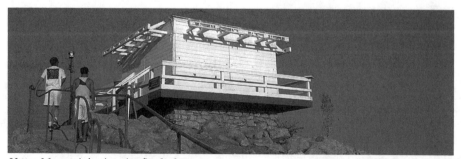

Vetter Mountain's pint-size fire lookout

closed to auto traffic and you may have to walk in to reach the trailhead. Otherwise, drive in, make an immediate right, and continue ½ mile to the start of the Vetter Mountain Trail, on your left. (Either way, remember that you must display a National Forest Adventure Pass on your parked car.)

Description: About 200 yards up the Vetter Mountain Trail, the Silver Moccasin Trail swings left—don't take it; this is your return route. Keeping straight, you ascend through mixed forest and then scattered pines, crossing service roads twice. A final, somewhat steep and eroded, switchbacking stretch of trail through chaparral leads to the lookout, 1.3 miles from the start.

Peering north and east from the lookout perch, you'll spot Pacifico Mountain, Mt. Williamson, Waterman Mountain,

Twin Peaks, Old Baldy, and other prominent peaks of the San Gabriel Mountains. The Front Range of the San Gabriels, which defines the north rim of the San Gabriel Valley and the L.A. Basin, sprawls west and south, blocking from view most of the city.

When it's time to descend, follow the dirt service road downhill instead of the trail. After 0.7 mile you'll meet a paved service road. Continue straight (east) on the pavement for another 0.6 mile and look carefully for the crossing of the Silver Moccasin Trail. Turn left on the trail, cross pavement again in a short while, and complete the final, mostly level stretch across a forested slope.

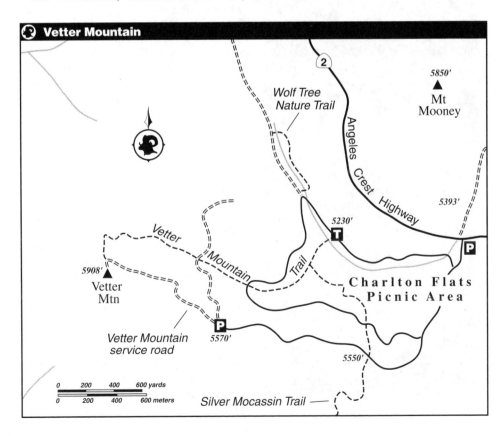

HIKE 25

Cooper Canyon Falls

Location	Central San Gabriel Mountains
Highlight	Beautiful, hidden waterfall
Distance	3.0 miles round trip
Total Elevation Gain/Loss	800'/800'
Hiking Time	1 ½ hours (round trip)
Optional Map	USGS 7.5-min *Waterman Mtn.*
Best Times	April through November
Agency	ANF/SCMRD
Difficulty	★★

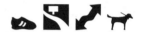

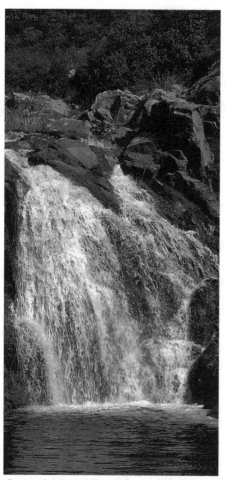

Cooper Canyon Falls

Cooper Canyon Falls roars with the melting snows of early spring, then settles down to a quiet whisper by June or July. You can cool off in the spray of the 25-foot cascade, or at least sit on a water-smoothed log and soak your feet in the chilly, alder-shaded pool just below the base of the falls. In the right season (April or May most years) these falls are one of the best unheralded attractions of the San Gabriel Mountains. Very little water can be found around here by the early fall season, but at least you can enjoy outstanding displays of autumn color along the chilly ravines.

The Burkhart Trail takes you quickly to the falls, downhill all the way, and then uphill all the way back. The forest traversed by the trail is dense enough to give plenty of cool shade for most of the unrelenting climb back up.

To Reach the Trailhead: From I-210 in La Cañada, drive 34 miles up Angeles Crest Highway to the Buckhorn Campground entrance road (mile 58.3 according to the roadside mile-markers). Drive all the way through the campground to the far (northeast) end, where a short stub of dirt road leads to the Burkhart trailhead. You must display a National Forest Adventure Pass.

Description: The Burkhart Trail takes off down the west wall of an unnamed, usually wet canyon garnished by two waterfalls. The first—a little gem of a cascade dropping 10 feet into a rock grotto—is easy to reach by descending from the trailside. The second, some 30 feet high, is dangerous to approach from above, but is reachable from below by scrambling up the canyon bottom from Cooper Canyon.

At 1.2 miles, the trail bends east to follow Cooper Canyon's south bank. Continue another 0.3 mile, down past the junction of the trail (Pacific Crest Trail) that doubles back to follow the north bank upstream. Look or listen for water plunging over the rocky declivity to the left. A rough pathway leads down off the trail to the alder-fringed pool below.

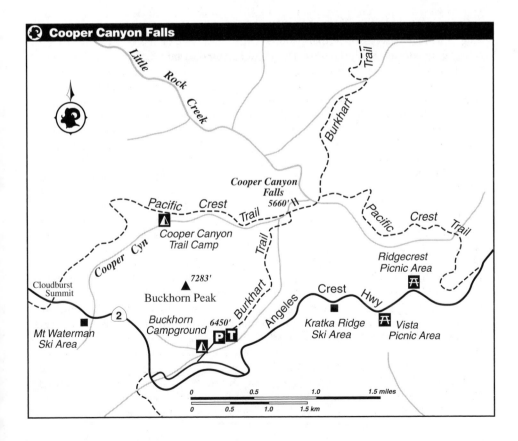

HIKE 26

Mt. Waterman Trail

Location	Central San Gabriel Mountains
Highlights	Vistas of yawning canyons; possible bighorn sheep sightings
Distance	7.8 miles
Total Elevation Gain/Loss	1400'/2250'
Hiking Time	4 ½ hours
Optional Map	USGS 7.5-min *Waterman Mtn.*
Best Times	May through November
Agency	ANF/SGRD
Difficulty	★★★

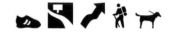

The Mt. Waterman Trail traverse across the north rim of San Gabriel Wilderness provides almost constant views of statuesque pines, yawning chasms, and distant, hazy ridges. You start near the entrance to Buckhorn Campground and you end up half-circling broad-shouldered Waterman Mountain by the time you arrive at Three Points, 5 miles away by car. Snow can linger on the easternmost mile of the trail until May, but it tends to disappear much earlier on the remaining (mostly south-facing) parts of the trail. This is one of the most popular High Country summer hikes—one that I can heartily recommend for all but the warmest days.

(If you prefer, you can shave some time, distance, and elevation gain from this hike by making use of the Mt. Waterman Ski Lift, which is open on summer weekends to cater to hikers and mountain bikers. The lift carries you 900 feet up from Angeles Crest Highway to a point about ¾ mile north of Waterman Mountain's summit. It helps to have the topographic map listed above if you are going to try to locate the Mt. Waterman Trail from there.)

To Reach the Trailhead: From I-210 in La Cañada, drive 34 miles up Angeles Crest Highway to the start of the Mt. Waterman Trail, where you'll find a parking lot and restrooms (mile 58.0 by the highway markers). Three Points trailhead, at the far end of the hike, is located a few miles west on Angeles Crest Highway, at the intersection of Santa Clara Divide Road (mile 52.8 on Angeles Crest Highway). Cars parked at either trailhead must display a National Forest Adventure Pass.

Description: From the Buckhorn end, follow the well-graded Mt. Waterman Trail—not the old road bed paralleling the trail at first—along a shady slope. After 1.0 mile of easy ascent through gorgeous mixed-conifer forest, you come to a saddle overlooking Bear Creek. The trail turns west, follows a viewful ridge, and then ascends on six long switchbacks to a trail junction, 2.1 miles. A trail to Waterman Mountain's summit goes right; you stay left and contour west about ½ mile, then zigzag south down to a second junction, 3.5 miles. Twin Peaks saddle, a spacious spot suitable for camping, lies below to the left. If you're day-hiking this stretch, then stay right (west).

The remaining 4+ miles take you gradually downhill (more steep at the very end) along a generally south-facing slope. You wind in and out of broad ravines, either shaded by huge incense cedars and vanilla-scented Jeffrey pines, or exposed to the warm sunshine on chaparral-covered slopes. The older cedar trees are gnarled veterans of past fires. The rugged topography of San Gabriel Wilderness below conceals the hangouts of herds of Nelson bighorn sheep. This area and another to the east, Sheep Mountain Wilderness, were classified as statutory wilderness areas in part to preserve the habitat of these magnificent animals.

Near the end of the Mt. Waterman Trail, you hook up briefly with the Pacific Crest Trail. You swing down to cross Angeles Crest Highway, and climb up on the other side to reach the parking lot at Three Points.

An excellent way to extend and embellish this hike is to tackle either or both summits of Twin Peaks. Getting to either involves considerable scrambling, though a decently worn-in use trail exists between Twin Peaks Saddle and the ridge between the two peaks. The east peak is easier to reach. There, on rock outcrops just below the summit, you can get a dizzying view of the canyons below. Quite often you can look out over a low-lying blanket of smog in the L.A. Basin and see Santa Catalina Island floating out at sea beyond the hazy dome of Palos Verdes. The Santa Ana Mountains, Palomar Mountain, the Santa Rosa Mountains, San Jacinto Peak and Old Baldy arc around the horizon from south to east.

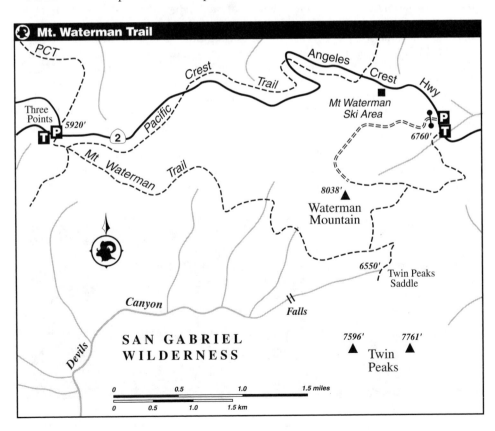

HIKE 27

Devil's Punchbowl

Location	San Gabriel Mountains, north slope
Highlight	Spectacular geological formations
Distance	1.0 mile
Total Elevation Gain/Loss	300'/300'
Hiking Time	½ hour
Optional Map	USGS 7.5-min *Valyermo*
Best Times	All year
Agency	DPNA
Difficulty	★

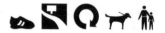

Tens of millions of years in the making, Devil's Punchbowl is without a doubt Los Angeles County's most spectacular geological showplace. Looking down into this 300-foot-deep chasm, you immediately sense the enormity of the forces that produced the tilted and tangled collection of beige sandstone slabs.

The Punchbowl is caught between two active faults—the main San Andreas Fault and an offshoot, the Punchbowl Fault—along which old sedimentary formations have been pushed upward and crumpled downward, as well as transported horizontally. Weathering and erosion have put the final touches on the scene, roughing out the bowl-shaped gorge of Punchbowl Canyon and carving,

in a host of unique ways, the rocks exposed at the surface.

Devil's Punchbowl Natural Area lies in the pinyon-juniper transition zone between the Mojave Desert and the richly forested slopes of the higher San Gabriels. The park features a superb nature center, a couple of short nature walks (including the loop trail described here), and the Punchbowl Trail—a part of the High Desert National Recreation Trail. South of the punchbowl are long-distance trails leading through Angeles National Forest to the high country along Angeles Crest Highway.

To Reach the Trailhead: To get Devil's Punchbowl from most parts of L.A., exit Antelope Valley Freeway (Highway 14) at

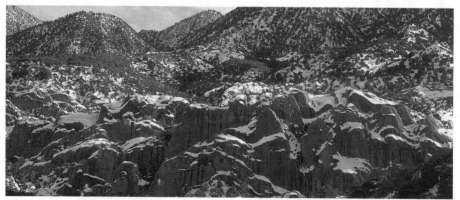

Inside the snow-dusted Punchbowl

Pearblossom Highway, and follow it east through the town of Littlerock to Pearblossom. At Pearblossom, turn right (south) on Longview Road (County N6) and follow signs for the park, 7 miles ahead. The park is open 7 days a week from sunrise to sunset, with no admission charge.

Description: The 1-mile Loop Trail is a perfect introduction to the Punchbowl area. It begins just behind the nature center, zigzags down off the rim to touch the seasonal creek in Punchbowl Canyon, and then climbs back out of the canyon opposite some of the tallest upright rock formations in the park. Near the start of the trail is a side path—the 0.3-mile Pinon Pathway—a self-guiding nature trail that loops through the pinyon-juniper forest along the Punchbowl rim.

During winter, occasional snowfalls dust the Punchbowl and leave a lingering, thicker mantle of white on the pine-dotted slopes above it. At these times the Loop Trail can become muddy and slippery, and therefore probably not suitable for small children.

Peripatetic walkers may wish to undertake the 6-mile-round-trip trek via the Punchbowl Trail to the Devil's Chair, which perches on the upper rim of the canyon complex that generally encompasses the Punchbowl. At the fenced viewpoint there, you can peer over what looks like frozen chaos—a vast assemblage of sandstone chunks and slabs tipped at odd angles, bent, seemingly pulled apart here, compressed there. There's a reason for this chaos: Devil's Chair sits practically astride the "crush zone" of the Punchbowl Fault.

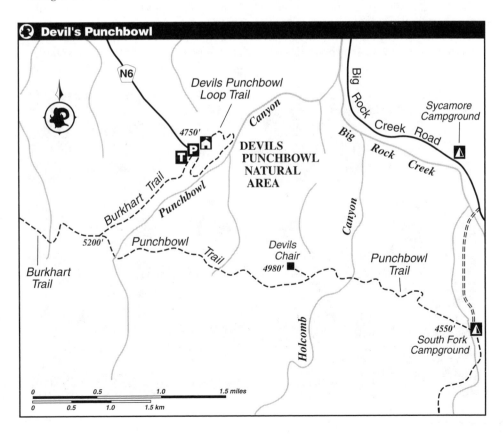

HIKE 28

Mt. Baden-Powell Traverse

Location	Eastern San Gabriel Mountains
Highlights	Subalpine habitat; panoramic views; possible bighorn sheep sightings
Distance	9.2 miles (includes Throop Peak and Mt. Burnham summits)
Total Elevation Gain/Loss	2400'/3700'
Hiking Time	5 hours
Optional Map	USGS 7.5-min *Crystal Lake*
Best Times	May through November
Agency	ANF/SGRD
Difficulty	★★★

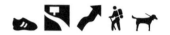

Massive Mt. Baden-Powell stands head and shoulders above the foggy or smoggy marine layer that often enshrouds the lowlands of the Los Angeles Basin and the Inland Empire. From Baden Powell's flattish top, the brown Mojave Desert floor stretches interminably inland toward some hazy vanishing point. The disembodied summit ridges of mountain ranges as far west as Ventura County and as far south as San Diego County seem to float over opaque blankets of haze. Santa Catalina, and sometimes other Channel Islands, are visible on an average early-summer morning.

Named in honor of Lord Baden-Powell, the British Army officer who started the Boy Scout movement in 1907. Baden-

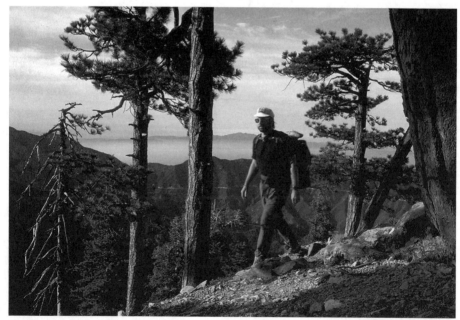

On the Baden-Powell Traverse

Powell soars higher (9399') than any other mountain in the San Gabriel mountain range—except for the Mt. San Antonio (Old Baldy) complex to the east. Many thousands of hikers troop to Baden-Powell's summit yearly, most of them by way of the trail from Vincent Gap on Angeles Crest Highway. Baden-Powell's summit is the last major milestone on the 52-mile trek from Chantry Flat to Vincent Gap known as the Silver Moccasin Trail. The 5-day-long Silver Moccasin backpack is a rite-of-passage for L.A.-area Scouts.

If you want to climb Mt. Baden-Powell without having to retrace your steps, you can try a one-way hike, described here, from Dawson Saddle to Vincent Gap. The effort is only bit more than what's involved in the usual round trip from Vincent Gap, and you'll visit two other peaks as well. All three peaks offer their own unique and panoramic perspective of the rugged Sheep Mountain Wilderness to the south. As the name suggests, this wilderness protects the habitat of the Nelson bighorn sheep, which number several hundred in the San Gabriel Mountains. Early-morning sightings of the bighorn are not unusual on and near Mt. Baden-Powell.

At a moderate pace, including a few short breaks and a stop for lunch, the 9-mile hike should take you about 6 hours. Snow accumulations can blanket the area until June. Thereafter, little or no water can be found on the route, so carry plenty of it. The start and end points of the hike are 5 miles apart by way of Angeles Crest Highway, so you should plan to bring either two cars for a car shuttle, or one car plus a bicycle (to be left near the end point for use in retrieving the car from the start point after the hike is over).

To Reach the Trailhead: From I-210 in La Cañada, drive 50 miles east on Angeles Crest Highway to reach the Vincent Gap trailhead (mile 74.8 according to the roadside mile markers). Alternately, you can approach this same trailhead from the east

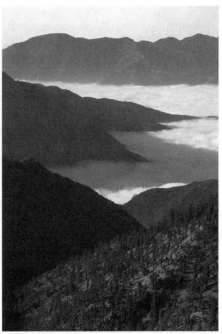

Marine-layer clouds below Mt. Baden-Powell

by way of I-15, Highway 138, and Angeles Crest Highway through Wrightwood. Vincent Gap is 10 miles west of Wrightwood via Angeles Crest Highway. Your hike will end at Vincent Gap—but it begins about 5 miles west of Vincent Gap at a point just east of Dawson Saddle (mile 69.6 on Angeles Crest Highway). There's room for parking along Angeles Crest Highway there, across from where the trail starts. Both trailheads require a National Forest Adventure Pass for any parked vehicle.

Description: Beginning at the highway near Dawson Saddle, the Dawson Saddle Trail goes immediately uphill (south), switchbacking up through pines and firs to gain the top of a long, gradually ascending ridge that culminates at Throop Peak. An impressive 3540 hours of volunteer labor by Boy Scouts were required to build this trail, which was completed in 1982. About halfway up the trail, lodgepole pines dominate the forest, but keen eyes will spot a few limber pines, which are relatively rare in Southern California. Look closely at the needles: Lodgepole-pine needles come in bundles of two, while limber pines have bundles of five.

After 1.8 miles you join the Pacific Crest Trail. From this junction, the first side trip takes you southwest on the PCT for 200 yards, then off-trail in the same direction another 300 yards to Throop Peak. You'll find a hikers' register there, as well as on the other two peaks you'll reach later.

Return to the Dawson Saddle Trail junction and continue northeast on the PCT, which follows the main, semi-shaded ridgeline. You descend to a saddle, then ascend to Mt. Burnham's north flank, from where switchbacks take you over to Burnham's east shoulder. That's

where you can double back (go west) for the easy side trip to Burnham's summit.

After bagging Burnham, continue east, climbing a breathless 400 feet more, to reach the next trail junction. Just above it is Baden-Powell's summit, and an impressive monument constructed by the Boy Scouts. Weather-beaten lodgepole and limber pines dot the summit area.

Return to the junction and take the main, heavily traveled trail that descends Baden-Powell's northeast ridge. After 40 switchbacks and 3.8 miles of steady descent you'll reach the end—the large Vincent Gap parking area at mile 74.8 on Angeles Crest Highway. About halfway down this trail, from the 25th switchback corner, a side trail leads about 200 yards east to a dribbling pipe at Lamel Spring. This is the only normally dependable source of water along the route.

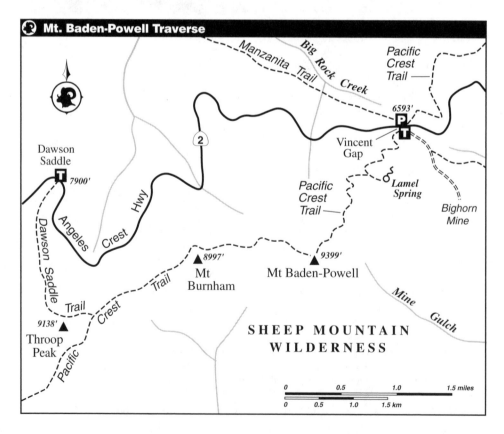

HIKE 29

Lightning Ridge Nature Trail

Location	Big Pines Recreation Area
Highlight	Botanical features; nice views
Distance	0.8 mile
Total Elevation Gain/Loss	250'/250'
Hiking Time	½ hour
Optional Map	USGS 7.5-min *Mount San Antonio*
Best Times	April through November
Agency	ANF/SCMRD
Difficulty	★

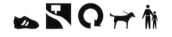

On the eastern Angeles Crest, not far above the L.A. Basin's smoggy blanket of air, lies Big Pines Recreation Area—a designated year-round recreation zone in Angeles National Forest. Blanketed by a heterogeneous mixture of pines, firs, and oaks, Big Pines boasts the clean, dry, evergreen-scented air and crystalline blue skies characteristic of the melding of mountain and desert environments. Winter and spring skiing (sometimes aided by the labors of snow-making machines) is offered at three sites in the Big Pines area. Several trails lace the area, including one of the finer interpretive trails around: the Lightning Ridge Trail.

To Reach the Trailhead: From most urban parts of Southern California, the fastest way to get to the Big Pines area is by way of I-10 and I-15 toward Cajon

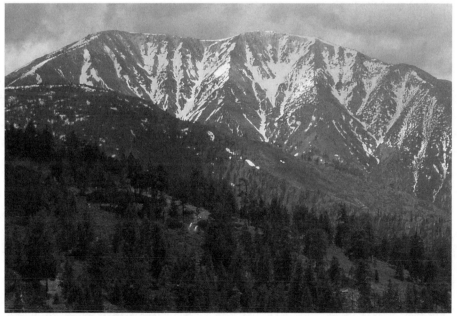

Long view of Old Baldy from the north

Pass. Before reaching the top of the pass, exit I-15 at Cajon Junction. Drive 8.6 miles west on Highway 138 to the junction of Highway 2 (Angeles Crest Highway). Turn left there, and continue uphill into the pine-clad San Gabriel Mountains and through the sprawling mountain town of Wrightwood. At a point 10 miles from Highway 138 you'll come to crossroads of Big Pines, where you can drop by the Forest Service's Grassy Hollow Visitor Center. Here you'll find leaflets, maps, and interpretive brochures for nearby trails, including the Lightning Ridge Trail. Continue another 2 miles west of Big Pines to reach the Lightning Ridge trailhead on the north side of Angeles Crest Highway, opposite Inspiration Point. You'll need to post a National Forest Adventure Pass on your parked car.

Description: The Lightning Ridge Trail contours through the cool precincts of a wooded northeast-facing slope, then switchbacks upward to meet the Pacific Crest Trail on a windblown crest. You'll see Jeffrey pines, sugar pines, and white firs, and pass right through a beautiful glade of black oaks called Oak Dell—very nice in October when the leaves turn crispy gold and acorns fall. Near the crest are a number of stunted and distorted

trees battered by winds and flattened by snow drifts that can pile up 10 feet high. On the crest itself you'll meet a segment of the 2600-mile-long Pacific Crest Trail. At this locale, some 14 percent of the PCT's winding course leads south to the Mexican border, and about 86 percent leads north to the Canadian border.

When you reach the PCT junction, try stepping off the trail and walking a short distance over to the top of the ridgecrest. The view from there is similar to that from Inspiration Point below, only a bit more panoramic. Old Baldy and Mt. Baden-Powell rise like massive sentinels, bracketing the rugged slopes and canyons of the Sheep Mountain Wilderness. To the south you look straight down the V-shaped, linear gorge of East Fork San Gabriel River.

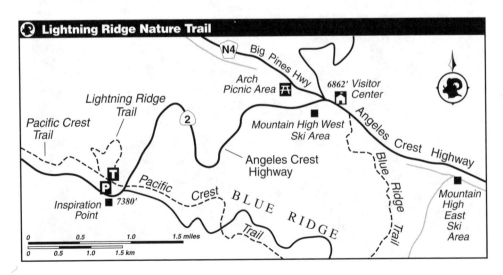

Lightning Ridge Nature Trail

HIKE 30

Lewis Falls

Location	San Gabriel Mountains, above Azusa
Highlight	Beautiful stream and cascades
Distance	0.8 mile round trip
Total Elevation Gain/Loss	300'/300'
Hiking Time	½ hour (round trip)
Optional Map	USGS 7.5-min *Crystal Lake*
Best Times	All year
Agency	ANF/SGRD
Difficulty	★

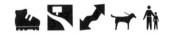

At the precipice called Lewis Falls, Soldier Creek shoots (or merely dribbles) some 50 feet down a two-tiered rock face. The volume of water splattering on rocks and sand below is seldom dramatic; but the cool spray and the sounds of falling water are refreshing. The hike to the base of the falls is short—only about 15 minutes, a manageable adventure (with some assistance) for small children.

To Reach the Trailhead: Lewis Falls is located off Highway 39—the road from Azusa into San Gabriel Canyon and the Crystal Lake Recreation Area. Use the roadside mileage markers to identify the starting point—a small, shaded turnout on the right at mile 34.8, where Soldier Creek tumbles through a culvert under the highway. Don't forget to display a National Forest Adventure Pass on your car.

Description: From the highway turnout, make your way up a well-beaten trail on the east side of the creek, under shade-giving oaks, laurels, and bigcone Douglas-firs. Nearly the entire Crystal Lake basin was burned in the 2002 Curve Fire, so the landscape will look a bit harsh and denuded for the next several years to come. As you approach the falls, the trail virtually disappears in the flood-scoured bed of Soldier Creek. A final, 200-yard scramble along the stream takes you to the base of the falls.

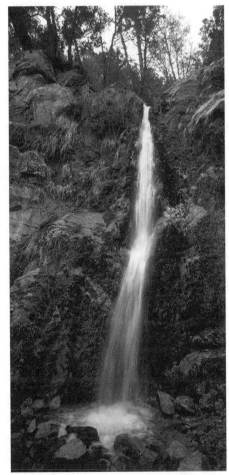

Lewis Falls

Most of the year Soldier Creek is a tame brook, easily jumped by the average adult. But a major storm, or a rapid thaw in the snowpack above, could produce runoff deep and swift enough to be hazardous—at least for kids.

Just above Lewis Falls, but not accessible by the route just described, is a beautiful stretch of Soldier Creek featuring half a dozen small cascades. This secret hideaway is also a short walk away from Highway 39. To go that way, drive to mile 36.8 on Highway 39, from where a wide, gated dirt road goes east. Park so as not to block the gate, and on foot follow the dirt road 0.5 mile east to its end. Find a narrow trail on the left, contouring through the brush. It leads 300 yards, sometimes precariously, across a steep slope to the cascades.

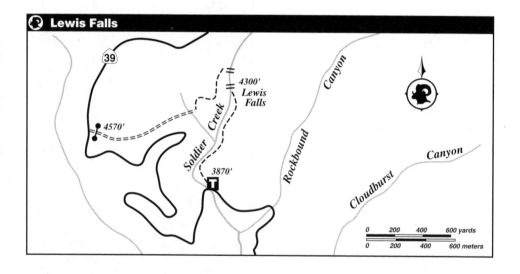

HIKE 31

Mt. Islip

Location	Crystal Lake Recreation Area
Highlight	Ocean to desert views
Distance	7.7 miles
Total Elevation Gain/Loss	2400'/2400'
Hiking Time	4 hours
Optional Map	USGS 7.5-min *Crystal Lake*
Best Times	May through November
Agency	ANF/SGRD
Difficulty	★★★

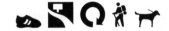

The south approach of Mt. Islip, one of the significant high points in the San Gabriel Mountains, feels a bit like real mountain climbing, despite the rather straightforward ascent by way of marked trails. You begin amid spreading oaks and tall conifers in Crystal Lake basin, rise through progressively smaller and sparser timber, and finally reach the nearly bald and often windblown summit. There, a comprehensive view, both north over the Mojave Desert and south over the metropolis, is offered on clear days. For the slight effort of an extra half mile on the way up or down, you can spend the night at Little Jimmy Campground, one of the nicest trail camps in the San Gabriels. The 2002 Curve Fire swept nearly the entire Crystal Lake basin, burning to the ground much of the low growing vegetation, and singeing or destroying most of the trees. How quickly and completely the forest recovers will depend largely on how wet or dry the coming winter rainy seasons prove to be.

To Reach the Trailhead: From I-210 in Azusa, drive north on Azusa Avenue, which becomes San Gabriel Canyon Road (Highway 39) as it passes flood-control basins at the mouth of San Gabriel Canyon. Continue 24 miles north through the canyon to the Crystal Lake Recreation Area turnoff. Drive a half mile past the Crystal Lake visitor center to the main hikers' parking lot, and don't forget to display a National Forest Adventure Pass on your parked car.

Description: Start hiking on the marked Windy Gap Trail. On the way to Windy Gap (2.5 miles), you cross the Mt. Hawkins Truck Trail twice (on the first crossing the road is paved, on the second it's dirt) and then tackle the steep, upper slopes of the cirquelike rim overlooking Crystal Lake basin. Windy Gap is the lowest spot on the north side of that rim.

At Windy Gap you meet the Pacific Crest Trail, which joins from the right (east). Continue briefly north on the PCT to the next junction. Going left takes you more directly to the summit of Mt. Islip, while going right would lead you to Little Jimmy Campground and a more roundabout ascent of the mountain. In either case, you'll end up on the trail that follows the sunny east ridge of Mt. Islip to its summit. [NOTE: Hard snow or ice can linger on the steep, north-facing slopes north of Windy Gap until sometime in May. You can avoid that stretch if need be by going straight up the east shoulder of Mt. Islip from Windy Gap; that route becomes snow-free earlier in the season.]

On the summit (3.5 miles) you'll discover the shell of an old stone cabin, and footings of a fire lookout tower that stood on Islip from 1927 until 1937, when the lookout was moved to a better site to the southeast—South Mt. Hawkins. That structure was completely destroyed in the 2002 Curve Fire, but plans are afoot to rebuild it, again on South Mt. Hawkins.

On your return, for the sake of variety, you can follow the Islip Ridge and Big Cienega trails. Two switchbacks below the summit of Mt. Islip, turn right on the Islip Ridge Trail, which goes down Islip's south ridge. A future extension of that trail will go south and east all the way to Crystal Lake. You, however, travel just 1.0 mile down Islip Ridge Trail and then veer east on Big Cienega Trail. After another 2.0 miles of gradual descent along wooded south-facing slopes, you join the Windy Gap Trail just north of the upper crossing of Mt. Hawkins Truck Trail. Turn right and return to the hikers' parking lot.

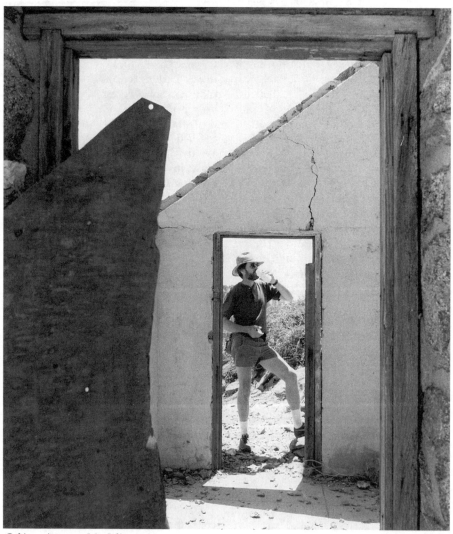

Cabin ruins atop Mt. Islip

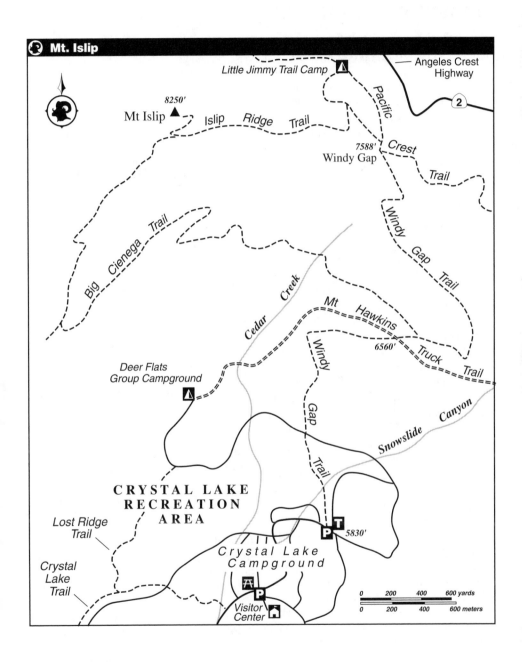

Mt. Islip

Little Jimmy Trail Camp

Angeles Crest Highway

Pacific

2

8250'
Mt Islip

Islip Ridge Trail

7588'
Windy Gap

Crest

Trail

Big Cienega Trail

Windy Gap Trail

Cedar Creek

Mt Hawkins

6560' Truck Trail

Deer Flats
Group Campground

Windy

Gap

Trail

Snowslide Canyon

CRYSTAL LAKE
RECREATION
AREA

Lost Ridge
Trail

P T 5830'

Crystal Lake
Campground

Crystal
Lake
Trail

P

Visitor
Center

| 0 | 200 | 400 | 600 yards |
| 0 | 200 | 400 | 600 meters |

HIKE 32

Down the East Fork

Location	San Gabriel River, San Gabriel Mountains
Highlights	An epic trek along a cascading stream; nearly a vertical mile of descent
Distance	14.5 miles
Total Elevation Gain/Loss	200'/4800'
Hiking Time	11 hours
Recommended Maps	USGS 7.5-min *Crystal Lake, Mount San Antonio, Glendora*
Best Times	May through November
Agency	ANF/SGRD
Difficulty	★★★★★

Born from snow-fed rivulets, the many tributaries of the East Fork San Gabriel River gather together to form one of the liveliest and most remote streams in the San Gabriels. At The Narrows of the East Fork, the water squeezes through the deepest gorge in Southern California. From the bottom of The Narrows, the east wall soars about 5200 feet to Iron Mountain, and the west wall rises about 4000 feet to the South Mt. Hawkins divide.

On this grand journey down the upper East Fork, you'll descend nearly a mile in elevation, travel from high-country pines and firs to sun-scorched chaparral, and cross three important geologic faults—the Punchbowl, Vincent Thrust, and San Gabriel faults. During the course of a single day you could experience a temperature increase of as much as 60°F.

You can do this hike in one incredibly long day with an early start, or you can camp overnight on one of the shaded streamside terraces near the mid-point of the trek. The better camping sites include former trail camps at Fish and Iron forks, and the lower part of The Narrows. Because the route passes through the Sheep Mountain Wilderness, check with the Forest Service to see if you need an overnight permit.

Navigation on the trip is easy throughout—you simply head down-canyon the whole way. Consult a detailed map often if you want to confirm exactly where you are. Heavy runoff after a storm or major snowmelt can create hazardous stream crossings, which is one of the reasons why this trip is only recommended for the late-spring through fall seasons. The other reason is the upper trailhead at Vincent Gap may be unreachable due to snow cover. Contact the rangers for more information about either issue.

It's practical to have someone drop you off at the starting point, Vincent Gap, and later pick you up at the hike's end, East Fork Station. That being said, it is important to note that the amount of time required to complete the trip can be highly variable due to problems with adverse weather or swift-flowing water, excessive bushwhacking along the banks of the upper river, how heavy backpacks are, and the hiking ability of the slowest member of your party. This is not a trip for hikers without plenty of successful experience in off-trail wilderness travel. Allow some flexibility in your planned time of arrival at the end.

Cars parked at either the start or the end point will need a National Forest Adventure Pass.

To Reach the Trailhead *(Vincent Gap)*: From I-210 in La Cañada, drive 50 miles east on Angeles Crest Highway to reach the Vincent Gap trailhead (mile 74.8 according to the roadside mile markers). Alternately, you can approach this same trailhead from the east by way of I-15, Highway 138, and Angeles Crest Highway through Wrightwood. Vincent Gap is 10 miles west of Wrightwood via Angeles Crest Highway.

To Reach the Trailhead *(East Fork Station)*: From the community of Azusa, just north of I-210, drive north on Azusa Avenue and San Gabriel Canyon Road (Highway 39) for 11 miles to East Fork Road. Continue up East Fork Road 6 miles to its terminus near the East Fork ranger station

Description: From the parking area on the south side of Vincent Gap, walk down the gated road to the southeast. After only about 200 yards, a footpath veers left, into Sheep Mountain Wilderness. Take it; the road itself continues toward the Bighorn Mine, an "inholding" of privately owned land inside the wilderness boundary.

Intermittently shaded by bigcone Douglas-firs, white firs, Jeffrey pines, and live oaks, the path descends along the south slope of Vincent Gulch. The gulch itself follows the Punchbowl Fault, a splinter of the San Andreas. At 0.7 mile, on a flat ridge spur, look for an indistinct path intersecting on the right. This leads about 100 yards to an old cabin believed to have been the home of Charles Vincent. Vincent led the life of a hermit, prospector, and big-game hunter in the Baden-Powell/Old Baldy area from 1870 until his death in 1926.

After a few switchbacks, the primitive trail crosses Vincent Gulch (usually dry at this point, wet a short distance below) at 1.6 miles. Thereafter it stays on or above the east bank as far as the confluence of Prairie Fork, a wide drainage coming in from the east at 3.8 miles from the start. You veer right (west) down a gravelly

wash, good for setting up a camp. Shortly after, at the Mine Gulch confluence, you bend left (south) into the wide bed of the upper East Fork. For several miles to come, there is essentially no trail. It may take several hours to traverse this stretch, depending on the energy and motivation of your group.

Proceed down the rock-strewn flood plain, crossing the creek (and battling alder thickets) several times over the next mile. The canyon becomes narrow for a while starting at about 5.0 miles, and you must wade or hop from one slippery rock to another. Fish Fork, on the left at 7.3 miles from the start, is the first large stream below Prairie Fork.

If you have the time for an intriguing side trip, Fish Fork canyon is well worth exploring. Chock full of alder and bay, narrow with soaring walls, its clear stream tumbling over boulders, the canyon boasts one of the wildest and most beautiful settings in the San Gabriels. About 1.6 miles upstream lies a formidable impasse: There, the waters of Fish Fork drop 12 feet into an emerald-green pool set amid sheer rock walls. A bigger waterfall, inaccessible by means of this approach, lies farther upstream.

Well below Fish Fork, you enter The Narrows. A rough trail, worn in by hikers, traverses this one-mile-plus section of fast-moving water. You'll pass swimmable (if chilly) pools cupped in the granite and schist bedrock, and cross the stream when necessary. Listen and watch for water ouzels (dippers) by the edges of the pools. Old mining trails once threaded the canyon walls here and to the north, but all are virtually obliterated now.

At the lower portals of The Narrows (9.7 miles), you come upon the enigmatically named Bridge to Nowhere. During the 1930s, road-builders managed to push a highway up along the East Fork stream to just this far. The arched, concrete bridge, similar in style to those built along Angeles Crest Highway, was to be a key

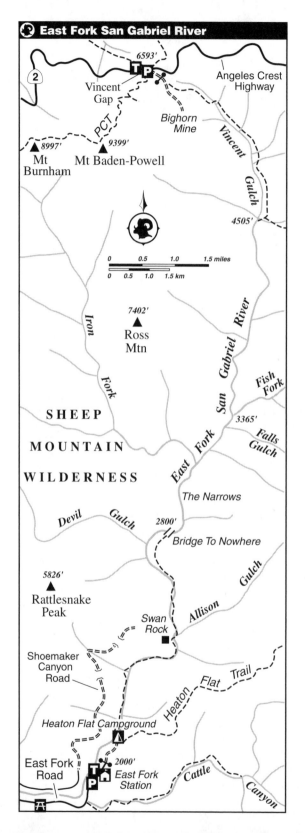

6593'

T P

Angeles Crest
Highway

Vincent
Gap

Bighorn
Mine

PCT

▲ 8997'
Mt
Burnham

▲ 9399'
Mt Baden-Powell

Vincent Gulch

4505'

0   0.5   1.0   1.5 miles
0   0.5   1.0   1.5 km

Iron

7402'
▲
Ross
Mtn

Fork

San Gabriel River

Fish Fork

SHEEP

3365'

MOUNTAIN

Falls Gulch

WILDERNESS

East Fork

The Narrows

Devil   *Gulch*

2800'

Bridge To Nowhere

Gulch

5826'
▲
Rattlesnake
Peak

Swan
Rock ■

Allison

Shoemaker
Canyon
Road

Heaton   Flat   Trail

Heaton Flat Campground ▲

East Fork
Road

2000'
T P
East Fork
Station

Cattle

Canyon

⌂

link in a route that would carry traffic between the San Gabriel Valley and the desert near Wrightwood. Fate intervened. A great flood in 1938 thoroughly demolished most of the road, leaving the bridge stranded. Another, later attempt to construct a road through the East Fork gorge also resulted in failure. High on the canyon's west rim lies Shoemaker Canyon Road—a "road to nowhere."

Below the bridge, on remnants of the old road washed out in 1938, you'll run into more and more hikers, fishermen, and other travelers out for the day. At 12.0 miles, Swan Rock—an outcrop of metamorphic rock branded with the light-colored imprint of a swan—comes into view on the right. At 14.0 miles you come upon Heaton Flat Campground. From there a final, easy 0.5-mile stroll takes you to the East Fork Station and trailhead at the end of East Fork Road.

HIKE 33

Fish Canyon Falls

Location	Foothills of the San Gabriel Mountains behind Duarte
Highlight	Arguably the most beautiful waterfall in Angeles National Forest
Distance	5.0 miles
Total Elevation Gain/Loss	900'/900'
Hiking Time	2 ½ hours
Optional Map	USGS 7.5-min *Azusa*
Best Times	November through June
Agency	ANF/SGRD
Difficulty	★★

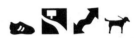

Time-traveling visitors from a century ago would have a hard time recognizing Fish Canyon today. Long gone are the dozens of vacation cabins lining the canyon and the dance hall at the canyon's mouth. Today, the lower canyon is being chewed apart on an astounding scale by rock quarrying operations. These operations, however, extend only as far into the canyon as the Angeles National Forest boundary. Beyond lies the perennially green Fish Canyon, its sparkling stream, and its magnificent, multi-tiered waterfall.

It is difficult to be definitive about how to hike into the upper canyon and visit the falls, because the means of access have changed frequently over the past 20 years. During the 1980s and most of the '90s, public access to the canyon was made difficult or impossible by operations at the Vulcan Materials quarry. The access issue was at least temporarily resolved in 1998, when the city of Duarte opened a new trail bypassing the quarry on the canyon's steep, west wall. Unfortunately, the devilish climb and descent on this trail (if accomplished twice during the round trip to and from the falls) occupies almost three fourths of the time and energy expended on the entire hike to the falls. The round trip to and from the falls via this route totals 9 miles with elevation gains

and losses of 3100 feet. To make things worse, the lower part of the bypass trail quickly fell into disrepair due to its unfavorable route across perpetually sliding, steep slopes. It is still passable, though some consider it to be excessively dangerous.

Currently, an easier solution is being implemented, although no one knows for how long. On Sundays, when quarry operations are suspended, hikers have been given permission to pass through quarry property and continue on up the canyon toward the falls.

To Reach the Trailhead: To reach Fish Canyon, drive east on Huntington Drive in Duarte to Encanto Parkway. Turn left and follow Encanto Parkway (and its extension, Fish Canyon Road) northeast for 1.4 miles. A trailhead parking lot for the bypass trail lies on the left. This is probably where you will leave your car. Just beyond, at the terminus of Fish Canyon Road, is the entrance to the quarry, where (if permission is granted to you, and probably only on Sunday) you may start your hike.

Description: The first half mile up the canyon is through a literal no-man's land of raw earth and gargantuan machinery flanked by dynamite blasted cliffs. Then, suddenly, you enter a delightful, alder-

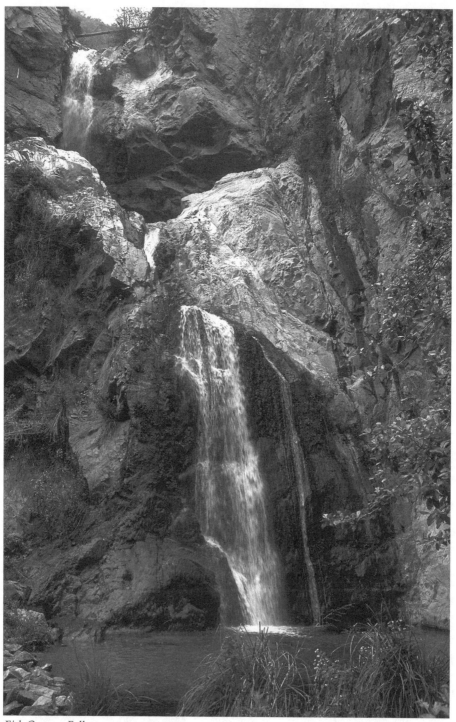

Fish Canyon Falls

lined riparian zone with the Fish Canyon stream alongside you and a trail to follow up the canyon. Around the first bend, the trail climbs to a bench on the left and the ugliness of the quarry is instantly forgotten.

The remainder of the route features a gentle ascent, superb scenery, and many historical reminders. Notice the old cabin foundations, rock and mortar walls, and rusty household equipment. Check out the botanical evidence: nonnative ivy, vinca, trees-of-heaven, agaves, and ornamental yuccas. Plenty of native vegetation thrives here, too. Live oaks, bigleaf maples, and bay laurels cling tenaciously to the canyon's precipitous walls, helping to hold together the structurally precarious miscellany of smashed-up granitic and metamorphic rock.

After about 1.1 miles of walking on the left bank, the trail crosses over the creek to the east bank—a foot- and leg-wetting exercise when the water's running high. A final 0.3-mile stretch leads to a point on the canyonside offering a fine but not intimately close view of Fish Canyon Falls. The water tumbles nearly 100 feet down a cliff with four separate tiers, slides through riparian vegetation a short way, and makes a final, small leap into a crystalline pool just below the trail.

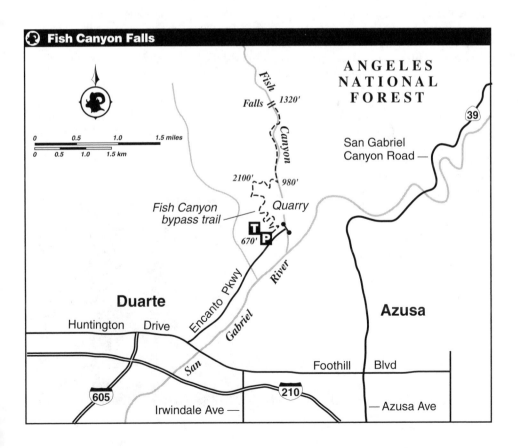

HIKE 34

Old Baldy

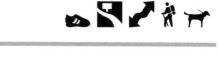

Location	Eastern San Gabriel Mountains
Highlights	Panoramic views along the Devils Backbone and atop L.A. County's highest point
Distance	6.4 miles round trip
Total Elevation Gain/Loss	2300'/2300'
Hiking Time	3 ½ hours (round trip)
Optional Map	USGS 7.5-min *Mount San Antonio, Telegraph Peak*
Best Times	May through November
Agency	ANF/SGRD
Difficulty	★★★

No Southland hiker's repertoire of experiences is complete without at least one ascent of Mt. San Antonio, or "Old Baldy." The east approach is the least taxing of the several routes to the summit, but it's by no means a picnic. You start at 7800 feet, with virtually no altitude acclimatization, and climb expeditiously to over 10,000 feet. Given the easy access, it's beguilingly easy to come unprepared for high winds or bad weather, which although fairly rare may come up suddenly. Ice, if present, can be a serious hazard as well.

To Reach the Trailhead: By mechanical means (a car) you can get to the upper terminus of Mt. Baldy Road in less than half an hour from the valley flatlands below. To do this, exit the 210 Freeway at Mills Avenue in Claremont, and follow Mills north toward the mountains. After about a mile Mills becomes Mt. Baldy Road. Continue all the way to the end of the road, where you enter the parking lot for the Mt. Baldy Ski Lift.

By further mechanical means—the ski lift—you ascend effortlessly to an elevation of 7800 feet at Mt. Baldy Notch, where you begin the hike. Although the ski lift caters mostly to skiers (7 days a week during the winter season), it remains open during the summer season on weekends (9 A.M. to 4:45 P.M.) for the ben-

efit of sightseers and hikers. If it's a weekday, or you don't like being dangled over an abyss, you can always walk up the ski-lift-maintenance road starting from Manker Flats. That option adds 3.6 miles and an elevation change of about 1600 feet both on the way up and on the way down. A lodge at the upper terminus of the lift offers food and beverages.

Description: From Mt. Baldy Notch, technically the spot about 200 yards northeast of the top of the ski lift, take the maintenance road to the northwest that climbs moderately, then more steeply through groves of Jeffrey pine and incense cedar. After a couple of bends, you come

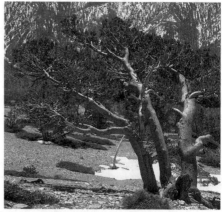

Lodgepole pines near timberline

to the road's end (1.3 miles) and the beginning of the trail along the Devil's Backbone ridge.

The stretch ahead, once a hair-raiser, lost most of its terror when the Civilian Conservation Corps constructed a wider and safer trail, complete with guard rails, in 1935–36. The guard rails are gone now, but there's plenty of room to maneuver, unless there are problems with strong winds and/or ice. Devil's Backbone offers grand vistas of both the Lytle Creek drainage on the north and east and San Antonio Canyon on the south.

The backbone section ends at about 2.0 miles as you start traversing the broad south flank of Mt. Harwood. Scattered lodgepole pines now predominate. At 2.6 miles you arrive at the saddle between Harwood and Old Baldy, where backpackers sometimes set up camp (no water,

no facilities here). Continue climbing up the rocky ridge to the west, past stunted, wind-battered conifers barely clinging to survival in the face of yearly onslaughts by cold winter winds. You reach the summit after a total of 3.2 miles.

On the rocky summit, barren of trees, you'll find a rock-walled enclosure and a register book that fills up with the names of hundreds of hikers on a fair-weather weekend. Most days you can easily make out the other two members of the triad of Southern California giants—San Gorgonio Mountain and San Jacinto Peak—about 50 miles east and southeast, respectively. On days of crystalline clarity, the Old Baldy panorama includes 90° of ocean horizon, a 120° slice of the tawny desert floor, and the far-off ramparts of the southern Sierra Nevada and Panamint ranges, as much as 160 miles away.

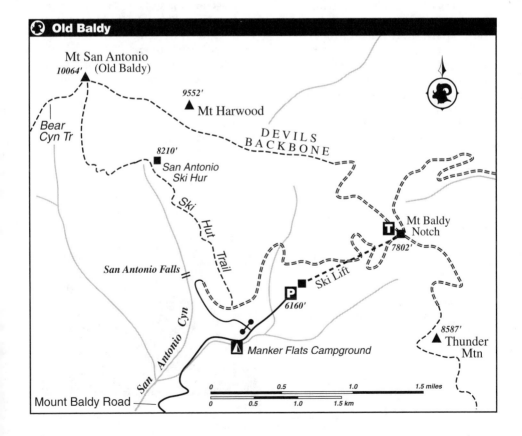

HIKE 35

Cucamonga Peak

Location	Eastern San Gabriel Mountains
Highlights	Alder-shaded stream; stupendous valley views during clear weather
Distance	12.0 miles round trip
Total Elevation Gain/Loss	4300'/4300'
Hiking Time	7 hours (round trip)
Optional Maps	USGS 7.5-min *Mt. Baldy, Cucamonga Peak*
Best Times	May through November
Agency	ANF/SGRD
Difficulty	★★★★

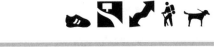

Cucamonga Peak's south and east slopes feature some of the most dramatic relief in the San Gabriel range. At 8859 feet, the peak stands sentinel-like only 4 miles from the edge of the broad inland valley region known as the Inland Empire. Go all the way to the top for the view, but don't be too disappointed if there's nothing below but haze and smog. So much beautiful high country can be seen along the way that reaching the top is just icing on the cake.

Most of the hike lies within Cucamonga Wilderness, requiring a permit for both day and overnight use. Near Cucamonga's summit you'll tackle a steep, north-facing gully that can retain snow into May. Be sure to discuss with a ranger the possible hazards of snow and ice if it's early or late in the year.

To Reach the Trailhead: Exit the 210 Freeway at Mills Avenue in Claremont, and follow Mills north toward the mountains. After about a mile Mills becomes Mt. Baldy Road. An 8-mile climb up through San Antonio Canyon on Mt. Baldy Road takes you to the small village of Mt. Baldy, and a national-forest ranger station on the left where you can pick up the needed wilderness permit. Continue 1.5 miles past the village to a short spur road on the right, signed NO OUTLET. Park

at the end of that spur, which is the trail-head for the Icehouse Canyon Trail, and don't forget to post a National Forest Adventure Pass on your car.

Description: Walk up the Icehouse Canyon Trail following the alder-shaded, boulder-filled streambed, which may be dry at its lowermost end. The first couple of miles along the canyon are a fitting introduction to a phase of Southern California scenery not familiar to a lot of visitors and newcomers. Huge bigcone Douglas-fir, incense cedar, and live oak trees cluster on the banks of the flowing stream, which dances over boulder and fallen log. Moisture-loving, flowering plants like columbine sway in the breeze. Some of old cabins along the lower canyon still survive, while others, destroyed by flood

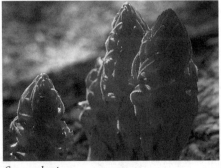

Snow plant

or fire, have left evidence in the form of foundations or rock walls.

Old newspaper reports suggest that an ice-packing operation existed in or near Icehouse Canyon during the late 1850s. The ice was packed down San Antonio Canyon on mules to a point accessible to wagons, whereupon it was carted, as quickly as possible, to Los Angeles for use in making ice cream and for chilling beverages. Whether ice was actually quarried in this canyon or in another, Icehouse Canyon's name is apt enough: Cold-air drainage produces refrigeratorlike temperatures on many a summer morning, and deep-freeze temperatures in winter.

Chapman Trail (a longer, alternate route) intersects on the left at 1.0 mile. At Columbine Spring (2.4 miles, last water during the warmer months), the trail starts switchbacking up the north wall.

After passing the upper intersection of the Chapman Trail at 2.9 miles, you continue to pine-shaded Icehouse Saddle, 3.5 miles, where trails converge from many directions. The trail to Cucamonga's summit contours southeast, descends moderately, and climbs to a 7654-foot saddle (4.4 miles) between Bighorn and Cucamonga peaks. Thereafter, it switchbacks up a steep slope dotted with lodgepole pines and white firs.

At 5.8 miles, the trail crosses a shady draw 200 feet below and northwest of the Cucamonga Peak summit. A signed but indistinct side path goes straight up to the top, 6.0 miles from your starting point at the Icehouse Canyon trailhead. Return the same way—or take the alternate route, the Chapman Trail, if you'd like to explore a longer but more gradual descent from Icehouse Saddle.

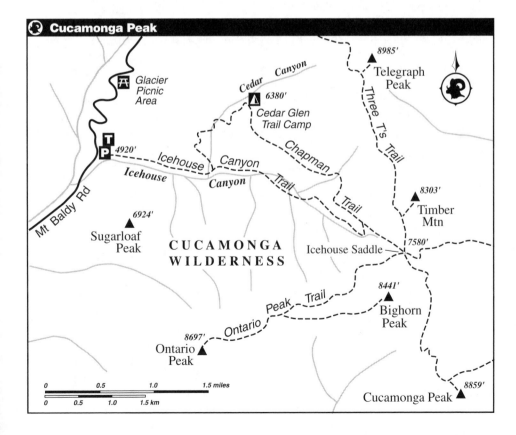

HIKE 36

Cougar Crest Trail

Location	Big Bear Lake, San Bernardino Mountains
Highlights	Pinyon-juniper forest; lake and mountain views
Distance	6.6 miles round trip (to Bertha Peak)
Total Elevation Gain/Loss	1450'/1450'
Hiking Time	3 ½ hours (round trip)
Optional Map	USGS 7.5-min *Fawnskin*
Best Times	April through November
Agency	SBNF/BBD
Difficulty	★★

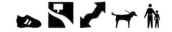

Big Bear Lake, with its popular resorts and ski areas, offers some fine hiking experiences for those willing to stretch their legs a bit. A number of old roads and trails lace the slopes south of Big Bear Lake (the mini-metropolis of that same name on the lake's south shore), but better hiking can be found on the sloping mountain rim that rises above the serene and mostly undeveloped north shore of the lake. Here, the Cougar Crest Trail ascends to a junction with the 2600-mile-long Pacific Crest Trail—the world's longest maintained footpath.

To Reach the Trailhead: Arriving at Big Bear by way of Highways 330 and 18 from the city of San Bernardino (the most common approach), turn left on Highway 38 as soon as you reach Big Bear Lake. Drive along the north shore for 5 miles to the large Cougar Crest trailhead on the left (north) side of the road. This same trailhead is located 4 miles west of Big Bear City via Highway 38. Be sure to display your National Forest Adventure Pass.

Description: From trailhead start heading up the Cougar Crest Trail, formerly an obscure dirt road. Traces of mining activity are evident as you climb upward along a shallow draw filled with a delightful mix of outsized pinyon pines and junipers, and occasional straight and tall Jeffrey pines. The mingling of the

sweet and pungent scents exuded by the wood and needles of these trees is intoxicating on a warm day.

After a long mile, the old road becomes a narrow trail and begins to curl and switchback along higher and sunnier slopes. Big Bear Lake comes into view occasionally, its surface azure in the slanting illumination of a spring or summer morning, or dotted with silvery pinpoints of light on a late fall day.

After about 2 miles, the trail reaches a divide, bends right, and for a short distance traverses a cool (or sometimes cold and icy), north-facing slope. At 2.2 miles, the Cougar Crest Trail joins the Pacific Crest Trail—the latter a path reserved for hikers and horses only (no mountain bikes or other mechanical conveyances are allowed on the entire PCT route between the Mexican and Canadian borders). You bear right and start contouring east, high on the sunny, south-facing slope. Spread before you now is the lake (technically a shallow reservoir), which half-fills a 10-mile-long trough in the mountains, and various resort and residential communities spread along the shore and beyond. Behind the lake and about 12 miles distant, the rounded, often-snow-mantled ramparts of San Gorgonio Wilderness gleam.

The southern view does not significantly improve as you press on, though the high point ahead, Bertha Peak, will furnish a better view in other directions. When the PCT crosses a rock-strewn service road (2.6 miles from the start), leave the nicely graded trail and start climbing east on the road. A sweaty, 0.7-mile ascent takes you to a small microwave relay station atop Bertha Peak. Outside the relay station's perimeter fence you'll find a peak baggers' register, plus fine views over the treetops into Holcomb Valley and the Mojave Desert to the north.

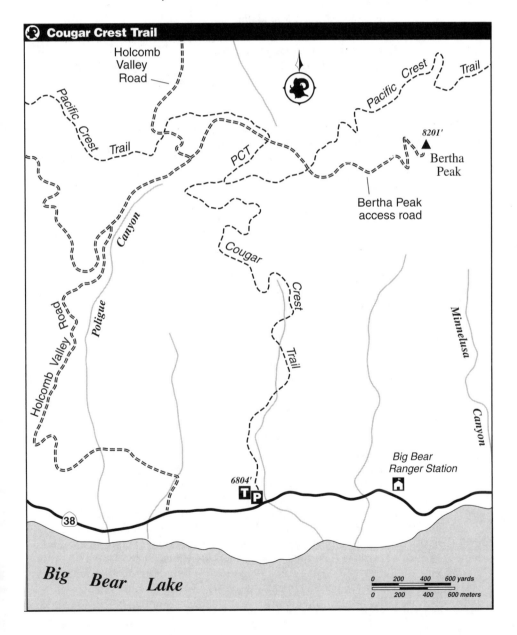

HIKE 37

Forsee Creek Trail

Location	San Gorgonio Wilderness, San Bernardino Mountains
Highlight	Peak bagging amid Southern California's highest mountains
Distance	12.6 miles round trip (to Trail Fork Camp)
Total Elevation Gain/Loss	3700'/3700'
Hiking Time	8 hours (round trip)
Recommended Map	Forest Service *San Gorgonio Wilderness* topographic map
Best Times	May through November
Agency	SBNF/SGD
Difficulty	★★★★

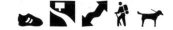

Tucked amid the tall, straight trunks of lodgepole pines at nearly 2 miles high, the wind-sheltered and mostly bug-free Trail Fork Camp is a peak bagger's delight. Just above the trail camp lies the lightning-tortured roof of Southern California—San Bernardino Mountain—containing four named highpoints within reach of an easy, half-day stroll. Farther east lies the big daddy of Southern California summits—San Gorgonio Mountain—within reach of an all-day (16-mile round trip) dayhike involving only moderate elevation change.

The trek to Trail Fork Camp and the crest beyond is itself a challenging dayhike. It's somewhat easier if you take one full day to hike in and a partial day to return. The high peaks of San Gorgonio Wilderness tend to create their own local storms in summertime, so be aware of thunderstorm forecasts before embarking on your journey. Raingear and a tent with waterproof fly are musts during such conditions; better yet, consider canceling or postponing your trip if there is tropical moisture in the area.

A wilderness permit for day or overnight use for all but the very beginning of this trip is required. Permits are available on a first-come, first-served basis at the Mill Creek Ranger Station, at Mill Creek Road (Highway 38) and Bryant

Street, east of the town of Mentone. The ranger station opens at 8 A.M. weekdays and 7 A.M. weekends; some permits may be available by self-registration outside the door before those hours. The station also sells a Forest-Service topographic map titled "Guide to the San Gorgonio Wilderness," which includes the Forsee Creek route.

To Reach the Trailhead: To reach the trailhead from I-10 at Redlands, take Highway 38 east through Mentone (and past the Mill Creek Station), up onto the forested highlands of the San Bernardino Mountains. At a point 18 miles beyond Mill Creek Station, turn right on Jenks Lake Road. After 0.3 mile turn right on a rough dirt road signed FORSEE CREEK TRAIL, and proceed cautiously another 0.6 mile to a large clearing used for parking. Do post a National Forest Adventure Pass on your car.

Description: From the trailhead, make your way steadily uphill under shade-giving Jeffrey pines, incense-cedars, white firs, and black oaks, and a few sugar pines, quickly passing a side trail to Johns Meadow. Most summers, thin streams of water cascade down two or three gullies traversed by the first 2 miles of trail. After an hour or two of unrelenting labor, you leave the "yellow-pine" vegetation behind and enter a zone dominated by lodgepole pines. Much higher up, the lodgepole pines (with two needles per cluster) are joined by limber pines (having five needles per cluster and rubbery branch tips).

At 4.2 miles, Jackstraw Springs trail camp (prone to mosquitoes in the summer) lies down a side path to the right. At 6.2 miles, the trail bends sharply right and arrives at a junction. Just below, hidden

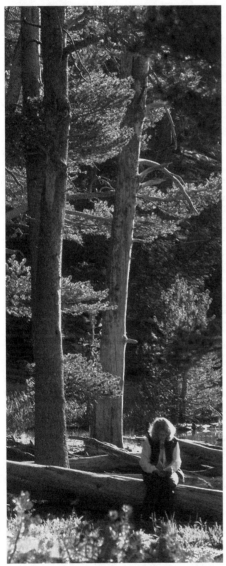

A quiet moment amid the high-country pines

in a clump of bushes, lies Trail Fork Springs—oftentimes the first trickle in the headwaters of Forsee Creek. Retrace your steps about 100 yards on the Forsee Creek Trail to find the steep, narrow side path leading east up to Trail Fork Camp. Several flat sites for camping can be found hereabouts amid the lodgepoles and weathered outcrops of banded metamorphic rock. A bald area on a flat ridge just northeast is the perfect spot to admire a view stretching north toward Big Bear Lake, and to toast the last rays of the setting sun.

If time and energy permit, pay a visit to nearby Shields and Anderson peaks, 0.7 mile and 0.4 mile away, respectively. On the crest between these peaks lie scraggly pines, many battered and stripped of their bark by lightning strikes. North of the crest, in protected pockets, uniformly spaced lodgepole pines grow tall and straight with dark "bathtub rings" around their waists indicating snow accumulations several feet deep.

An optional peak-bagging foray to the west might include both of the San Bernardino peaks, plus the historic Colonel Henry Washington Monument, which commemorates the original San Bernardino baseline and meridian survey point, established in 1852. (The monument lies off-trail; you'll find it by walking 160 yards straight up the ridge from the southwesternmost switchback in the San Bernardino Peak Divide Trail.) For over 150 years, all land surveys of Southern California have referred to Colonel Washington's initial baseline. Due west of the monument, starting from the foot of the mountain, today's Base Line Road stretches radially outward many miles across the flat, alluvial plain occupied by San Bernardino and several of its satellite cities. As viewed from the monument on clear days, Base Line Road seems to point toward a vanishing point in or beyond the San Gabriel Valley.

It is possible to return to the trailhead via a much longer (17.5 miles total) route that loops around via Johns Meadow. Descend the San Bernardino Peak Divide Trail north to an 8270-foot trail junction near Manzanita Springs. Then head northeast on the often-steep, unmaintained, partially obscure trail toward Johns Meadow. East of Johns Meadow, the trail is maintained.

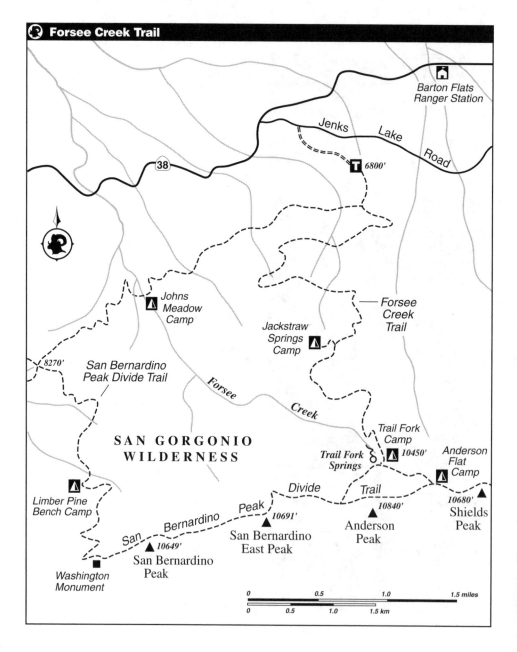

HIKE 38

Dollar Lake

Location	San Gorgonio Wilderness, San Bernardino Mountains
Highlight	Sparkling glacial tarn
Distance	12.6 miles round trip
Total Elevation Gain/Loss	2700'/2700'
Hiking Time	7 hours (round trip)
Optional Map	Forest Service *San Gorgonio Wilderness* topographic map
Best Times	May through November
Agency	SBNF/SGD
Difficulty	★★★★

Sparkling and silvery like a freshly minted silver dollar, Dollar Lake lies cupped amid a talus-frosted natural bowl, not far below the great divide of San Bernardino Mountain. Snow lingers late on the steep slopes overlooking the lake, sometimes into August. It's hard to believe this splendid landscape, reminiscent of the High Sierra, exists here in Southern California, only 20 air-miles from the suburban housing tracts of San Bernardino.

A dayhike to Dollar Lake (via the South Fork Trail) in the San Gorgonio Wilderness is not only possible but rather straightforwardly easy for any well-conditioned Southern Californian willing to rise early and get to the trailhead by 8 or 9 in the morning. A wilderness permit for day or overnight use of all but the lower part of the trail is required. A limited number of permits are available on a first-come, first-served basis at the Mill Creek Ranger Station, at Mill Creek Road (Highway 38) and Bryant Street, east of the town of Mentone. The station opens at 8 A.M. weekdays and 7 A.M. weekends; some permits may be available by self-registration outside the door before those hours. The station also sells a Forest-Service topographic map titled "Guide to the San Gorgonio Wilderness," which includes the Dollar Lake route.

To Reach the Trailhead: To reach the trailhead from I-10 at Redlands, take Highway 38 east through Mentone (and past the Mill Creek Station), up onto the forested highlands of the San Bernardino Mountains. At a point 18 miles beyond Mill Creek Station, turn right on Jenks Lake Road. Proceed 3 miles to the large South Fork Trailhead parking lot on the left. You'll need to display a National Forest Adventure Pass on your parked car.

Description: The South Fork Trail crosses Jenks Lake Road, heading south, and commences a moderate ascent up a shady canyon. Soon, the trail switches back, climbs out of the canyon and climbs southeast toward a bracken-filled clearing—Horse Meadows. Near the meadow's upper edge, you cross a dirt road (1.5 miles). That road, now closed to traffic, leads to a spot known as "Poopout Hill," an earlier trailhead higher on the mountain that used to save hikers about 2 miles of hiking each way as compared to the South Fork route they now must follow.

Continue your ascent through the typical mid-elevation yellow-pine belt, consisting here of mostly of ponderosa pines and white firs. At around 4.0 miles, the trail draws close to the South Fork Santa Ana River. Remain on the right bank of the creek, staying right at the signed junction with the Dry Lake Trail. Off to the left is South Fork Meadows, where many small tributaries combine and funnel into the South Fork. Days or weeks later some of this water will be traveling down the wide Santa Ana River flood-control channel through Anaheim and Santa Ana. Much of the water seeps into gravelly or sandy soils downstream, recharges underground aquifers, and never reaches the ocean. You stay to the right and do not cross the South Fork.

Your ascent continues on the crooked, mostly shaded Dollar Lake Trail. The yellow-pine belt fades while stout and straight lodgepole pines appear in greater numbers. At 5.9 miles, just past a large, manzanita-covered patch on the mountainside, you'll come to junction where a side trail starts slanting down toward Dollar Lake, a short half mile away. The San Bernardino Mountains are the only range of mountains within Southern California to show evidence of glaciation (prior to about 10,000 years ago), and the depression occupied by Dollar Lake is suggestive of this.

If your trip involves backpacking, the trail campground at Dollar Lake is a pleasant enough overnight stop. One mile above Dollar Lake (by trail) is Dollar Lake Saddle, and 4 miles southeast of that is the summit of San Gorgonio Mountain. Prior to the closing of the Poopout Hill trailhead in 1988, northern ascents of Gorgonio via either Dollar Lake or Dry Lake were the easiest, if not quite the shortest. Since then, the easiest and fastest way up the mountain has been by way of Vivian Creek (see Hike 39).

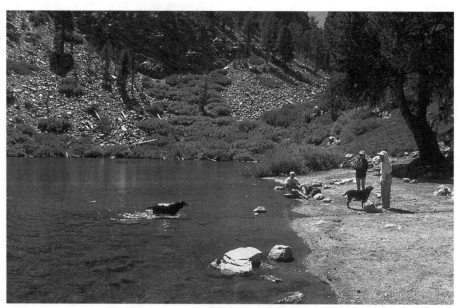

Dollar Lake

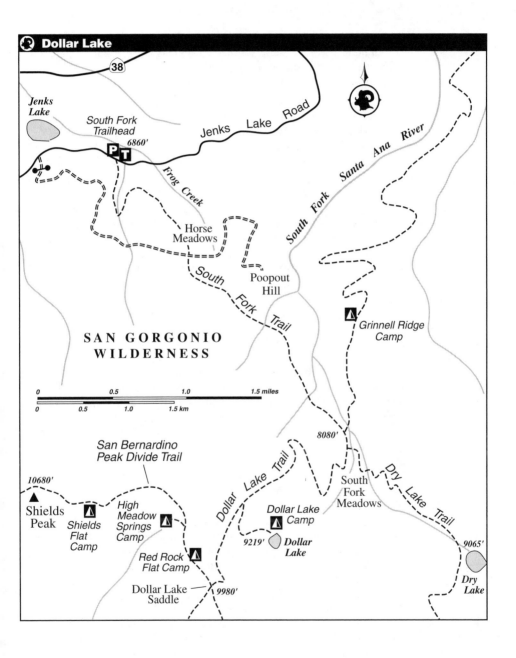

HIKE 39

San Gorgonio Mountain

Location	San Gorgonio Wilderness, San Bernardino Mountains
Highlight	Standing atop Southern California's highest spot
Distance	15.6 miles round trip
Total Elevation Gain/Loss	5700'/5700'
Hiking Time	10 hours (round trip)
Optional Map	Forest Service *San Gorgonio Wilderness* topographic map
Best Times	April through November
Agency	SBNF/SGD
Difficulty	★★★★

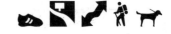

The barren, talus-strewn summit of San Gorgonio Mountain (or "Greyback," after its steely gray appearance from the valleys below) receives dozens of hikers on most fine-weather weekends. No hiker, however, ever has an easy time of it. Either variation of the popular northern approach (via Dollar Lake or Dry Lake) requires over 20 miles of round-trip hiking. On the southern approach by way of the Vivian Creek Trail, described here, you begin hiking at a point several hundred feet of elevation lower than the northern (South Fork) trailhead, but you save at least 5 miles of distance on the round trip.

The Vivian Creek Trail is the original path to the top of San Gorgonio, built around the turn of the 20th Century. Today, about eight distinct routes (or variations on routes) culminate at the summit. After 1988, when the north-side "Poopout Hill" trailhead closed, the Vivian Creek route once again become the fastest and easiest way up the mountain. The south-facing Vivian Creek route also has the advantage of a longer season; most snow on the upper parts of the trail is gone by May or June, a month or more before the northern routes are similarly clear.

Of those people who approach the summit by way of Vivian Creek, perhaps half do so over a two- or three- day period, hauling their overnight gear to

camps such as Halfway or High Creek, and dayhiking from there. Others, in excellent condition and traveling lightly, have taken as little as 7 hours total, with a half-hour spent at the top and some jogging on the way down. At a leisurely pace with plenty of breaks, a day-long summit hike could take a mind- and leg-numbing 14 hours. This is okay in June or July (assuming you start hiking at dawn), but not good during November, when daylight lasts 11 hours or less.

San Gorgonio Mountain lies within the heart of the San Gorgonio Wilderness. Whether dayhiking or backpacking, you must secure a wilderness permit from the Mill Creek Ranger Station, at Mill Creek Road (Highway 38) and Bryant Street, east of the town of Mentone. The station opens at 8 A.M. weekdays and 7 A.M. weekends. Some permits may be available by self-registration outside the door before those hours. Others may be available in advance by mail. The station also sells a Forest-Service topographic map titled "Guide to the San Gorgonio Wilderness," which includes the entire Vivian Creek route.

To Reach the Trailhead: To reach the trailhead from I-10 at Redlands, take Highway 38 east through Mentone to Mill Creek Station, and up Mill Creek Canyon for another 6.2 miles beyond the station to the intersection of Valley of the Falls Boulevard (a.k.a. Forest Home Road, on the right). Continue driving uphill through the cabin community of Forest Falls, all the way to the end of Valley of the Falls Boulevard, which is where you can find a spacious trailhead parking lot. Be sure to display a National Forest Adventure Pass on your car.

Description: From the trailhead, walk east (uphill) past a vehicle gate and follow a dirt road for 0.6 mile to its end. Go left across the wide, boulder wash of Mill Creek and find the Vivian Creek Trail going sharply up the oak-clothed canyon wall on the far side. The next half mile is excruciatingly steep; and this pitch is worse on the return, when your weary quadriceps muscles must absorb the punishment of each lurching downhill step.

Mercifully, at the top of the steep section, the trail levels momentarily, then assumes a moderate grade up alongside Vivian Creek. A sylvan Shangri-La unfolds ahead. Pines, firs, and cedars reach for the sky. Bracken fern smothers the banks of the melodious creek, which dances over boulders and fallen trees. After the first October frost, the bracken turns a flaming yellow, made all the more vivid by warm sunlight pouring out of a fierce blue sky.

Near Halfway Camp (2.5 miles) the trail begins climbing timber-dotted slopes covered intermittently by thickets of manzanita. Dobbs Peak, just below timberline, comes into view in the north, though the nearly treeless San Bernardino Mountain divide remains hidden. After several zigs and zags on north-facing slopes, you swing onto a brightly illuminated south-facing slope. Serrated Yucaipa Ridge looms in the south, rising sheer from the depths of Mill Creek Canyon. Soon thereafter, the sound of bubbling water heralds your arrival at High Creek (4.8 miles) and the trail camp of the same name. Be ready for a chilly night if you stay here; cold, nocturnal air often flows down along the bottom of this canyon from the 10,000-foot-plus peaks above.

Past High Creek Camp the trail ascends gently on several long switchback segments through lodgepole pines, and at

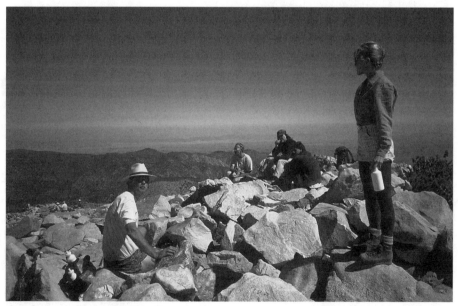

San Gorgonio Mountain summit

length attains a saddle on a rocky ridge. The pines thin out and appear more decrepit as you climb crookedly up along this ridge toward timberline. At 7.2 miles, the San Bernardino Peak Divide Trail intersects from the left. Stay right and keep climbing on a moderate grade across stony slopes dotted with cowering krummholz pines. Soon, nearly all vegetation disappears.

On the right you pass Sky High Trail, which bends around the mountain and descends toward Dry Lake and South Fork Meadows in the north. Don't give up! Keep straight and keep going. A final burst of effort puts you on a boulder pile marking the highest elevation in Southern California (7.8 miles from your starting point). From this vantage, even the soaring north face of Mt. San Jacinto to the south appears diminished in stature.

Several campsites surrounded by enclosures of piled-up stones are scattered on the summit plateau. These comprise Summit trail camp, a fine place to stay overnight if the weather is calm and clear (most typically in September and October). At night, planets and stars gleam overhead, but they must compete for attention with the glow of millions of lights below.

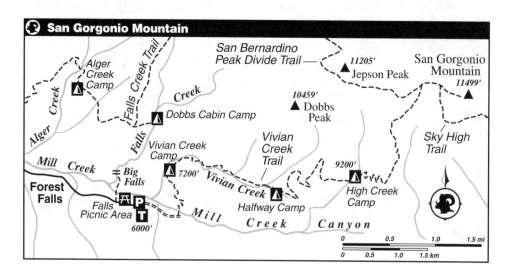

HIKE 40

Deep Creek

Location	Near Hesperia; north slope of the San Bernardino Mountains
Highlights	Natural hot-spring pools alongside a mountain stream
Distance	3.8 miles round trip
Total Elevation Gain/Loss	950'/950'
Hiking Time	2 ½ hours (round trip)
Optional Map	USGS 7.5-min *Lake Arrowhead*
Best Times	March through November
Agency	SBNF/AD
Difficulty	★★

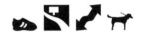

Deep Creek Hot Springs in the San Bernardino National Forest has been a minor magnet for hikers and other nature lovers—eccentric and otherwise—for decades. Volunteers have spent years fashioning rock-bound basins that impound water ranging from about 96°F to about 102°F. Water flowing out of those basins quickly reaches chilly Deep Creek, which has carved a deep cleft in the north slope of the San Bernardino Mountains.

To Reach the Trailhead: To get to the most convenient portal for the hot springs hike, which lies outside the national forest boundary, go north on I-15 over Cajon Pass and through the high desert community of Hesperia. Exit at Bear Valley Road and turn right. Travel east for 10 miles to Central Avenue. Turn right on Central, and drive 3 miles south to Ocotillo Way. Turn left on Ocotillo, and proceed 2.3 miles east to Bowen Ranch Road. Turn right on this unpaved but well graded road, and continue 8.0 miles (mostly southwest, more or less parallel to a high-voltage powerline) to a toll gate and 1920s-vintage cabin at the rustic, private Bowen Ranch. Pay the $4-per-person day-use fee at the gate, and be sure to pick up a copy of the hand-drawn "treasure" map which may help you navigate to the hot-springs site. Park your car at the ranch's overnight camping/parking area

a short distance past the toll gate. Since the ranch lies outside the San Bernardino National Forest boundary, there's no need to display a National Forest Adventure Pass.

If you want to pitch a tent or stay in a vehicle overnight at Bowen Ranch, the charge is $5 per person. Note that Forest Service regulations do not allow camping at the destination for this hike: Deep Creek Hot Springs. For the purposes of planning your trip, note that Bowen Ranch has no phone, no e-mail, and no website. Typically, the Forest Service has no definitive information about either the Bowen Ranch or about stream or weather conditions at Deep Creek.

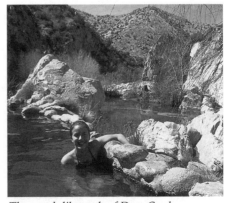

The womb-like pools of Deep Creek Hot Springs

Description: Now you're ready to head out on foot toward the springs, almost 2 miles away and nearly 1000 feet lower in elevation. After an initial 0.5 mile of downhill hiking, briefly jog left on a dirt road, then veer right on a signed trail entering San Bernardino National Forest land. You'll lose about 700 feet of elevation as you descend for another 1.3 miles into Deep Creek's canyon bottom. About halfway down this stretch, where the trail splits, take the right fork to ensure an easier, more gradual descent. Once you reach the canyon bottom you must decide how to cross the creek to reach the hot pools on the far side. In winter, the water is often swift and bone-chillingly cold. By spring, the shallowest wading route, through sluggishly moving water, might be only 1 or 2 feet deep.

Forest service regulations allow nude bathing in the Deep Creek Hot Springs drainage area, and typically about half of the visitors do so. Camping, campfires, and glass containers are strictly prohibited. Other regulations and rules of etiquette and behavior are listed in a leaflet available along the trail leading to the hot springs site.

Do realize that the uphill, post-soak hike back to the car can be enervating and possibly exhausting in the summer heat. Bring plenty of drinking water (not alcohol, which dehydrates the body) if the weather is warm! Inexperienced hikers have also gotten into deep trouble here when cold rain or snow is falling. The pools may be plenty warm, but inadequately equipped persons who can't get dry after a visit to the pools are at risk for hypothermia.

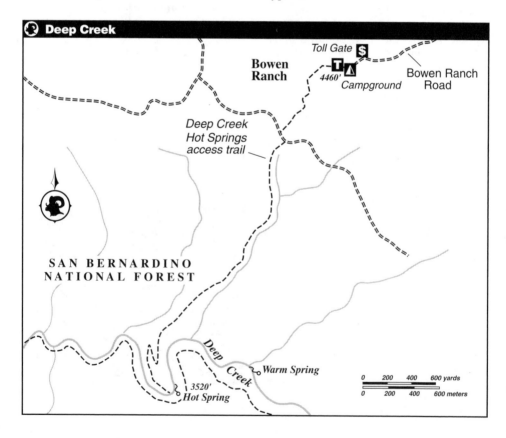

HIKE 41

Big Morongo Canyon

Location	Big Morongo Canyon Preserve, north of Palm Springs
Highlights	Riparian splendor amidst the desert; excellent birding
Distance	1 to 3 miles
Total Elevation Gain/Loss	50' to 300', depending on exact route
Hiking Time	½ to 2 hours
Optional Map	USGS 7.5-min *Morongo Valley*
Best Times	October through May
Agency	BMCP
Difficulty	★

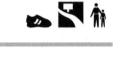

Nearly 300 species of birds have been spotted along a 6-mile stretch of Big Morongo Canyon, just outside the town of Morongo Valley. Wildlife frequenting the canyon includes bighorn sheep, bobcat, mountain lion, and mule deer. The 4500-acre Big Morongo Canyon Preserve, administered by the federal Bureau of Land Management, encompasses the wettest parts of the canyon. The preserve sits astride a melding of coastal chaparral and desert habitats and is regarded as one of the most important wildlife oases in the California desert. The exotic freshwater marsh found here owes its existence to seepage of water up along a geologic fault associated with a great rift between tectonic plates—the San Andreas Fault Zone—not far to the south.

The uppermost (wet) part of Big Morongo Canyon Preserve lies about 2000 feet above low-lying Palm Springs and the Coachella Valley, so the summer heat is intense but rarely intolerable here. Still, it's best to stick with the cooler months, or else confine your visit to early-morning or late-afternoon hours. The preserve is open daily from 7:30 A.M. to sunset.

To Reach the Trailhead: From I-10 near Palm Springs, drive 11 miles north on Highway 62 to Morongo Valley. Just past the business district turn right on East Drive, and look for the preserve entrance on the left.

Description: For a rewarding 1-mile stroll through contrasting habitats, walk past the visitor information display and pick up the Desert Wash Trail on the left.

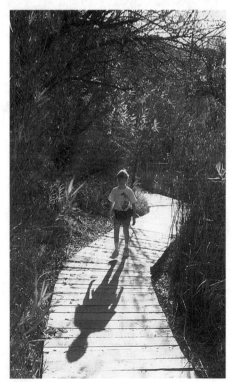

Willow Trail

It guides you over a sun-blasted terrace dotted with prosaic-looking shrubs such as honey mesquite, desert willow, and yerba santa. The latter exudes an unmistakable sweet-pungent odor. You dip to cross the Big Morongo Wash, and pass a spur trail, the Yucca Ridge Trail, over a half mile from the start. Continue on the Willow Trail, which will take you through the heart of Big Morongo's riparian oasis and back toward the start. You meander on boardwalks amid a junglelike assemblage of willows, cottonwoods, alders, and fan palms (the latter two apparently introduced, though they lie not far from the edge of their normal range). Watercress and water parsnip have overrun the surface of the shallow waters below your feet.

After a short half mile on the Willow Trail, you come to a trail intersection. Off

to the right a short distance is your parked car. To the left, on the Mesquite and Canyon trails, you can follow the waters of Big Morongo Canyon down as far as you like. About 1 mile down, just as the canyon begins to veer decidedly left (east), look for a short path on the left leading to a small metal dam and artificial waterfall. Downstream a bit farther you can descend to another, shady spot along the stream bank, sit for a while, and watch the silvery water slide by. For casual hiking, this is about as far as it's worth going.

If you're so inclined, and arrange for transportation on the far end, you can hike another 5 miles down the canyon all the way to Indian Avenue, northwest of Desert Hot Springs. The trail becomes poorer as you go. At some point, the stream goes underground and your remaining travel is in a dry wash.

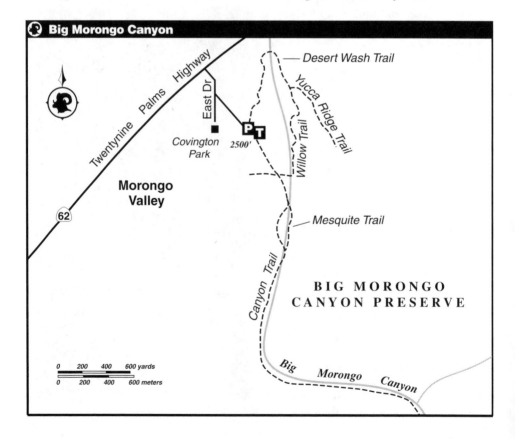

HIKE 42

Wonderland of Rocks Traverse

Location	Joshua Tree National Park
Highlight	Scrambling amid gigantic boulders
Distance	5.7 miles
Total Elevation Gain/Loss	200'/1200'
Hiking Time	6 hours
Recommended Map	USGS 7.5-min *Indian Cove*
Best Times	October through April
Agency	JTNP
Difficulty	★★★★

More than a hundred million years ago, a molten mass of rock lay several miles underground, cooling and crystallizing by agonizingly slow degrees. As the mass solidified, it contracted slightly, and fractures developed within it. Over geologic time, this mass moved upward while older, overlying layers of rock were eroded away. As the younger rock neared the surface, groundwater seeping into the fractures chemically transformed some of the rock crystals into clay. Large, more-or-less rectangular blocks of rock with rounded corners became isolated from each other in a matrix of loose clay. Once exposed above the surface, the clay quickly washed away, leaving open crevices between the blocks. Also, various mechanical forces and chemical weathering chipped away at boulders and rounded them even further.

The products of all this uplift and shaping are the monzogranite boulders we see today spectacularly exhibited in the Wonderland of Rocks section of Joshua Tree National Park. Everywhere you look, your mind is dazzled by huge, pancake- or loaf-like stacks of rocks (where horizontal fractures predominate), by rocks in columns or spires (where vertical fractures predominate), and by huge domes. Each structure is unique, having

been fashioned by a particular set of events occurring over millions of years.

Here we profile a one-way traverse across the Wonderland of Rocks known

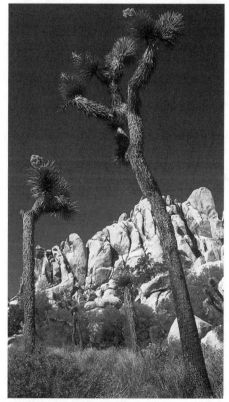

Joshua trees in Wonderland

by some as the "Wonderland Connection." Make no mistake, this is no easy stroll. Its four-star rating is solely on account of the fiercely jumbled landscape you must cross during the latter part of the trip. You should be adept at both boulder hopping and scrambling across tilted rock surfaces. Much of the travel involves meticulously lowering yourself downward over angular boulders—not recommended for the faint of heart. No camping is allowed in the Wonderland area, so this must be a daytrip only.

To Reach the Upper Trailhead: From Highway 62 in the community of Joshua Tree, take Park Boulevard (a.k.a. Quail Springs Road) into Joshua Tree National Park. Pay the national park entry fee (or show your yearly pass) when you reach the park boundary. Continue southeast a total of 11 miles from Highway 62 to reach the Wonderland backcountry board (kiosk) on the left (north) side of the road. This point is 0.7 mile east of Quail Springs Picnic Area and 2.3 miles northwest of Hidden Valley Campground.

To Reach the Lower Trailhead: The hike ends at the Indian Cove camp/picnic area, just south of Highway 62, 8 miles east of Joshua Tree and 5 miles west of Twentynine Palms. Drive all the way to the end of the road to the picnic ground at the mouth of Rattlesnake Canyon, where the one-way hike ends.

Description: From the Wonderland backcountry board, follow the Boy Scout Trail (a dirt road) 1.4 miles north across sandy flats dotted with Joshua trees to the Willow Hole Trail, intersecting on the right. Follow the Willow Hole Trail northeast to where it enters a dry wash, then continue downhill in the wash. The wash soon becomes a canyon bottom flanked by stacks of boulders. At 3.5 miles you arrive at Willow Hole—large pools flanked by a screen of willows.

Following a beaten-down path, you then work your way through the willows on the right, over a low ridge, and across a gap between two rock piles. Follow the narrow canyon bottom below, which carries water draining from the pools at Willow Hole during the wetter parts of the year. The remaining travel is entirely downhill, but progress is soon impeded as you negotiate a canyon section clogged with boulders.

At 0.7 mile beyond Willow Hole, a north-flowing tributary joins on the right. Stay in the main canyon as it veers north and descends sharply for 0.3 mile to join Rattlesnake Canyon. Exercise care while descending this hazardous stretch. (It was here, during a prearranged rendezvous and car-key exchange between my party and a party traveling in the opposite direction, that one set of keys was dropped into the boulder maze and almost irretrievably lost. The lesson: Always have an extra key in a magnetic box on the car frame or hidden nearby.)

Once you reach Rattlesnake Canyon, only a bit more than a mile of hiking remains. The going is easy for a while as you follow the sandy wash downhill (northeast). Some cottonwood trees brighten the otherwise desolate scene of sand and soaring stone walls. As the canyon bends left for a final descent to the flats of Indian Cove below, you face more episodes of serious scrambling. Keeping to the left-side canyon wall, work your way around a slotlike canyon worn in the granitic rock. Down in the bottom of the slot are potholes worn by the abrasive action of flash flooding. Only a bit more scrambling and a short walk down the canyon's sandy wash takes you to the end of the hike—the picnic area at Indian Cove.

A good resource for hiking routes and other features in the Wonderland of Rocks area is Patty Furbush's book, *On Foot in Joshua Tree National Park*, available at the park's visitor centers. The book includes a topographic map of the route just described.

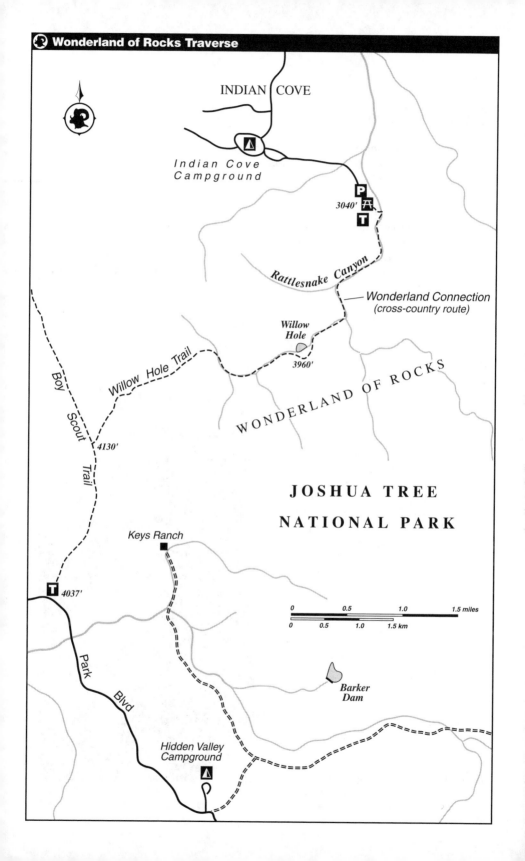

INDIAN COVE

Indian Cove
Campground

P
3040'
T

Rattlesnake Canyon

Wonderland Connection
(cross-country route)

Willow
Hole
3960'

Boy

Scout

Trail

Willow Hole Trail

4130'

WONDERLAND OF ROCKS

JOSHUA TREE

NATIONAL PARK

Keys Ranch

T 4037'

0	0.5	1.0	1.5 miles
0	0.5	1.0	1.5 km

Barker
Dam

Park

Blvd

Hidden Valley
Campground

HIKE 43

Ryan Mountain

Location	Joshua Tree National Park
Highlights	Panoramic mountain and desert views
Distance	3.0 miles round trip
Total Elevation Gain/Loss	1000'/1000'
Hiking Time	2 hours (round trip)
Optional Maps	USGS 7.5-min *Indian Cove, Key's View*
Best Times	September through May
Agency	JTNP
Difficulty	★★

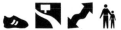

Elongated Ryan Mountain rises above the boulder-studded plains of Lost Horse and Queen Valleys in Joshua Tree National Park. The view from the top is arguably the best in the national park, encompassing the blocky summits of San Jacinto and San Gorgonio, the intricately dissected Wonderland of Rocks, and a succession of shimmering basins and skeletal mountain ranges stretching east toward the Colorado River and south toward Baja California. The popular trail from the mountain's base to its top is well worn, yet steep and rocky enough to be a potential hazard for young children (and others) prone to tripping or stumbling.

To Reach the Trailhead: From the national park's headquarters and main visitor center outside Twentynine Palms, drive 16 miles southwest on Utah Trail and Park Boulevard. Alternately, starting from the town of Joshua Tree, drive 17 miles southeast on Park Boulevard (a.k.a. Quail Springs Road). Your hike begins at the Ryan Mountain parking area, on Park Boulevard, 1 mile west of the entrance to Sheep Pass Group Camp.

Description: The trail takes you straightforwardly uphill along the north and west flanks of the mountain, amid scattered juniper and pinyon pine. Very soon, the geologic character of the rock underfoot changes. You cross the bound-

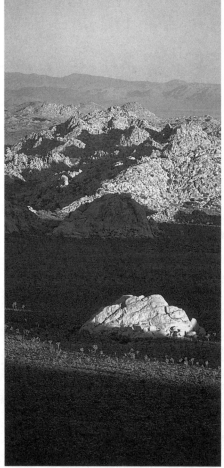

Lost Horse Valley and Wonderland of Rocks

ary between the White Tank monzogranite, the same rock you see exposed in
boulder piles in the valleys below, and the
Pinto gneiss, a much older rock into
which the monzogranite rock was in-
truded (many miles underground) some
130 million years ago. The Pinto gneiss,
which is foliated with layers of dark minerals, was metamorphosed (changed in
form by intense heat and pressure)
around 1.5 billion years ago, during an era
when life on Earth consisted of nothing
more than one-celled organisms.

If you can swing it, try a morning-twi-
light ascent of Ryan Mountain in the late
fall or early winter. As the sun rises, look
down and watch the interplay of light and
shadow across the Joshua-tree dotted
plains and on the monzogranite boulder
piles, which rise like battlements out of
the alluvium.

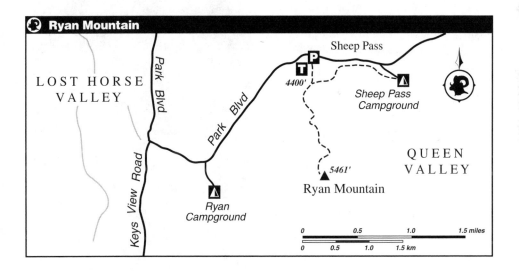

HIKE 44

Ladder Canyon

Location	Mecca Hills, north of the Salton Sea
Highlights	Slot canyon; fault-churned landscape
Distance	4.3 miles
Total Elevation Gain/Loss	750'/750'
Hiking Time	3 ½ hours
Optional Map	USGS 7.5-min *Mecca, Mortmar, Cottonwood Basin*
Best Times	October through April
Agency	BLM/PS
Difficulty	★★★

Ladder Canyon is the informal name given to a slot-like ravine incised into the sedimentary strata of the Mecca Hills on the eastern fringe of the Coachella Valley. Several ladders have been placed at strategic spots within the canyon, either to assist or to make feasible passages over abrupt "dry falls" (dropoffs) along the bottom. On rare occasions—mostly during summer thundershowers—these dropoffs come briefly alive with cascading, muddy water.

Ladder Canyon is a tributary of the superbly scenic Painted Canyon, which worms it way into the Mecca Hills Wilderness administered by the Bureau of Land Management. The famed San Andreas Fault Zone passes right through here, giving a glimpse of what hundreds of miles of horizontal displacement and tens of miles of stretching (over many millions of years) can do to a landscape consisting of little else but stark rock formations.

To Reach the Trailhead: The Mecca Hills lie about 120 miles east of Los Angeles and south of I-10. As you travel east from Palm Springs on I-10, note exits for Indio. Just beyond Indio, veer right onto Highway 86S, a new 4-lane expressway that takes you rapidly south, bypassing the towns of Coachella and Thermal. At a point 12 miles from the exit off I-10, turn left on Avenue 66 (State Highway 195)

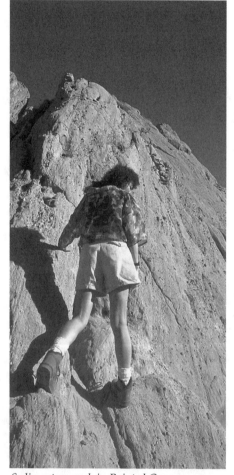

Sedimentary rock in Painted Canyon

and proceed east 1 mile toward the community of Mecca. Make a left turn just before you reach railroad tracks, and go right at the next intersection in order to cross those tracks. On the far side, turn right again, remaining on Highway 195. Go 0.2 mile through the town center of Mecca, and veer left staying on Highway 195. You are again traveling east on Avenue 66. Proceed 4 miles farther east through irrigated cropland, and cross over the Coachella Canal. (The road ahead, now called Box Canyon Road, continues through bone-dry desert hills toward I-10 and the southern border of Joshua Tree National Park.)

You drive only a short distance past the canal and look for the dirt road on the left signed PAINTED CANYON. The graded track ahead is normally suitable for most passenger cars, but road damage due to heavy rain could render it impassable for all but high-clearance, 4-wheel-drive vehicles. Continue 4.7 miles on the Painted Canyon road, entering the canyon itself in the last mile and a half. All around are fantastic formations of sandstone and shale (former sea bottom) that have been tilted upward at steep angles due to tensional forces along the San Andreas Fault. The road ends at a turnaround and parking area at a junction between two major canyons.

Description: On foot, start hiking into the narrow canyon with sheer sandstone walls on the right (northeast), which is upper Painted Canyon. During the cooler part of the year, low-angle sunlight partially illuminates the canyon bottom, spotlighting scattered smoke trees growing in the sandy wash, making them appear like gray puffs of smoke when seen from a distance.

At 0.4 mile, a slot-like ravine nearly blocked by fallen sandstone boulders (and possibly marked by a LADDER CANYON sign) can be seen along the canyon wall to the left. Some mild scrambling and clambering up several near-vertical lad-

ders allow you to gain elevation quickly. The original wooden ladders placed here are gradually being replaced by aluminum ones. Of course, all ladders will probably be swept away during the next major flood, probably years or decades away.

At 0.8 mile (from the start), there's a fork where the now-wider ravine divides into two nearly equal tributaries. Take the left fork for the easier route. (Using the right-fork tributary you would quickly climb to the west rim of Painted Canyon, and later rejoin the main route.) By 1.5 miles you reach the head of the left-fork ravine and find yourself just below and west of a rounded ridge (a large rock cairn lies on a knoll to the left). An informal trail

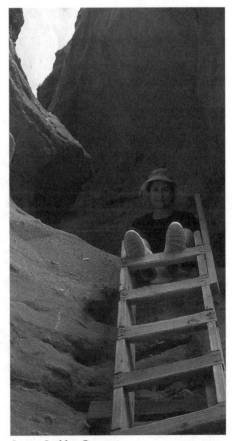

Lower Ladder Canyon

swings up that ridge and follows its course steadily uphill in the direction of some radio towers about 2 miles north.

In the direction opposite the radio towers, a gorgeous view of the Coachella Valley and Salton Sea unfolds as you climb. The below-sea-level Salton Sea is the largest inland body of water in California—blue and inviting from a distance, but not especially picturesque or sweet-smelling up close. The Sea has been the recipient of nearly a century's worth of irrigation runoff from the Coachella and Imperial valleys (and more recently waste water from the Mexicali region of northern Baja California), which has created a noxiously polluted body of water plagued by ever-increasing salinity levels. The vast, sunken landscape before you, flanked by mountains on both the east and west sides resulted from tensional forces that continue to pull apart the Pacific and North American tectonic plates in this part of California.

At 2.0 miles, in a saddle on the ridge, the trail turns abruptly right and darts down a rocky slope into the wide, sandy wash of upper Painted Canyon. Make a right and start to enjoy the entirely downhill remainder of the hike. Painted Canyon deepens as you descend, exposing a geological wonderland of primarily dark metamorphic rocks. At 2.7 miles a deep tributary canyon comes in from the left—offering a good side trip of a half-mile or more if you are curious and energetic. At 3.3 miles, a ladder facilitates easy passage over an otherwise frightening descent over a dry fall in the main canyon. The rest is easy going, on a wide bed of coarse sand past the Ladder Canyon turnoff and back to your car.

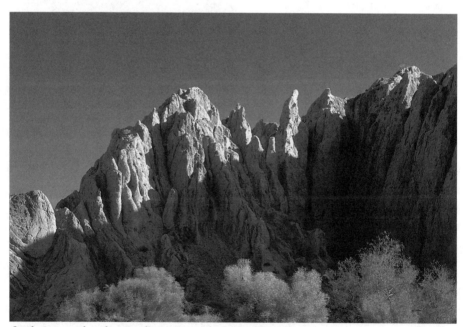

Smoke trees and upthrust sedimentary rock, Painted Canyon

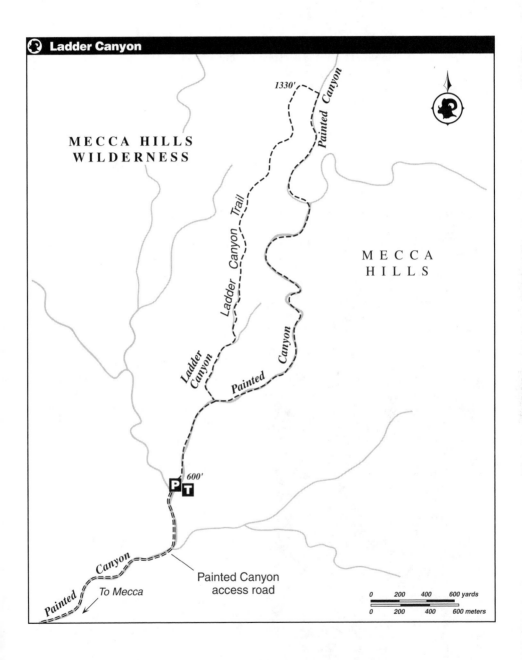

Ladder Canyon

1330'

Painted Canyon

MECCA HILLS
WILDERNESS

Ladder Canyon Trail

MECCA
HILLS

Ladder
Canyon

Painted Canyon

Painted

600'

P **T**

Painted Canyon
access road

Canyon

To Mecca

Painted

| 0 | 200 | 400 | 600 yards |
| 0 | 200 | 400 | 600 meters |

HIKE 45

Tahquitz Canyon

Location	Palm Springs
Highlights	Waterfall, spring wildflowers
Distance	2.0 miles
Total Elevation Gain/Loss	300'/300'
Hiking Time	2 hours
Optional Map	USGS 7.5-min *Palm Springs*
Best Times	November through April
Agency	ACBCI
Difficulty	★★

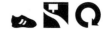

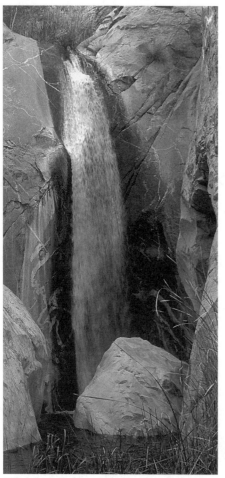

Tahquitz Falls

The Disneyesque guided hiking tour of lower Tahquitz Canyon, right on the edge of Palm Springs, is a far cry from the scene here in the 1970s and 80s, when scores—sometimes hundreds—of hippies and impromptu squatters occupied the canyon's idyllic glades. Flush with income from casinos and associated businesses, the canyon's owner, the Agua Caliente Band of Cahuilla Indians, turned the situation around during the 1990s. After a massive eviction and cleanup effort, the Indians opened a visitor center at the mouth of the canyon and started offering hiking tours up to as far as Tahquitz Falls. These guided hikes are the only way to visit the canyon today, and they are offered only during the cooler months of the year.

Although "tame" by most hikers' standards, the tour is an excellent introduction to the native riparian and desert flora of the low desert. A great deal effort has gone into eradicating nonnative invasive vegetation, which had degraded the biological quality of the canyon as much as grafitti and trash had earlier ruined the visual quality of the place. In March and April, after a wet winter rainy season, the canyon can be awash with wildflowers, and the 60-foot waterfall you visit at the midpoint of the tour thunders impressively.

To Reach the Trailhead: The Tahquitz Canyon visitor center, starting point for the hike, is located at the west end of Mesquite Avenue, off Palm Canyon Drive in the southwestern corner of Palm Springs, about two miles south of the commercial district of Palm Springs. The 2-hour hiking tours, offered between 8 A.M. and 3 P.M., depart on the hour (or less often depending on demand). The cost of admission to the visitor center, which includes a video presentation and the hike, is $12.50 for adults and $6 for children.

Description: The route of the guided tour may vary slightly, but generally covers a figure-8 route along both banks of the perennially flowing canyon stream. Expect to see, sniff, and learn about the Native American use of several varieties of native vegetation, including the distinctively aromatic creosote bush, yerba santa, and white sage. There's a prehistoric rock-art site along the way, with subtle painted designs and figures. You'll pass a small diversion gate and ditch where water in the canyon stream once flowed northeast toward the valley of Palm Springs. Tahquitz Falls, at the midpoint of the tour, features a shallow pool at its base. With the permission of your guide you many be able to take your

shoes off and wade some distance out toward the base of the falls. A hot tip: Store shoes well away from the stream; otherwise they may end up rafting quickly down the canyon.

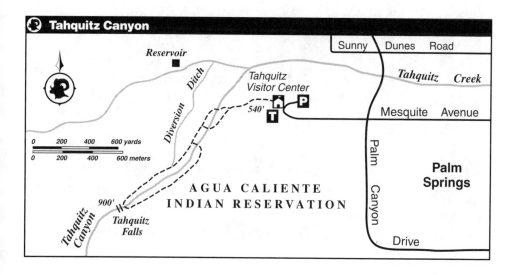

HIKE 46

San Jacinto Peak (The Easy Way)

Location	Above Palm Springs
Highlight	Broad view of Southern California from summit
Distance	11.0 miles round trip
Total Elevation Gain/Loss	2600'/2600'
Hiking Time	6 hours (round trip)
Optional Map	USGS 7.5-min *San Jacinto Peak*
Best Times	May through November
Agency	MSJSW
Difficulty	★★★

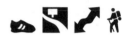

San Jacinto Peak is a close second after San Gorgonio Mountain on the roster of Southern California high points, but its more sharply defined and imposing bulk makes it instantly identifiable from almost anywhere. Upon witnessing the sunrise from the summit one morning, the famed naturalist John Muir exclaimed, "The view from San Jacinto is the most sublime spectacle to be found anywhere on this earth!"

Despite his propensity for superlatives, Muir may have been right. We may never know. Since his visit over a century ago, more than 20 million people have come to settle within a 150-mile radius around the mountain. Air pollution dims today's view, even on the clearest days. Still, hundred-mile visibility is not uncommon—out to the Channel Islands in the west, down to the northern sierras of Baja California to the south, and east into

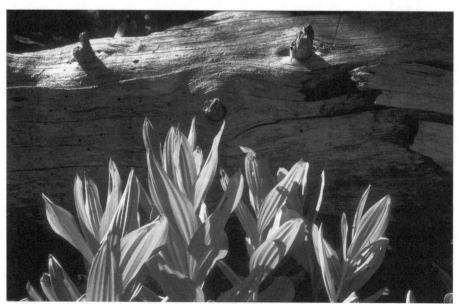

Skunk Cabbage near Round Valley

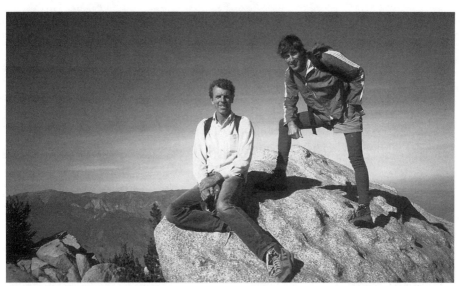

San Jacinto Peak summit, looking north

Arizona. San Gorgonio and the San Bernardino Mountains rear up in the north, 15 to 20 miles away, blocking vistas of the Mojave Desert.

The north face of San Jacinto, which at one point soars 9000 feet up in four horizontal miles, is one of the most imposing escarpments in the United States. Expert climbers have made the grueling ascent from the north in as little as 9 hours. Fortunately several easier, well-graded trails let you bag the summit from other directions with a lot less effort. Every summer, thousands of people take advantage of the easiest route of all, the 5.5-mile trail between the mountain station of the Palm Springs Aerial Tramway (8516 feet) and the top of San Jacinto (10,804 feet). Well-conditioned hikers accustomed to high altitudes will find this a moderate trip. Others, including those with modest or no goals, can still get plenty of pleasure out of shorter trips that don't stray very far from the mountain station. The slopes hereabouts feature some of the most inviting high-country forests and meadows south of the Sierra Nevada.

To prepare for you trip, call the Palm Springs Aerial Tramway, (760) 325-1391, or visit www.pstramway.com, for information and operating hours. The tramway closes for a few days in August for maintenance; otherwise, it normally operates 7 days a week year round.

To Reach the Trailhead: From eastbound I-10, take the Palm Springs exit (Highway 111), and drive 8.5 miles to Tramway Road, on the right. Drive 4 miles up Tramway Road to where it ends in the parking lot for the lower terminus (valley station) of the Palm Springs Aerial Tramway. Purchase a round-trip ticket, and ride the tramway to the mountain station, which includes visitor amenities such as restaurant and gift shop.

Description: A paved pathway leads 0.2 mile down from the mountain station to the San Jacinto State Wilderness ranger hut in Long Valley, where you must obtain a wilderness permit for travel beyond Long Valley. From the ranger hut, follow the wide trail leading steadily uphill for 2 miles to Round Valley—mostly through a coniferous forest of Jeffrey pine, sugar pine, and white fir. Backpacking campsites are located in the Round Valley area and at Tamarack Valley, ½ mile north of Round Valley via a side trail. Continue your ascent, somewhat steeper now, through thinning lodgepole pines to a trail junction at Wellman Divide, 3.2 miles from the start. This is where you get your first impressive view—south over tree-covered summits, foothills, and distant desert and coastal valleys.

After an almost obligatory (common, anyway) water or snack break at Wellman Divide, continue your leisurely uphill grind toward San Jacinto Peak. You traverse north for more than a mile across a boulder-strewn slope covered by scattered lodgepole pines and a carpet of low growing alpine shrubs. Abruptly, you change direction at a switchback corner, climb southwest for a while, and arrive (2 miles from Wellman Divide) in a saddle just south of the peak itself. Veer right, follow the path up along the right (east) side of the summit, pass a stone hut, then scramble from boulder to boulder for a couple of minutes to reach the top.

Hopefully the weather will allow you to rest a spell in the warm sun, cupped amid the jumbo-sized rocks, and savor the lightheaded sensation of being on top of the world. Make sure that you leave the summit of San Jacinto Peak in time to catch the last downhill tram ride.

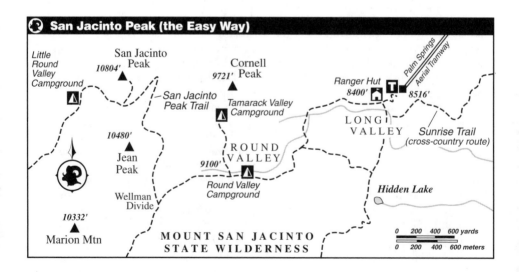

HIKE 47

San Jacinto Peak (The Hard Way)

Location	Palm Springs
Highlights	Greatest elevation gain of any dayhike in the Lower 48
Distance	20.0 miles
Total Elevation Gain/Loss	10,600'/2600'
Hiking Time	13 hours or more
Recommended Maps	USGS 7.5-min *Palm Springs, San Jacinto Peak*
Best Times	May through early June; October through early November
Agency	BLM/PS
Difficulty	★★★★★

This hike, known as the Cactus-to-Clouds Hike by Palm Springs hiking enthusiasts, is an absolute hoot—if you survive. For three decades now, ever-increasing numbers of adventurers have set foot in Palm Springs on a former Indian trail hacked into the east slope of Mt. San Jacinto. For some, the goal has been San Jacinto Peak, 14 trail-miles away and 10,400 feet higher. Other hikers have settled for Long Valley, where the mountain station of the Palm Springs Aerial Tramway sits—a "mere" 9 miles and 8000 feet higher.

You must prepare for this hike with plenty of vigorous physical conditioning. Fortunately there are many good routes on San Jacinto and in the nearby San Bernardino and San Gabriel mountains on which to practice. Conditioning hikes should include 5000 feet or more of elevation gain, plus exposure to elevations of 9000 feet or more.

Because the climate encountered on the full climb ranges from a low-desert type to an arctic-alpine type, you should try this hike only during the most moderate seasons—either late spring or early

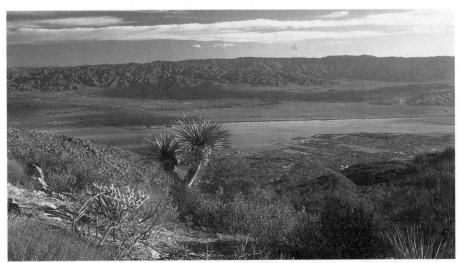

High-desert vegetation at the 5000-foot level

fall. If you go too early in the spring season, you might encounter treacherous patches of icy snow below Long Valley. In fall, you must wait till typical morning temperatures on the lower trail sink to less than lethally hot levels. The first snows usually arrive in November or December. For stable weather, it's hard to beat late October.

On a cool day during these moderate-season periods, you'll probably consume the better part of a gallon of water before your first dependable fill-up at Long Valley. In warm weather, you'll surely need a gallon or more. If you go all the way to San Jacinto Peak, remember that you must return to Long Valley and the tram station for a ride back down the mountain. The statistics quoted above in the capsulized summary include the round trip from Long Valley to the peak and back. When you arrive at the mountain station, you may need to purchase a one-way ticket for the tram ride down. Once you arrive at the bottom of the tram, you can call a taxi to get back to the starting point. Call the Palm Springs Aerial Tramway, (760) 325-1391, or visit www.pstramway.com, for information about the tramway and its operating schedule.

A predawn start on the trail is mandatory, preferably two hours before sunrise, to beat the worst of the heat and ensure enough daylight on your return.

To Reach the Trailhead: Ramon Road, a major east-west thoroughfare through the south side of Palm Springs, intersects that city's main north-south drag, Palm Canyon Drive, just south of the main business district. From that intersection, go 0.4 mile west on Ramon Road to where it dead-ends against the foot of Mt. San Jacinto. Parking space can be found on the nearby residential streets, but carefully note any signs regulating curbside parking.

Description: Follow a dirt road north from the end of Ramon Road, and almost immediately you'll see the Carl Lykken

Trail on the left. Climb about 1 mile and 1000 feet up this maintained riding and hiking trail to reach a rocky saddle. A rougher trail, originating at the Palm Springs Desert Museum, comes up from the east and joins the saddle as well. Another trail, also rough, takes off up the ridge to the west, past inscriptions that warn of the arduous ascent ahead.

That ridge-running trail is variously known as the Chino Canyon Trail, the Sunrise Trail, and the Outlaw Trail. Other than some improvements made by a labor gang in 1933, and light-duty maintenance by contemporary users, the trail remains sketchy in places, especially near the top. The name Outlaw Trail refers to the quasi-disapproval of its use by some rangers. Rescue attempts have been mounted in response to hikers getting into serious trouble, especially those attempting to hike the trail in the downhill direction. Do not hike the trail downhill from the top. You could lose your way and wander down the wrong ridge, and besides, a downhill ascent during the daytime means a temperature increase of as much as 60°F. Also, because the trail is so steep, the trail is at least as punishing on the leg muscles in the downhill direction as it is in the uphill direction.

Vistas of the Coachella Valley and the vast sweep of the Colorado Desert expand as you trudge uphill, step after step, curling up along one side of the sinuous ridge, then along the other. In a matter of a few hours, you will ascend through low-desert, high desert, and chaparral plant associations into a boreal zone of pines and firs.

At about 5 miles (from Ramon Road), the trail becomes more obscure and partly overgrown amid the manzanita chaparral. If you lose the trail, back up immediately and try to find it. You must stay on the route in order to negotiate the steep, rocky, brushy terrain ahead. At about 6.5 miles (elevation 5800 feet), the trail crosses a shallow ravine, veers left, traverses through some oaks just above the creek, crosses the ravine again, and then climbs out of the ravine toward a ridge. It wanders up this ridge, sparsely dotted with timber to about 7600 feet, where it veers right (northwest) and traverses several steep gullies on a deeply shaded (in the fall, at least) northeast-facing slope. The section ahead is very dangerous if covered by hard-packed snow or ice and you don't have an ice ax and crampons. As you near a sheer rock outcropping, the trail abruptly bends left (southwest) and climbs almost straight up a steep slope to the "lip" of terracelike Long Valley, elevation 8400 feet.

You've come 9 miles from Ramon Road and gained 8000 feet. If you choose to bail out at this point, simply head north through Long Valley a few hundred yards to the tramway station. Otherwise, pick up a wilderness permit at the Long Valley ranger hut below the tramway station.

From the ranger hut, follow the wide trail leading steadily uphill for 2 miles to Round Valley—mostly through a coniferous forest of Jeffrey pine, sugar pine, and white fir. Continue the somewhat steeper ascent beyond Round Valley through thinning lodgepole pines to a trail junc-tion at Wellman Divide, 3.2 miles from the start.

Beyond Wellman Divide, a more leisurely uphill grind takes you inexorably upward toward San Jacinto Peak. You traverse north for more than a mile across a boulder-strewn slope covered by scattered lodgepole pines and a carpet of low growing alpine shrubs. Abruptly, you change direction at a switchback corner, climb southwest for a while, and arrive (2 miles from Wellman Divide) in a saddle just south of the peak itself. Veer right, follow the path up along the right (east) side of the summit, pass a stone hut, then scramble from boulder to boulder for a couple of minutes to reach the top. The view is dizzying, not only because of the sheer height, but also because you have ascended into thin air to a level where about one-third of Earth's atmosphere lies below you.

Your journey is not over yet! Make sure that you leave the summit of San Jacinto Peak in time to catch the last downhill tram ride.

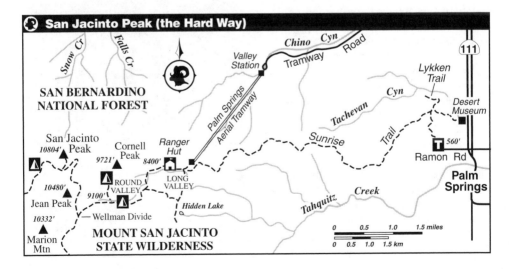

HIKE 48

San Jacinto Peak (The Middle Way)

Location	Idyllwild
Highlights	Broad vistas; Sierra Nevada-like atmosphere
Distance	15.4 miles
Total Elevation Gain/Loss	4400'/4400'
Hiking Time	9 hours
Optional Map	USGS 7.5-min *Idyllwild, San Jacinto Peak*
Best Times	April through November
Agency	SBNF/SJD
Difficulty	★★★★

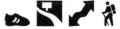

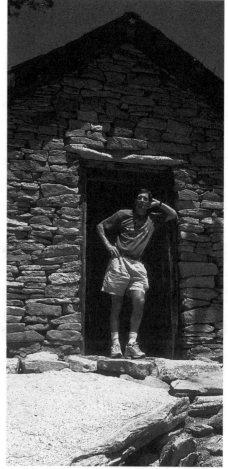

Stone hut below San Jacinto Peak

The San Jacinto Mountains, like many other units of the Peninsular Ranges (and much of the Sierra Nevada range to the north) have gradually sloping west slopes, and more steeply plunging east faces. Hike 47 in this book tackled the desert-facing east slope of San Jacinto range. This route meanders in a far more leisurely fashion up the forested west slope of the San Jacinto Mountains. The comparison to the Sierra Nevada is an apt one: The climb from the yellow-pine botanical zone in Idyllwild toward the arctic-alpine zone atop San Jacinto Peak is similar to many trips in the western Sierra Nevada that take hikers up through various forest belts to timberline.

This hike (midway in difficulty compared to the previous two in this book) to San Jacinto Peak, utilizes the popular Devil's Slide Trail out of the resort community of Idyllwild. To control excessive usage, the Forest Service has established quotas for this trail on summer weekends and holidays. Quotas or not, all users must obtain a wilderness permit (for either hiking or backpacking the route) at the Forest Service ranger station in the center of Idyllwild. The station is located on the east side of Highway 243, one block north of North Circle Drive. You will be driving past or very near this station on your way to the trailhead at Humber

Park. The phone number for the station is (909) 659-2117.

To Reach the Trailhead: Exit I-10 at Banning, and follow Highway 243 south for 25 miles to reach Idyllwild's town center, and North Circle Drive on the left (east). Drive ¾ mile northeast on North Circle Drive, veer right on South Circle Drive (crossing over Strawberry Creek), and take the first left—Fern Valley Road. Continue nearly 2 miles to the end of the road, where you will find parking space (perhaps not on weekends, unless it's early!) in the large lot at Humber Park.

Description: Two trails diverge from the upper part of the parking lot, the Ernie Maxwell Scenic Trail descending to the right (south), and the Devil's Slide Trail ascending to the left (east and north). You waste no time on that ascent as you switch back and forth along a zigzagging course, intermittently enjoying the shade cast by oak, pine, fir and cedar foliage. Two rock-climbing destinations are in view as you climb: Suicide Rock generally on the left or west, and the more imposing Lily Rock (or "Tahquitz") on the right. During spring and early summer, rivulets of ice-cold water flow down several of the small ravines you cross on your way up.

At the top of the ridge, Saddle Junction (2.5 miles), you can take a breather on a nearby rock or fallen log. Five trails converge in this flat space. Opportunities for wilderness camping are east of here in the Skunk Cabbage Meadow and Tahquitz Valley areas. These wilderness camping sites could be utilized as "base camp" for

a two- or three-day expedition to the peak and back.

For the next leg, follow the Pacific Crest Trail left (north) from Saddle Junction toward Wellman Divide. You ascend along a bouldered ridge, through statuesque Jeffrey pines and white firs, enjoying intermittent vistas east, south, and west. At a junction at 4.4 miles, the PCT swings left (west), contouring more or less across the south flank of Marion Mountain. Strawberry Cienaga, a permanently soggy area in the upper Strawberry Creek drainage, lies 1 mile down that trail—a possible side trip. Our way, however, continues north through scattered lodgepole pines and white firs, past a soggy, grassy spot called Wellman Cienaga, and reaches Wellman Divide (5.4 miles).

At Wellman Divide, the trail to the right descends to Round Valley and Long Valley, while our way stays left (north), climbing moderately but inexorably toward San Jacinto Peak. You traverse north for more than a mile across a boulder-strewn slope covered by scattered lodgepole pines and a carpet of low growing alpine shrubs. Abruptly, you change direction at a switchback corner, climb southwest for a while, and arrive (2 miles from Wellman Divide) in a saddle just south of the peak itself. Veer right, follow the path up along the right (east) side of the summit, pass a stone hut, then scramble from boulder to boulder for a couple of minutes to reach the top.

When it's time to go, retrace your route to the trailhead.

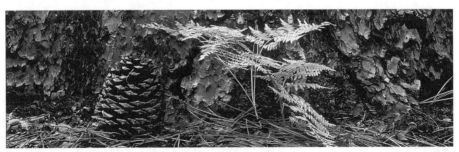

Bracken fern and pine near Saddle Junction

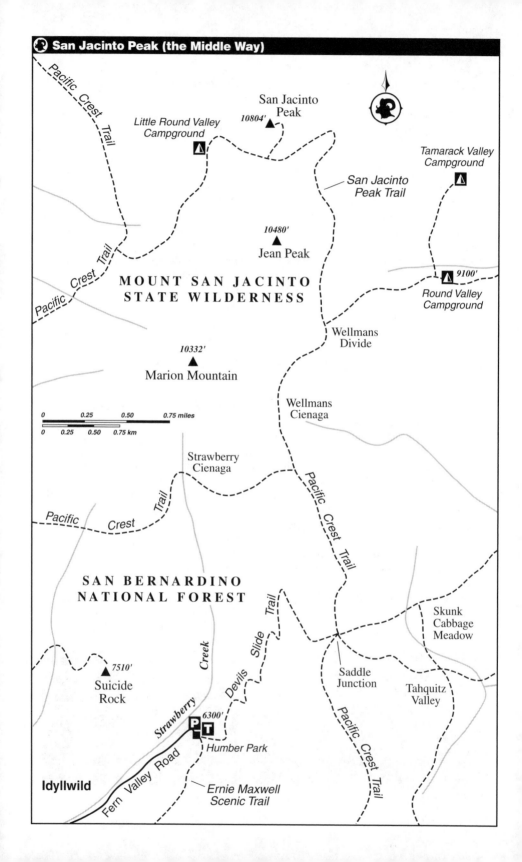

Pacific Crest Trail

San Jacinto Peak

Little Round Valley Campground

10804'

Tamarack Valley Campground

San Jacinto Peak Trail

Pacific Crest Trail

10480'
Jean Peak

MOUNT SAN JACINTO
STATE WILDERNESS

9100'
Round Valley Campground

Wellmans Divide

10332'
Marion Mountain

Wellmans Cienaga

0   0.25   0.50   0.75 miles
0   0.25   0.50   0.75 km

Strawberry Cienaga

Pacific   Crest   Trail

Pacific Crest Trail

SAN BERNARDINO
NATIONAL FOREST

Skunk Cabbage Meadow

Slide Trail

7510'
Suicide Rock

Devils Slide Trail

Creek

Saddle Junction

Tahquitz Valley

Strawberry

6300'

P T

Humber Park

Idyllwild

Fern Valley Road

Ernie Maxwell Scenic Trail

Pacific Crest Trail

HIKE 49

Tahquitz Peak

Location	Idyllwild
Highlight	Visiting a remote fire lookout
Distance	7.0 miles round trip
Total Elevation Gain/Loss	2000'/2000'
Hiking Time	4 hours (round trip)
Optional Map	USGS 7.5-min *Idyllwild*
Best Times	April through November
Agency	SBNF/SJD
Difficulty	★★★

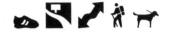

Tahquitz Peak celebrates a legendary demon who, in the oral tradition of the Cahuilla Indians, used to dine on maidens and create crackling bolts of lightning over the San Jacinto Mountains when displeased. At an elevation of 8828 feet, the forest lookout tower perched atop the peak commands a view westward over haze and smog to the crests of the Santa Ana and San Gabriel Mountains. On rare days of crystalline visibility, the coastline at Santa Monica and Malibu may be glimpsed, as well as the offshore islands of Santa Catalina and San Clemente.

A direct approach to Tahquitz Peak can be mounted by way of the South Ridge Trail out of the mountain hamlet of Idyllwild. First, you'll have to obtain a wilderness permit from the Forest Service station in Idyllwild's town center.

To Reach the Trailhead: Exit I-10 at Banning, and follow Highway 243 south for 25 miles to reach Idyllwild's town center on the left, where you will find the Forest Service station one block north of North Circle Drive. Continue south on Highway 243 for 1 mile and turn left on Saunders Meadow Road. Continue to Pine Street, turn left (north), go two blocks, turn right (east) on Tahquitz View Drive, and go right on South Ridge Road, Forest Road 5S11. If your car is sturdy enough, drive up this potholed road for 1.5 miles to the South Ridge trailhead.

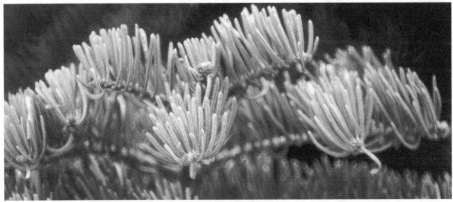

White-fir bough

Description: The no-nonsense South Ridge Trail ahead takes you steadily uphill along a viewful ridge, first through Jeffrey pine, live oak, and fir, then past thickets of low-growing chinquapin and stalwart lodgepole pines. Off to the left (north of the trail), you may see or hear some of the many rock climbers who gingerly make their way up the sheer face of Lily Rock (colloquially known as "Tahquitz"). Finally, after many switchbacks, you reach the fire lookout structure atop Tahquitz Peak, which may be staffed when you arrive. Visitors may or may not be invited to view the landscape from the tower itself. The summit view encompasses the timbered slopes of the southern San Jacinto Mountains and innumerable valleys and ridges spilling west and south toward Southern California's coast.

After taking in the view, descend from the lookout the way you came. The following longer, looping return is possible—perhaps a more suitable way to enjoy the mountain's charms on a two-day backpack: Head northeast, join the Pacific Crest Trail after 0.5 mile, and follow the PCT 1.3 miles north to Saddle Junction. (Nearby, to the east, are suitable wilderness campsites.) Descend Devil's Slide Trail 2.5 miles to Humber Park. There, you can arrange to be picked up. Or you can hoof it 2.6 miles down the gently descending Ernie Maxwell Scenic Trail to Tahquitz View Drive, not far away from the dirt road leading to your starting point.

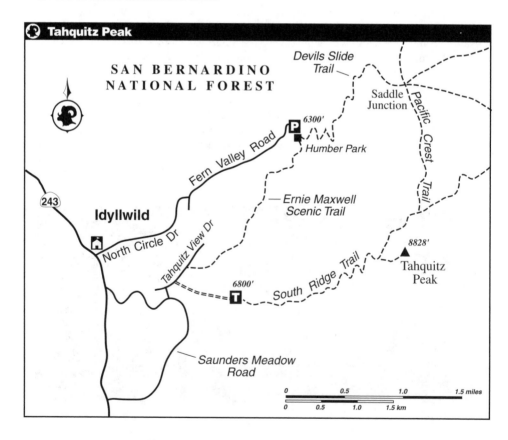

HIKE 50

Toro Peak

Location	Santa Rosa Mountains
Highlight	A forested sky-island overlooking the shimmering desert
Distance	3.0 miles round trip
Total Elevation Gain/Loss	800'/800'
Hiking Time	1 ½ hours (round trip)
Optional Map	USGS 7.5-min *Toro Peak*
Best Times	May through November
Agency	SBNF/SJD
Difficulty	★★

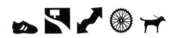

At 8716 feet Toro Peak crowns the Santa Rosa Mountains, an elongated complex of ridges running for some 35 miles between Palm Springs in Riverside County and Borrego Valley in San Diego County. Perhaps nowhere else in Southern California does the juxtaposition of mountain and desert seem so dramatic.

To Reach the Trailhead: Driving up the tortuous road toward Santa Rosa Mountain and Toro Peak is at least half the battle. From a point on Pines to Palms Highway (Highway 74) about 20 miles south of Palm Desert and 5 miles east of the Highway 371 junction above Anza, turn south on the Santa Rosa Mountain Road, Forest Road 7S02. For more than 12 miles you ascend on a progressively more rugged dirt roadway (best suited for 4-wheel-drive vehicles) to a locked gate below Toro Peak. Park so as not to block the gate. [NOTE: The entire length of the road from Highway 74 to Toro Peak can be used as a challenging mountain-bike

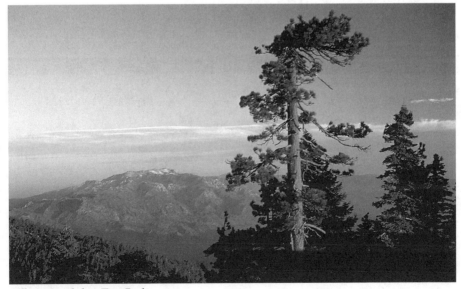

Jeffrey pines below Toro Peak

route, though the final stretch near the top is extremely steep for cyclists going either up or down.]

Description: Starting from the gate, follow the road ahead—a no-nonsense, heart-palpitating exercise, until you reach the peak This last segment of bulldozed road was cut into the mountain some four decades ago to service a microwave relay station that, unfortunately, sits squarely on the mountain's now blasted, flattened top. You can't complain about the view, though. From the summit, the timbered landscape quickly falls away—to barren slopes, then lower still to the flat Coachella Valley on the east, the saline wasteland of the Salton Sea to the southeast, and the shimmering peaks and valleys of the Anza-Borrego Desert to the south.

Considering the tedious drive in, you might as well make a two-day trip out of an outing to the Santa Rosas. Opportunities for car camping abound along the upper, forest-fringed parts of the road. Winter snows may clog the uppermost 5 miles of the road, down to about Santa Rosa Spring, until sometime in April. If they do, your trek to Toro Peak may be much longer, but rewarding nonetheless as the snow-covered road passes through

a gorgeous timberland of Jeffrey pine, sugar pine, and white fir. Within a day or two after a fresh dusting of snow, the gently graded Santa Rosa Mountain Road can be used as a superb cross-country ski route.

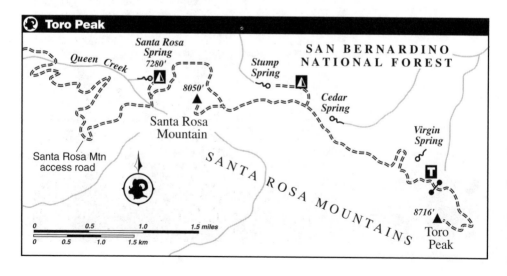

HIKE 51

Lone Tree Point on Catalina

Location	Santa Catalina Island
Highlights	Island and sea vistas
Distance	5.5 miles
Total Elevation Gain/Loss	1500'/1500'
Hiking Time	3 hours
Optional Map	USGS 7.5-min *Santa Catalina East*
Best Times	All year
Agency	CIC
Difficulty	★★

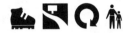

Santa Catalina Island, "twenty-six miles across the sea" as the song goes, stretches 21 miles in length and up to 8 miles at maximum width. The town of Avalon snuggles against a cove near the eastern end of the island, protected from prevailing winds that come out of the west and northwest. Avalon experiences the same almost-frost-free climate as the most even-tempered areas of the Southern California coastline, and enjoys possibly the cleanest air of any spot near the Southern California coast. In the hills above Avalon you can find wild mountainsides smothered in Catalina's own unique assemblage of chaparral, spectacular ocean views, and the some of the finest hiking in all of California.

Catalina was for most of this century owned by the Wrigley family (of chewing-gum and Chicago Cubs fame). In 1972 management of most of the island passed into the hands of the Catalina Island Conservancy, whose function is to preserve and protect the island's wild lands. Recreational use of the island today, including camping, hiking, backpacking, and mountain biking (on selected routes), is allowed on most of the island.

The languid pace of life on Catalina reflects its aloofness from the increasingly frantic business of living on the Southern

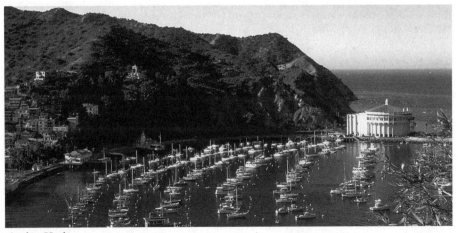

Avalon Harbor

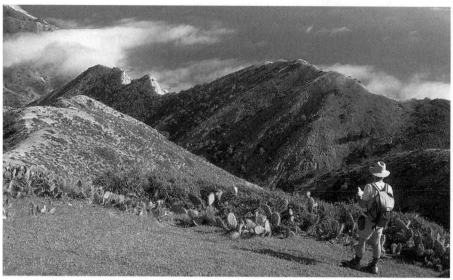

Palisades below Lone Tree Point

California mainland. An overnight visit here is truly relaxing, whether you choose to lodge in Avalon or prefer to rough it at one of the several campgrounds spread around the island's coast and interior.

To Reach the Trailhead: Ferries to Catalina depart terminals at San Pedro, Long Beach, and Newport Beach. Air service is also available from Long Beach. For more information about camping, lodging, hiking and biking on the island, and transportation to the island, the following two phone numbers are most useful: Catalina Island Conservancy, (310) 510-2595; and Santa Catalina Island Company, (310) 510-2800. You may also visit Catalina Island Conservancy's extensive website www.catalinaconservancy.org, for information and links to other websites.

The hike described here, excellent during the spring wildflower season and on crisp fall or winter days, begins at Hermit Gulch Campground near Avalon and loops over the top of the hills overlooking Avalon and the ocean. (You'll need a free permit for this, available at the Catalina Conservancy office at 125 Claressa Avenue in Avalon.) The highlight of the hike is a side trip over to Lone Tree

Point, which commands an unparalleled view of the clifflike Palisades falling sheer to the ocean. You'll encounter a couple of very steep grades on the old fire break leading to Lone Tree Point, so be sure to wear running shoes or boots with a studs or lugs to ensure plenty of traction. Small children will probably need some assistance on that stretch.

Buffalo, boar, deer, and goats—all introduced to the island at one time or another—may be seen on various parts of the island. Recent efforts to remove many of these non-indigenous and often destructive animals have been quite successful. Spotting great herds of goats on the island is a thing of the past.

Description: From Hermit Gulch Campground, start your hike by following the recently reworked Hermit Gulch Trail up the ravine to the west. Before long, you leave the trickling stream in the canyon bottom and begin a twisting ascent up along a shaggy slope. During the springtime, red monkeyflower, shooting star, lupine, and other native wildflowers dot the trailside and adorn small clearings amid the tangles of chaparral. After 1.5 miles and an elevation gain of 1200 feet, you meet Divide Road, the fire road along the eastern spine of the island.

Turn right, walk a few paces, and then climb the steep embankment to the left. Ahead you'll see an old fire break heading southwest, up and over several rounded, barren summits. Continue for 0.7 mile or more, passing over the peaklet designated "Lone Tree" on most maps. That's where you'll find the best view of the ocean and shoreline. Sometimes you can gaze south over shore-hugging fog and spy the low dome of San Clemente Island, some 40 miles across the glistening Pacific. During the best visibility you can trace the mainland coast down as far as San Diego, and also spy the long crest of the Peninsular Ranges—the chain of mountains running through Riverside and San Diego counties into Baja California.

After taking in the visual feast, backtrack to Divide Road. From there you loop back to the starting point via a longer but more gradually descending route. Head south down Divide Road for 0.8 mile, then veer left on Memorial Road. Easy walking down this crooked dirt road takes you along a cool, north-facing slope covered by tall and luxuriant (by mainland standards) growths of scrub oak, manzanita, and toyon. At the bottom of the hill you come upon Wrigley Memorial. Below that, you pass through the botanical gardens started by Wrigley's wife in the 1920s. Because of the virtually frost-free climate, an extensive array of California natives and exotics from distant corners of the world are able to thrive here. Once beyond the garden gates, it's but a couple hundred yards back to the campground.

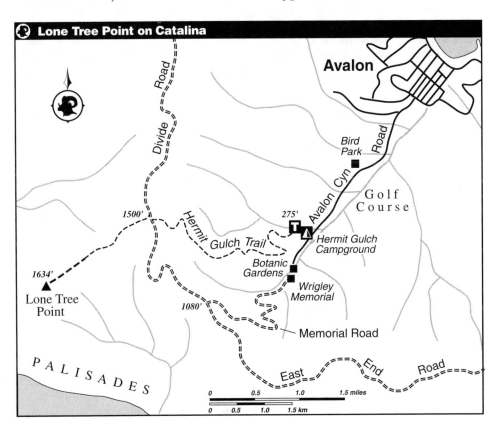

Lone Tree Point on Catalina

HIKE 52

Water Canyon

Location	Chino Hills
Highlight	Secluded woodsy canyon
Distance	4+ miles round trip
Total Elevation Gain/Loss	500'/500'
Hiking Time	2 hours (round trip)
Optional Map	USGS 7.5-min *Prado Dam*
Best Times	November through May
Agency	CHSP
Difficulty	★★

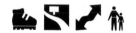

Little known even among local people, who number in the millions, Chino Hills State Park can at least lay claim to being California's most expensive state park. The state spent some $60 million to acquire more than 12,000 acres of rolling hills midway between the teeming L.A.-Orange County urban plain, and the rapidly urbanizing "Inland Empire" region surrounding Riverside and San Bernardino.

The park is dominated by rolling, grassy hills of a sensuous and classically Californian nature. Down in the moist, hidden hollows, the southern oak woodland plant community thrives. Some of the best remaining stands of California walnut, a tree whose native range is confined to the Los Angeles Basin and surrounding foothills, are found in the park's larger ravines. The park serves as a wildlife refuge as well, hosting mule deer, foxes, rabbits, coyotes, bobcats, badgers, and rattlesnakes. Several rare or endangered species of birds may visit the park, including the southern bald eagle, peregrine falcon, and least Bell's vireo.

If you're searching for the single most intriguing spot in the Chino Hills, you may find it in the upper reaches of Water Canyon. Concealed in the inky depths of this steep-walled ravine, massive sycamores and oaks reach skyward, casting a perennial chill. Except for the occasional buzz of a small aircraft and the rustle of leaves in the breeze overhead, the silence and stillness are absolute.

To Reach the Trailhead: Chino Hills State Park has a temporary main entrance that is as obscure as the park itself. From the Riverside Freeway (Highway 91) drive north on Highway 71 seven miles to the Soquel Canyon Parkway exit. From the Pomona Freeway (Highway 60) drive south on Highway 71 five miles south to the same exit. Head west on Soquel Canyon Parkway 1.0 mile to Elinvar Drive. Turn left, left again after 0.2 mile, and then immediately right on the gravel road signed CHINO HILLS STATE PARK. The road ahead is open during park hours, 8 A.M. to sunset. After 2 miles the road becomes paved and bends sharply right. There's an equestrian campground on the left, an equestrian staging area with lots of parking space on a knoll to the right, and a pay station by the road, where you can pay day-use or camping fees. More parking space can be found at the Rolling M Ranch (park office), a little farther ahead along the paved road

Description: From the equestrian campground, start heading south on the wide trail (dirt road) along the shallow valley known as Lower Aliso Canyon. About 0.5 mile from the campground, you dip to cross Aliso Canyon's small stream, which can be wet or dry. On the other side, you join another road at a T-intersection. Turn right, go about 100 yards, and go right again on the narrow trail going up Water Canyon. This is one of the few trails in the park reserved exclusively for hikers. Equestrian and bike traffic is prohibited.

Lining Water Canyon is a narrow finger of riparian willow and sycamore growth, flanked by grizzled oaks and well-proportioned walnut trees. After a short mile you pass a thicket of prickly pear cacti so dense it forms a trailside wall. The trail, which may or not have benefited from recent maintenance, may be partially hidden beyond this point by seasonal grasses, especially after a wet winter season. Intrepid hikers can continue another half mile up along the shady

canyon bottom and reach the darkest heart of the canyon, flanked by steep slopes on both sides. Watch out for poison oak, stinging nettles, and rattlesnakes. The pristine little patch of wilderness in upper Water Canyon is as close—and as far—from modern civilization as you will find anywhere around the L.A. metropolitan area.

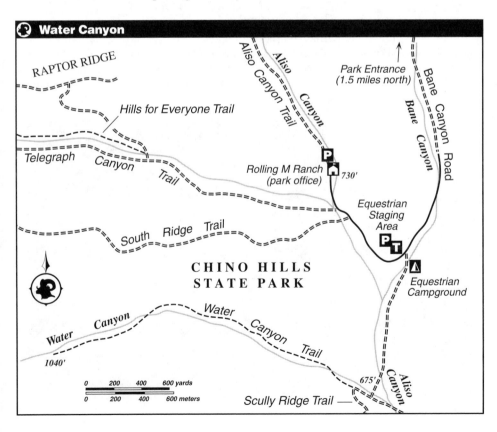

HIKE 53

Santiago Oaks Regional Park

Location	City of Orange
Highlights	Oak woodland and trickling stream
Distance	1 to 3 miles
Total Elevation Gain/Loss	100′ to 400′, depending on exact route
Hiking Time	½ to 1 ½ hours
Optional Map	USGS 7.5-min *Orange*
Best Times	All year
Agency	SORP
Difficulty	★

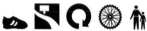

What Santiago Oaks Regional Park lacks in sheer size is more than adequately compensated for by its rare beauty. The core of the park is made up of two former ranch properties acquired in the mid-1970s. A small Valencia orange grove and many acres of ornamental trees planted around 1960 on these properties complement the natural riparian and oak-woodland communities along Santiago Creek.

To Reach the Trailhead: From the Costa Mesa Freeway (Highway 55) in the city of Orange, exit at Katella Avenue and proceed east. Katella becomes Villa Park Road and again changes its name to Santiago Canyon Road on the eastern outskirts of Orange. At 3 miles east of Highway 55, turn left on Windes Drive, which leads straight into Santiago Oaks Regional Park. As you approach the park entrance, subdivisions quickly fade from sight and a lush strip of riparian vegetation—willows and sycamores—comes into view on the left. Beyond the entrance

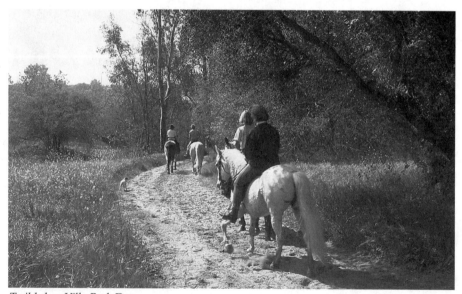

Trail below Villa Park Dam

(day-use fee collected here) and the parking lot, you can stroll up past some oak-shaded picnic sites to the superb nature center which is housed in a nicely refurbished 70-year-old ranch house.

Description: The park is laced with several miles of trail, the best of which stay close to the wooded bottomlands of Santiago Creek. You might begin with the self-guiding Windes Nature Trail and its extension—the Pacifica Loop—starting alongside the nature center. Though only about 0.7 mile long, the trail is very steep in places; it meanders up to the northern summit of Rattlesnake Ridge, an isolated, erosion-resistant block of mostly conglomerate rock. A slice of Pacific coastline can be glimpsed from the high point of the trail, and a fenced lookout point nearby offers a view almost straight down on Santiago Creek and the rest of the park.

Back down by the nature center, you can walk upstream along the shaded creek bank to reach a small rock-and-cement dam dating from 1892. This dam replaced an earlier one, built in 1879, that was part of one of Orange County's first irrigation systems. Today, the surviving dam is a historical curiosity, dwarfed by the large Villa Park flood-control dam a short distance upstream, and Santiago Reservoir farther upstream.

West of the nature center, you can ford Santiago Creek and stroll along several paths amid the eucalyptus, pepper, and other exotic trees rooted to the gently sloping bench on the creek's far side. Because of the diversity of its habitats, Santiago Oaks is a delightful birding spot, with species ranging from the tree-dwelling western bluebird and acorn woodpecker to the water-loving great

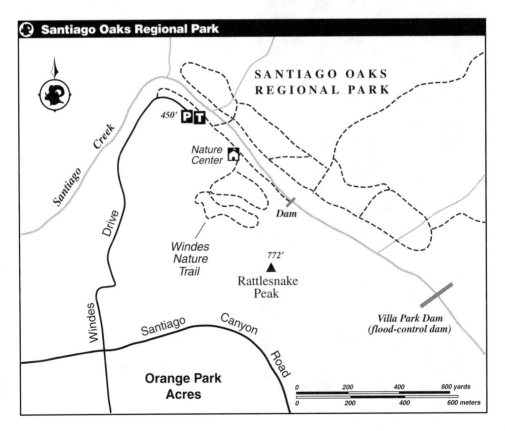

Santiago Oaks Regional Park

SANTIAGO OAKS
REGIONAL PARK

450' P T

Nature
Center

Santiago Creek

Drive

Dam

Windes
Nature
Trail

772'
▲
Rattlesnake
Peak

Windes

Santiago Canyon Road

Villa Park Dam
(flood-control dam)

**Orange Park
Acres**

0   200   400   600 yards
0   200   400   600 meters

blue heron. On occasion, vultures and ospreys, as well as some common hawks,
may be seen soaring overhead.

Longer-distance trails radiate outward
from Santiago Oaks Regional Park toward
Irvine Park to the southeast, and up the
slope east and northeast into Weir Canyon
Park. Massive suburban development is
taking place on and beyond these slopes,
but many hundreds of acres here are
being earmarked as future open-space
parkland as well.

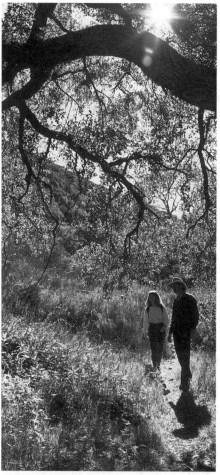

Oaks of Santiago Oaks

HIKE 54

El Moro Canyon

Location	Crystal Cove State Park
Highlights	Unspoiled coastal hills and canyon
Distance	6.8 miles round trip
Total Elevation Gain/Loss	900'/900'
Hiking Time	3 ½ hours (round trip)
Optional Map	USGS 7.5-min *Laguna Beach*
Best Times	All year
Agency	CCSP
Difficulty	★★

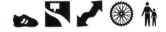

Crystal Cove State Park preserves one of the last large, undisturbed parcels of open space along the Orange County coast, near Laguna Beach. Besides containing a 3-mile stretch of bluffs and ocean front, the park reaches back into the San Joaquin Hills to encompass the entire watershed of El Moro Canyon—over 4 square miles of natural ravines, ridges, and marine terrace formations. In the backcountry (El Moro Canyon) section of the park alone, visitors can explore about 20 miles of dirt roads and paths open to hikers, equestrians, and mountain bicyclists. The entire section was swept by wildfire in October 1993, but several wet winter seasons since promoted a vigorous regrowth of sage-scrub, chaparral, and oak-woodland vegetation.

Upper El Moro Canyon is far and away the most beautiful attraction in the park's backcountry. You stroll past thickets of willow, toyon, elderberry, and sycamore, all brightly illuminated by the sun; then you suddenly plunge into cool, dark, cathedral-like recesses overhung by the massive limbs of live oaks. In one such recess, several shallow caves, adorned with ferns at their entrances, pock a sandstone outcrop next to the road. Before the establishment of the California missions, coast-dwelling Indians gathered acorns, seeds, and wild berries in this canyon.

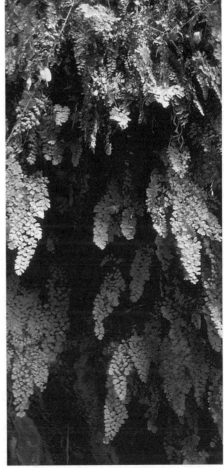

Fern grotto, El Moro Canyon

These foods, coupled with the abundant marine life nearby, provided a balanced and healthy diet.

To Reach the Trailhead: From a point on Pacific Coast Highway about 3 miles north of Laguna Beach and 4 miles south of Corona del Mar, turn east onto an access road leading toward Crystal Cove State Park's office and backcountry trailhead, open 8 A.M. to sunset. A fee is charged for parking in the large lot there.

Description: Take the trail leading from the parking-lot entrance southwest across a grassy flat and down into shallow El Moro Canyon. There you join a wide trail which goes up the canyon. Turn left and walk uphill on a mostly easy gradient. Other trails intersect left and right; you simply stay in the canyon bottom. At a point about 3 miles up the canyon, the canyon-bottom trail leaves the lushness of

the canyon floor and starts climbing very sharply to a ridge above. This is a good spot to turn around and head back the way you came—the easy way. Should you wish to extend your hike, you can loop north and return to your starting point using any of several ridge-running trails.

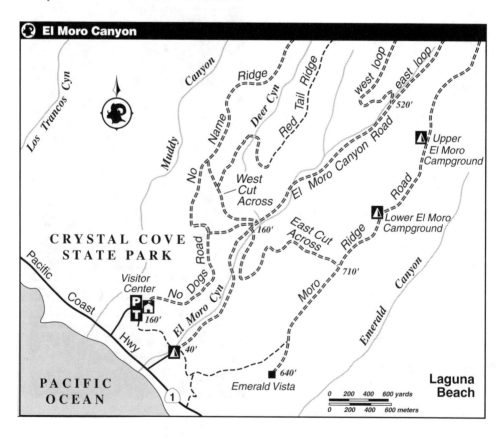

HIKE 55

Whiting Ranch

Location	Lake Forest/El Toro
Highlight	Orange County's "mini-Grand Canyon"
Distance	4.0 miles round trip
Total Elevation Gain/Loss	500'/500'
Hiking Time	2 hours (round trip)
Optional Map	USGS 7.5-min *El Toro*
Best Times	October through June
Agency	WRWP
Difficulty	★★

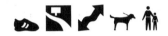

In 1991, Orange County opened to the public its newest large open-space preserve—Whiting Ranch Wilderness Park. Currently encompassing some 1500 acres along the rim of the communities of Lake Forest and El Toro, the park will grow dramatically in the next decade when thousands of acres of Irvine Company land to the north will pass into public ownership in exchange for that company's development rights elsewhere in the county.

Whiting Ranch's rounded hills look a bit nondescript when viewed from the suburbs below, but up close they conceal some pleasant surprises. You can prove this for yourself by trekking 4 miles (out and back) to Red Rock canyon, the site of a spectacular erosional feature—sandstone cliffs banded with layers of ancient

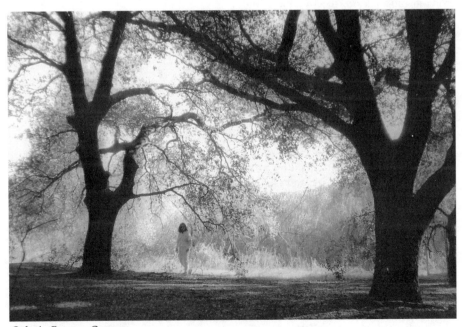

Oaks in Borrego Canyon

sand and mud. Late in the day, the sun's warm glow brings out a reddish tint in the rock.

To Reach the Trailhead: To reach the park's main entrance from I-5 in southern Orange County, take Lake Forest Drive east and north for 5 miles to Portola Parkway, turn left, and follow Portola northwest for another half mile. Look for a trailhead parking area on the right, just beyond a shopping center. The lot is open from 7 A.M. to sunset. If you are using the Foothill Transportation Corridor (Highway 241) toll road, exit at either Lake Forest Drive or Portola Parkway.

Description: Like most trails in the Whiting Ranch Wilderness Park, the wide path ahead is open to mountain biking and horse riding, as well as hiking. You immediately plunge into a densely shaded ravine called Borrego Canyon, following a trickling stream. For a while, suburbia rims the canyon on both sides, but soon enough it disappears without a trace. The trek up the canyon feels Tolkienesque as you pass under a crooked-limb canopy of live oaks and sycamores, and sniff the damp odor of the streamside willows. Often in the late fall and winter, frigid air sinks into these shady recesses overnight, and by early morning frost mantles everything below eye-level.

After no more than about 40 minutes of walking, you come to Mustard Road, a fire road that ascends both east and west to ridgetops offering long views of the ocean on clear days. Turn right on Mustard Road, pass a picnic site, and take the second trail to the left, into Red Rock canyon.

Out in the sunshine now, you follow the Red Rock Trail (for travelers on foot only) up the bottom of a sunny canyon that becomes increasingly narrow and steep. Presently, you reach the base of the eroded sandstone cliffs, formed of sediment deposited on a shallow sea bottom about 20 million years ago. This type of

rock, which contains the fossilized remains of shellfish and marine mammals, underlies much of Orange County. Rarely is it as well exposed as here.

A brochure and trail map for the entire park is available at the trailhead, and maps or directional signs can be found at several of the trail junctions. After visiting Red Rock canyon, you might decide to return via a more roundabout and lengthy route. If a half day's hike sounds about right, I'd suggest circling east on Mustard Road, then south on Whiting Road down to Serrano Canyon. The woodsy descent through Serrano Canyon takes you back to Portola Parkway, and from there you follow the sidewalk a mile back to your starting point.

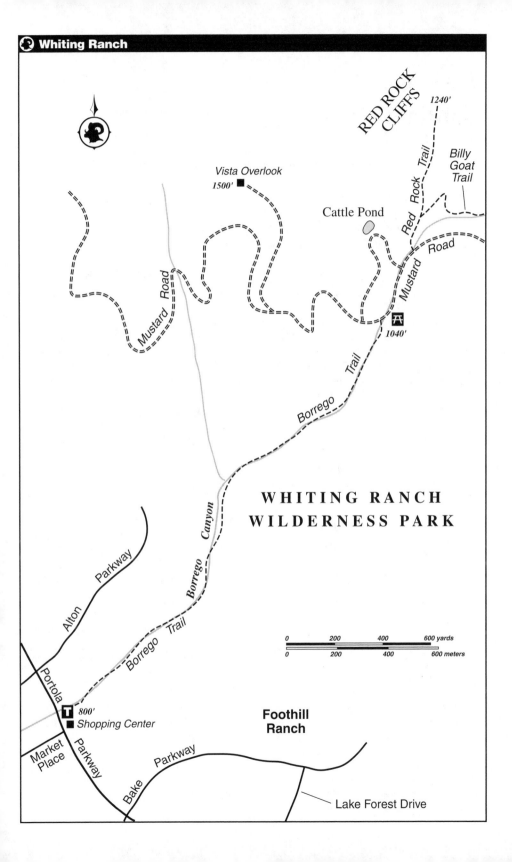

RED ROCK CLIFFS

1240'

Billy Goat Trail

Red Rock Trail

Vista Overlook
1500'

Cattle Pond

Mustard Road

Mustard Road

1040'

Borrego Trail

WHITING RANCH
WILDERNESS PARK

Borrego Canyon

Alton Parkway

Borrego Trail

| 0 | 200 | 400 | 600 yards |
| 0 | 200 | 400 | 600 meters |

Portola

Borrego Trail

800'
Shopping Center

Foothill Ranch

Market Place

Bake Parkway

Parkway

Lake Forest Drive

HIKE 56

Santiago Peak

Location	Santa Ana Mountains
Highlight	Best urban/mountain/ocean view in Southern California
Distance	15.0 miles round trip
Total Elevation Gain/Loss	3950'/3950'
Hiking Time	8 hours (round trip)
Optional Map	USGS 7.5-min *Santiago Peak*
Best Times	October through May
Agency	CNF/TD
Difficulty	★★★★

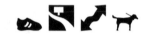

To the Indians, it was *Kalawpa* ("a wooded place"), the lofty resting place of the deity Chiningchinish. Early settlers and surveyors named it variously Mt. Downey, Trabuco Peak, Temescal Mountain, and Santiago Peak. Finally, mapmakers decided on the name that eventually stuck: Santiago. Today's 'dozer-scraped summit overrun with telecommunications antennae hardly pays just homage to the peak's historic and scenic values. Witness, for example, this record of its first documented ascent in 1853, by a group of lawmen pursuing horse thieves up a canyon from the east:

> After an infinite amount of scrambling, danger and hard labor, we stood on the very summit of the Temescal mountain, now by some called Santiago... where we beheld with pleasure a sublime view, more than worth the journey and ascent...

In 1861, while making a geologic survey of the Santa Anas, William Brewer and Josiah Whitney reached the same summit on their second try, using a northeast ridge. Their impressions echoed the sentiments of the earlier climbers: "The view more than repaid us for all we had endured."

The view so enthusiastically described by these early climbers is equally spectacular today—given, perhaps, a clearer-than-average winter day. Under good conditions, you can trace the coastline from Point Loma to Point Dume, spot both Santa Catalina Island and San Clemente Island, and scratch your head trying to identify the plethora of mountain ranges and lesser promontories filling the landscape inland.

Clockwise around the compass from northwest to southeast the major ranges on the horizon are the Santa Monica, San Gabriel, San Bernardino, Little San Bernardino, San Jacinto, Santa Rosa, Palomar, and Cuyamaca mountains. To the south you might see several of the lower ranges along the Mexican border and perhaps glimpse the flat-topped summit of Table Mountain, a few miles inland from the Baja California coast. In the west and northwest, smog permitting, the flat urban tapestry spreads outward, spiked by the glass skyscrapers of downtown Los Angeles.

Don't underestimate the time required to bag Santiago Peak by way of today's most scenic approach, Holy Jim Trail. In winter, you'll need an early start to ensure a daylight return. With summit temperatures roughly 20°F cooler than below, you should pack along some extra clothing. Plenty of water is a good idea too: Bear Spring, on the way to the summit, should not be considered a potable source.

To Reach the Trailhead: From the Foothill Transportation Corridor Toll Road (Highway 241) in Rancho Santa Margarita, exit at Santa Margarita Parkway. Drive 1.5 miles east and turn left on Plano Trabuco Road. Plano Trabuco Road becomes Trabuco Canyon Road 0.6 mile ahead at a sharp bend to the left. Curve downward into Trabuco Canyon, and at the bottom turn right on the unpaved Trabuco Canyon road, which leads east toward Cleveland National Forest lands.

Driving this unpaved road may be an adventure itself, not one to be undertaken by low-slung cars. Rocks and potholes are the rule. Proceed 4.7 miles east up the canyon, taking care not to blunder up someone's dirt driveway, to the Holy Jim trailhead on the left. You will need to display a National Forest Adventure Pass on your car.

Description: Proceed on foot (north) up along the east bank of Holy Jim Canyon's small stream, passing a number of cabins. More than a century ago this shady hollow was home to settlers who eked out a living by raising bees. One beekeeper—James T. Smith—became so famous for his cursing habit that he was variously nicknamed "Cussin' Jim," "Lyin' Smith," "Greasy Jim," and "Salvation Smith." Dignified government cartographers invented a new name, "Holy Jim."

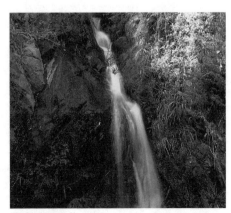

Holy Jim Falls

After passing a gate at 0.5 mile, you continue upstream another 0.7 mile, fording the stream seven times. Presently the trail switches back sharply to the left, while a lateral trail continues straight, going another 400 yards up along the stream to Holy Jim Falls. This little gem of a waterfall is worth the side trip if the stream is flowing decently.

Our way zigzags upward through dense chaparral on the west wall of Holy Jim Canyon. Well traveled but minimally cleared of encroaching vegetation, the trail offers intimate glimpses of the immediate surroundings flashing by at eyeball level. There's a sense of motion and accomplishment as you ascend this trail.

Soon a few antenna structures atop Santiago Peak come into view, tantalizingly close, but about 3000 feet higher. At 2.7 miles, the trail crosses the bed of Holy Jim Canyon at elevation 3480 feet, well above the falls. You may be tempted at this point to follow the line of scattered trees that struggle up toward the head of the canyon, or to try another short cut to the summit by way of the scree-covered slopes left or right; however, loose rock and thickets of thorny ceanothus would surely cost you more time, effort, and grief than you ever imagined.

So continue ahead on the trail, where soon you make a delicate traverse over a section prone to landsliding. After another mile on sunny, south-facing slopes, you contour around a ridge and suddenly enter a dark and shady recess filled with oaks, sycamores, bigleaf maples and bigcone Douglas-firs. By 4.5 miles, you come upon Main Divide Road, opposite Bear Spring.

From now on you simply follow the Main Divide Road (dirt road) uphill. Three more miles of steady climbing in sun and in shade bring you to Santiago's summit.

You must walk around the antenna installation on the summit to take in the complete panorama. Modjeska Peak, 1 mile northwest and about 200 feet lower, isn't high enough to block the view of any far-horizon features. Collectively, Santiago and Modjeska peaks form a familiar notch-like feature visible for miles around known as "Old Saddleback." The fine-grained rock of Old Saddleback is the prototype of the "Santiago Peak volcanics" exposed on many of the coastal mountain ranges extending south through San Diego County into Baja California. These metamorphosed volcanic-rock formations were originally part of a chain of volcanic islands that collided with our continent some 80 million years ago.

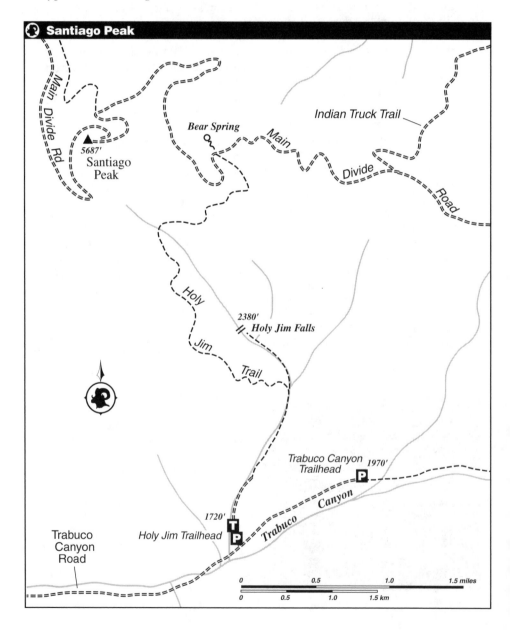

HIKE 57

Trabuco Canyon Loop

Location	Santa Ana Mountains
Highlights	Spring wildflowers, autumn color, views
Distance	10.0 miles
Total Elevation Gain/Loss	2700'/2700'
Hiking Time	5 ½ hours
Optional Maps	USGS 7.5-min *Santiago Peak, Alberhill*
Best Times	November through May
Agency	CNF/TD
Difficulty	★★★

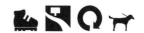

Wide-open views atop the Main Divide (Santa Ana Mountains), plus passages through pockets of dense chaparral and timber make this one of the more varied and interesting hikes in this book. Depending on the level of maintenance the trails receive, there may be passages over-grown by brush and poison oak. Wear long pants, or at least have them handy in your pack.

To Reach the Trailhead: From the Foothill Transportation Corridor Toll Road (Highway 241) in Rancho Santa Margarita, exit at Santa Margarita Parkway. Drive 1.5 miles east and turn left on Plano Trabuco Road. Plano Trabuco Road becomes Trabuco Canyon Road 0.6 mile ahead at a sharp bend to the left. Curve downward into Trabuco Canyon, and at the bottom turn right on the unpaved Trabuco Canyon road, which leads east toward Cleveland National Forest lands. To reach the trailhead, continue 5.7 miles—all the way up this poorly maintained dirt road, a job for autos with high clearance and sturdy shock absorbers. A National Forest Adventure Pass is required for parking at the road end, which is where the hike begins.

Description: A trace of the now-retired road continues up-canyon—for hikers, equestrians, and skilled mountain bikers only. You travel past Orange County's biggest alder grove; fine specimens of live oak, bay laurel, and maple; a tiny community of madrone trees; and a wide variety of spectacular spring wildflowers. In late March and April, look for colorful displays of bush lupine, matilija poppy, paintbrush, wild sweet pea, red and sticky

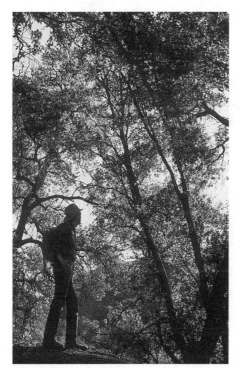

Upper Trabuco Canyon

(yellow) monkeyflowers, prickly phlox, Mariposa lily, wild hyacinth, and penstemon along the sunnier spots traversed by the trail. Historically, Trabuco Canyon is significant for its mining activity, and as the site of the killing of one of California's last wild grizzly bears in 1908.

After 1.0 mile the trail passes close to an old adit, one of several reminders of gold-and-silver-mining activity, which persisted until about 1925. Some scraggly big-cone Douglas-fir trees can be seen on a darkly vegetated slope to the south. Early miner Jake Yaeger built his cabin in the shade of a spreading maple down near the creek.

At 1.8 miles you come to a junction with the West Horsethief Trail branching to the left. Take it. Earlier, you may have spotted switchbacks carving up the treeless slope that now lies ahead. This improved section of the West Horsethief Trail replaces the original, straight-up-the-ridge route used by Indians in prehistoric times and by horse thieves in the Spanish days. After following a ravine bottom for a short while, the West Horsethief Trail begins it climb in earnest, zigzagging through dense chaparral. During the coolness of the morning, diligent effort will get you to the top of this tedious stretch fast enough; later in the day this could be a hot, energy-sapping climb.

After 1100 feet of elevation gain the trail straightens, begins to level out atop a ridge, and enters a vegetation zone dominated by manzanita and blue-flowering ceanothus. Cool "mountain" air washes over you, perhaps bearing the scent of the pines that lie ahead. Nearly coincident with the change of vegetation is a change in the rocks and soils underfoot. As you climb higher, light-colored granitic boulders and soil replace the dark-brown, crumbly metasedimentary rocks seen earlier. Although the younger granitic rock doesn't crop out below, you may remember having seen granitic boulders down in the bed of Trabuco Canyon. These resistant blocks, originally weathered out of the granitic mass above, were swept down during flash floods.

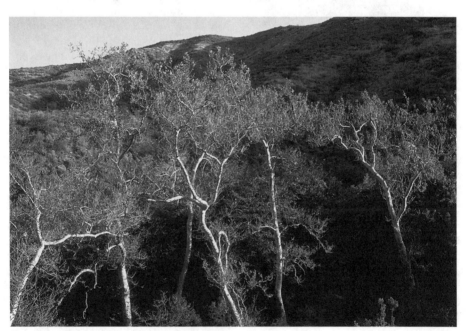

Sycamores in late winter, Trabuco Canyon

At 3.3 miles from the Trabuco Canyon roadhead, the West Horsethief Trail joins Main Divide Road (a truck trail) in a sparse grove of Coulter pines. Turn right and commence an easygoing, 2.5 mile passage along the "roof line" of Orange County. To the west lies Orange County's urban plain; to the east lies the more sparsely populated yet rapidly urbanizing Riverside County. The linear trough lying below you, north and east, was produced by movements along the Elsinore Fault.

At 5.8 miles, amid a patch of Coulter pines and incense-cedars, you come to Los Pinos Saddle. At the northwest corner of a large, cleared area in the saddle itself, find and follow the Trabuco Canyon Trail, which angles downward along the uppermost reaches of Trabuco Canyon's main fork. Thick stands of live oak and big-cone Douglas fir keep the upper part of the trail dark and gloomy during the fall and winter months, and delightfully cool at other times. Flowering currant and ceanothus shrubs at the trailside brighten things up in the spring.

One mile below the saddle, the trail veers left, crosses a divide, and begins descending along a tributary of Trabuco Canyon. You walk by thickets of California bay (bay laurel), which exude an enigmatically pleasant/pungent scent. After crossing the tributary ravine twice, the trail clings to a dry and sunny south-facing slope. Down below, in an almost inaccessible section of the ravine, you may hear water trickling and tumbling over boulders half-hidden under tangles of underbrush and trees. Before long, you arrive back at the junction of the Horsethief Trail in shady Trabuco Canyon, and continue down to the trailhead.

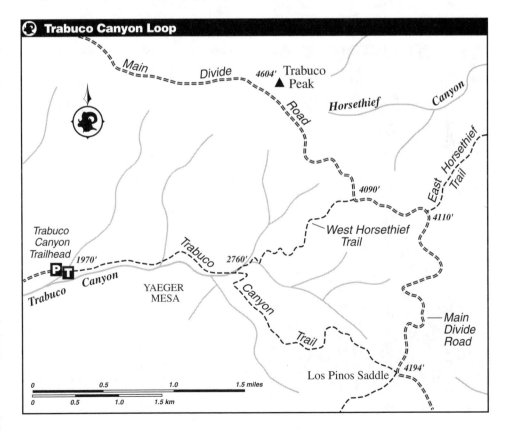

HIKE 58

Bell Canyon Loop

Location	Caspers Wilderness Park, Santa Ana Mountains foothills
Highlights	Interesting geologic features; wide variety of botanical features
Distance	3.3 miles
Total Elevation Gain/Loss	400'/400'
Hiking Time	1 ½ hours
Optional Map	USGS 7.5-min *Canada Gobernadora*
Best Times	October through May
Agency	CWP
Difficulty	★★

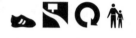

Caspers Wilderness Park is the crown jewel of Orange County's regional park system. It is the county's largest park (8000 acres), the least altered by human activities, and the most remote from population centers. ("Remote," of course, is a relative term in Orange County. The county is more than two-thirds urbanized).

To Reach the Trailhead: Caspers Park is easy to find. From I-5 at San Juan Capistrano, drive east on Ortega Highway (Highway 74) 7.6 miles to the park entrance station on the left. Pay the day-use (or camping) fee here and drive past (or visit) the park's visitor center, which houses a small museum and an open-air loft offering an expansive view of the Santa Ana Mountains. Continue 1 mile to the trailhead at the site of an old windmill, which will be your starting point for this looping hike.

Description: The hike touches upon the best features of Caspers Park, starting with a rather dizzying passage across the top of some curious white sandstone formations, rather like the breaks along the upper Missouri River or the barren cliffs of the South Dakota badlands. You'll loop up and over the main ridge defining the west edge of the park, enjoying views of much of Orange County's remaining rural and wild areas.

Start off on the path signed NATURE TRAIL. Follow it across the wide bed of Bell Canyon and into the dense oak woodland on the far side. After 0.3 mile, you'll spot a park bench beneath a gorgeous, spread-

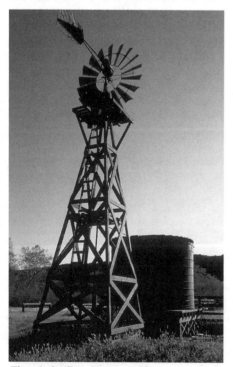

The windmill at Caspers Park

ing oak tree. A little farther on, veer left on the Dick Loskorn Trail. This path meanders up a shallow draw and soon climbs to a sandstone ridgeline that at one point narrows to near-knife-edge width. At one point you step within a foot of a modest but unnerving abyss. The sandstone is part of a marine sedimentary formation, called the Santiago Formation (roughly 45 million years old), which crops out along the coastal strip from here down to mid-San Diego County.

After climbing about 350 feet, you reach a dirt road—the West Ridge Trail. Turn right (north), skirting the fence line of Rancho Mission Viejo, a vast landholding that encompasses much of southern Orange County. Before World War II, it included all of Camp Pendleton as well. To the left you look down on Cañada Gobernadora ("Canyon of the Governor's Wife"—though a less literal meaning refers to the invasive chamise, or greasewood, that used to fill the canyon). The

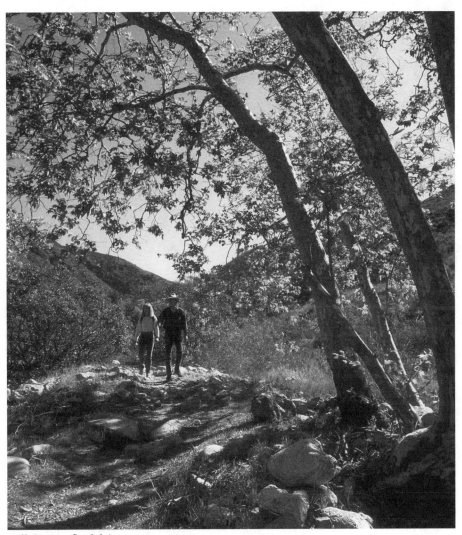

Bell Canyon floodplain

wide floor of Cañada Gobernadora is gradually being overtaken by luxury housing development.

After 0.7 mile on the West Ridge Trail, turn right on the trail named Star Rise. You descend back into Bell Canyon, which is lined with oaks and sycamores. Nearing the bottom, veer right on the Oak Trail. On this delightful trace of a trail you meander past California sycamores as well as ancient coast live oaks. In the late autumn, you crunch through the crispy leaf litter beneath the sycamores and watch golden sunbeams dance amid the thousands of fluttering leaves overhead. In early spring, when these leaves are emerging, the sunlight filtering through them bathes the ground shadows in a jungle-green luminance.

The Oak Trail will return you to the Nature Trail, and then your starting point.

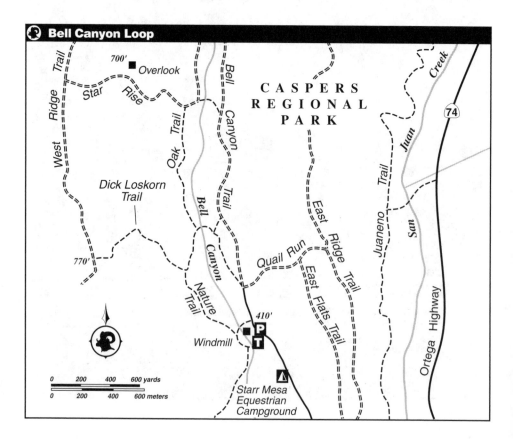

San Juan Loop Trail

Location	Santa Ana Mountains
Highlights	Trickling stream; small waterfall and pool
Distance	2.1 miles
Total Elevation Gain/Loss	350'/350'
Hiking Time	1 hour
Optional Map	USGS 7.5-min *Sitton Peak*
Best Times	November through June
Agency	CNF/TD
Difficulty	★

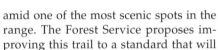

From San Juan Capistrano to Lake Elsinore, two-lane Ortega Highway stretches like a snake over the midriff of the Santa Ana Mountains, giving road warriors a taste of Orange County's wild, unfamiliar side. Even the most casual traveler can get to know the rugged and circumspect beauty of these corrugated mountains better by trying out the San Juan Loop Trail, right off the highway amid one of the most scenic spots in the range. The Forest Service proposes improving this trail to a standard that will make it suitable for wheelchairs.

To Reach the Trailhead: From I-5 in San Juan Capistrano drive 19.5 miles east on Ortega Highway (Highway 74) to reach the starting point, a well-marked trailhead parking lot on the left. (On the right is a humble but noted local land-

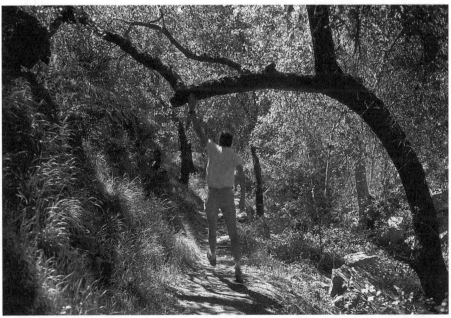

San Juan Loop Trail

mark—the Ortega Oaks Store, or "Candy Store.") You'll need to post a National Forest Adventure Pass on you car.

Description: From the trailhead lot, a well-worn path takes off north along a slope overlooking the highway. Around a bend to the left, the trail starts threading the side of a narrow gorge that re-sounds—after the rainy season begins in fall or winter—with echoes of falling water. A spur path leads down toward the lip of the falls; from there you can boul-der-hop over to the edge of a reflecting pool. A single gnarled juniper clings sen-tinel-like to a rock face overlooking this pool, very far from its normal, high-desert habitat 50 or more miles north or east. If the mood strikes you, rest your bones amid the smooth contours of the water-polished granite, and settle in for a mo-ment's quiet meditation.

Past the falls, you descend on ramp-like switchbacks through dense chaparral and presently reach the oak-dotted flood-plain of San Juan Creek. Stay left at the Chiquito Trail junction to remain on the loop trail. Ahead, you'll plunge into a ver-itable thicket of centuries-old coast live oak trees. The overarching limbs mute the glare of the sun and sky. In the soft, fil-tered light, the ground glows with the sea-sonal greens, browns, and reds of ferns, poison oak, and wild grass.

Touching briefly upon the perimeter of Upper San Juan Campground, the trail veers sharply left to gain an open slope, again parallel to the highway. Continue for another 0.5 mile across this sun-struck slope, dotted with wildflowers in the spring, and arrive back at the trailhead.

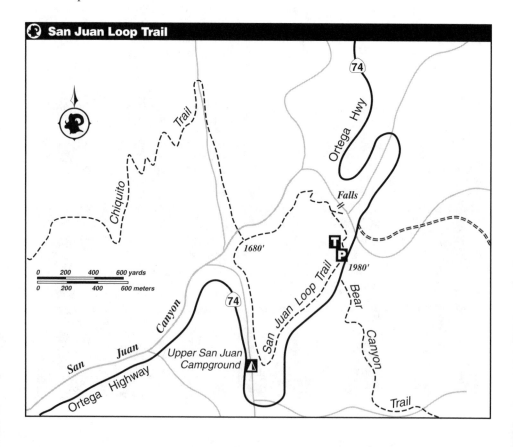

San Juan Loop Trail

HIKE 60

Sitton Peak

Location	Santa Ana Mountains
Highlights	Coast and mountain views
Distance	9.5 miles round trip
Total Elevation Gain/Loss	2150'/2150'
Hiking Time	5 ½ hours (round trip)
Recommended Map	USGS 7.5-min *Sitton Peak*
Best Times	October through May
Agency	CNF/TD
Difficulty	★★★

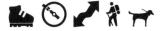

From below, Sitton Peak looks unimposing—a bump atop the rambling Santa Ana Mountains. On the summit, though, the feeling is decidedly "top of the world." When an east or north wind blows, cleansing the sky of water vapor and air pollution, fifty-mile vistas in every direction are not uncommon.

To Reach the Trailhead: From I-5 in San Juan Capistrano drive 19.5 miles east on Ortega Highway (Highway 74) to reach the starting point, a well-marked trailhead parking lot on the left. On the right is the Ortega Oaks Store, or "Candy Store." You'll need to post a National Forest Adventure Pass on you car.

Description: You begin this hike by taking the Bear Canyon Trail south from the Ortega Oaks Store. After 1.0 mile of moderate ascent, you come to a trail junction in a patch of oak woodland. Go right (the Morgan Trail forks left) and begin climbing more steeply along a chaparral-clothed slope. At about 2.0 miles, you reach a dirt road, the old Verdugo Truck Trail, which to the right is now part of our Bear Canyon Trail. You can either cross the old road and go straight on a newer footpath, or go right on the road (the old road is a bit more scenic). You are now well inside the boundary of the San Mateo Canyon Wilderness, part of Cleveland

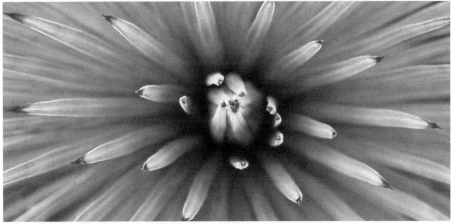

Lord's candle yucca below Sitton Peak

National Forest, where trailside camping is permitted (by permit only).

By following the old road south, you soon pass (at 2.7 miles) oak-shaded Pigeon Spring, a seasonal trickle of water at the head of Bear Canyon. An old watering trough is here, with seeps nearby. Enjoy the shade—you won't find much more of it on the road ahead.

Continue south another half-mile to reach a saddle called Four Corners (3.2 miles), where four old roads and the newer footpath join together. Swing right on the road that climbs northwest—a disused section of the Sitton Peak Road. After a steady ascent of about 300 vertical feet, you reach a flat area (4.0 miles) just below a boulder-studded ridge (3250 feet elevation) to the north. Easily climbed, the ridge summit offers a view somewhat similar to the one seen from Sitton Peak.

The flat area by the road (just inside the wilderness boundary) makes a good overnight campsite for those who backpack in.

Beyond the flat area the road descends another 0.5 mile to a saddle just below Sitton Peak. From this saddle, you leave the road and follow a steep, informal trail up through scattered manzanita and chamise on the east slope of the peak.

The view from the top is especially impressive to the west. Here the foothills and western canyons of the Santa Anas merge with the creeping suburbs of southern Orange County. Beyond lies the flat, blue ocean punctuated by the profile of Santa Catalina Island. Some 2000 feet below, toylike cars on the highway make their way down the sinuous course of San Juan Canyon.

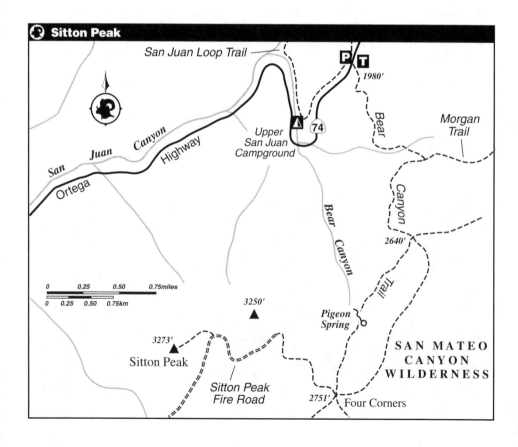

HIKE 61

Tenaja Falls

Location	San Mateo Canyon Wilderness
Highlight	Beautiful, multilevel waterfall
Distance	1.4 miles round trip
Total Elevation Gain/Loss	300'/300'
Hiking Time	1 hour (round trip)
Optional Map	USGS 7.5-min *Sitton Peak*
Best Times	December through June
Agency	CNF/TD
Difficulty	★

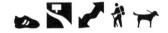

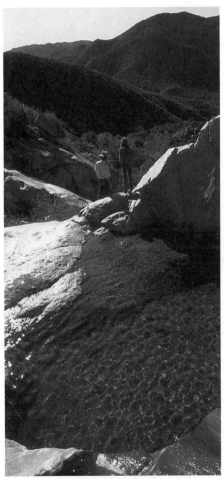

Upper pool, Tenaja Falls

With five tiers and a total drop of about 150 feet, Tenaja Falls is the most interesting natural feature in the San Mateo Canyon Wilderness section of Cleveland National Forest. In late winter and spring, water coursing down the polished rock produces a kind of soothing music not widely heard in this somewhat dry corner of the Santa Ana Mountains.

The only easy way to reach Tenaja Falls on foot is from the south, though the driving route to that trailhead is rather lengthy by way of any approach.

To Reach the Trailhead *(from I-5)*: From I-5 in San Juan Capistrano drive 23 miles east on Ortega Highway (Highway 74) to reach the paved Killen Trail (a.k.a. South Main Divide Road) on the right. Proceed south to Wildomar Campground and ORV area. Beyond, new asphalt has transformed many miles of bone-shaking former truck trail into a decently paved if narrow paved road. Continue a total of 16 miles (from Ortega Highway) to a large turnout on the right, overlooking the tree-covered bottom of San Mateo Canyon. This is the Tenaja Falls trailhead, and you will need a National Forest Adventure Pass to park there.

To Reach the Trailhead *(from I-15)*: Exit I-15 at Clinton Keith Road in Murrieta. Proceed 6 miles south on Clinton Keith Road and 1.7 miles west on Tenaja Road to a marked intersection, where you must turn right to stay on Tenaja Road. Continue west on Tenaja Road for another 4.2 miles, then go right on the one-lane, paved Cleveland Forest Road. Proceed another mile, passing the Tenaja trailhead and ranger station, and continue 4.6 miles farther along the newly paved Old Tenaja Road to reach the Tenaja Falls trailhead, a large turnout on the left, overlooking the tree-covered bottom of San Mateo Canyon. Don't forget to post a National Forest Adventure Pass on your parked car.

Description: On foot, from the Tenaja Falls trailhead, head down to the canyon bottom, veer left a little, and cross the creek on remnants of a old concrete ford. Balance on rocks or wade on through the water. Continue north on a steadily rising old roadbed—now a wilderness trail—and you'll soon be treated to a fairly distant view of the falls. After 0.7 mile the road passes near the upper lip of the falls, where a few large oaks provide welcome shade.

Further exploration of the falls requires rock-climbing skills and extreme caution. The flow of water has worn the granitic rock almost glassy smooth. While scouting the middle tiers and pools, I found that slightly wet bare feet provided much more traction than the soles of my running shoes. Don't be lured into dangerous situations though.

A somewhat safer way of approaching the lower falls is to scramble over the rough-textured rocks well away from the water. You might also backtrack down the road and then scramble down the slope into the brush-choked creekbed down near the base of the falls.

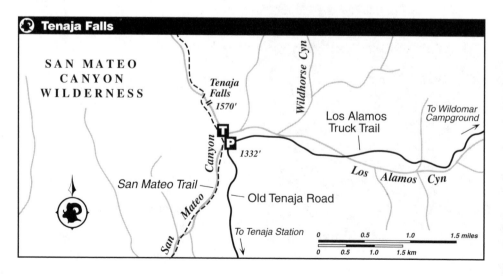

HIKE 62

Tenaja Canyon

Location	San Mateo Canyon Wilderness
Highlight	Riparian- and oak-woodland in a steep canyon
Distance	7.4 miles round trip (to Fishermans Camp)
Total Elevation Gain/Loss	1300'/1300'
Hiking Time	3 ½ hours (round trip)
Optional Map	USGS 7.5-min *Wildomar, Sitton Peak*
Best Times	November through May
Agency	CNF/TD
Difficulty	★★★

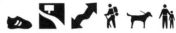

As the gloom of a late afternoon descended upon the deep-cut, linear furrow of Tenaja Canyon, dozens of orange-bellied newts waddled determinedly uphill and across the trail, oblivious to my footfalls. The cute faces and beady eyes of these little amphibians mirrored a mindless desire I cannot fathom: Sex in a bower of leaf litter and ferns? A bellyful of succulent tree-dwelling insects, ripe for the taking?

The Tenaja Trail rambles along a 10-mile stretch of the 62-square-mile San Mateo Canyon Wilderness, the largest parcel of designated wilderness near the Southern California coast. The Wilderness consists mostly of steep, rough and rocky chaparral country, yet it is softened by strips of oak woodland and riparian vegetation that thrive along the larger canyon bottoms. This hike explores the south end of the Tenaja Trail, which follows Tenaja Canyon down to its confluence with San Mateo Canyon. Unlike all other hikes in this book, the route takes you down and later all the way back up, so remember that if the day is warm or you feel fatigued, you can always reverse your course at any time.

To Reach the Trailhead: To reach the Tenaja trailhead, exit I-15 at Clinton Keith Road in the community of Murrieta. Proceed 6 miles south on Clinton Keith Road

and 1.7 miles west on Tenaja Road to a marked intersection, where you must turn right to stay on Tenaja Road. Continue west on Tenaja Road for another 4.2 miles, then go right on the one-lane, paved Cleveland Forest Road. Proceed another mile to the trailhead parking area, which is just north of the Tenaja ranger station. Don't forget your National Forest Adventure Pass.

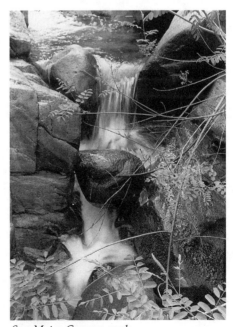

San Mateo Canyon creek

Description: An old-fashioned hand pump dispenses cold, sweet water at the trailhead. Sign in at the self-registration box, and head downhill on the trail going west. A few minutes' descent takes you to the shady bowels of V-shaped Tenaja Canyon, where huge coast live oaks and pale-barked sycamores frame a limpid, rock-dimpled stream. Mostly the trail ahead meanders alongside the stream, but for the canyon's middle stretch it carves its way across the chaparral-blanketed south wall, 200–400 feet above the canyon bottom.

After 3.7 miles of general descent, you reach Fishermans Camp, a former drive-in campground at one time accessible by many miles of bad road. Today the site, distinguished by its parklike setting amid a live-oak grove, serves as a fine wilderness campsite for an overnight backpack trip (a wilderness permit is required for this). The name of the place hints of the fishing opportunities afforded by nearby San Mateo Canyon creek during and after the rainy season. A native species of steelhead trout was recently discovered in this drainage, surprising experts who thought that steelhead might be extinct south of Los Angeles County.

At Fishermans Camp, three other trails diverge. Fishermans Camp Trail (the old road to the camp) travels east uphill to Old Tenaja Road. The San Mateo Trail, a narrow footpath, continues upstream to meet Old Tenaja Road and the continuation of the Tenaja Trail, and downstream many miles to the east boundary of Camp Pendleton. Your quickest return, however, is back the way you came.

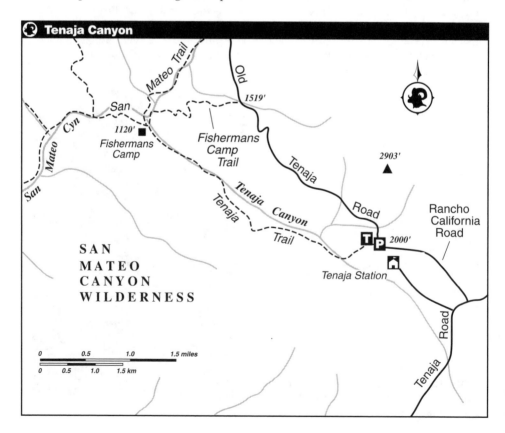

HIKE 63

Santa Rosa Plateau Ecological Reserve

Location	Near Temecula and Murrieta
Highlights	Green and golden hills, rare oaks, spring wildflowers, vernal pools
Distance	6.0 miles
Total Elevation Gain/Loss	650'/650'
Hiking Time	2 ½ hours
Optional Map	USGS 7.5-min *Wildomar*
Best Times	November through June
Agency	SRPER
Difficulty	★★

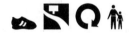

A circle, 100 miles in radius, centered on the Santa Rosa Plateau Ecological Reserve in the southwest corner of Riverside County, encompasses a megalopolis of some 20 million people. File this fact away in your mind, and then try to fathom its truth while walking amid the green and golden hills of this exquisitely beautiful reserve. Here is a classic California landscape of wind-rippled grasses, swaying poppies, statuesque oak trees, trickling streams, vernal pools, and a dazzling assortment of native plants (nearly 500 at last count) and animals. All who visit the reserve are struck by its timelessness and its insularity.

Starting with a nucleus of 3100 acres, purchased by The Nature Conservancy in 1984, the Santa Rosa Plateau reserve has expanded to enclose nearly 8300 acres—about 13 square miles—today. The west half of the reserve is laced with new hiking trails and well as old ranch roads, while much of the eastern part of the reserve lies off-limits to all visitation due to its ecologically sensitive nature. The 6-mile looping hike described here visits the major accessible highlights of the reserve,

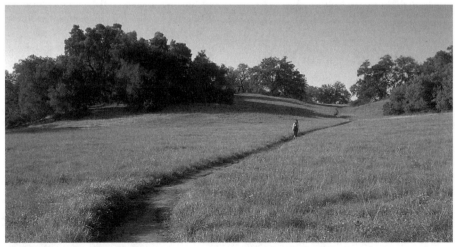

On the Trans-Preserve Trail

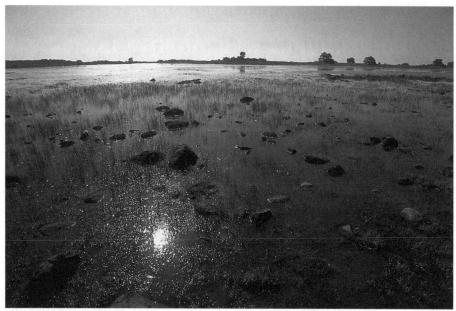

Vernal Pool, near maximum capacity

which are most beautifully presented in the green months of March and April.

To Reach the Trailhead: The reserve can be reached in less than 90 minutes from either central Los Angeles or San Diego. Take I-15 to the Clinton Keith exit in Murrieta. Drive south on Clinton Keith Road, passing the reserve's visitor center (open weekends) at 5 miles. Keep going, and note the sharp rightward bend at 6 miles where the road's name changes to Tenaja Road. At 0.7 mile past this sharp bend, park at the Hidden Valley Trailhead parking area (on either side of the road). There's a small day-use fee, payable here. Trails in the reserve are open from sunrise to sunset.

Description: From the Hidden Valley Trailhead, head southeast on the Coyote Trail. After 0.5 mile, turn right on the Trans Preserve Trail. Follow it for 1.5 miles over rolling and sometimes wooded terrain, passing through part of the reserve's 3000 acres of remnant native "bunchgrass prairie." Reserve managers have been implementing controlled burns to discour-

age the growth of nonnative grasses and encourage the recovery of native plants.

The last half mile of the Trans Preserve Trail rises to a plateau called Mesa de Colorado. At the top of the mesa, you turn left on the Vernal Pool Trail and soon visit one of the largest vernal pools in California (39 acres at maximum capacity). The hardpan surface underneath vernal pools is quite impervious to water, so once filled during winter storms the pools dry out mostly by evaporation. Unusual and sometimes unique species of flowering plants have evolved in and around this and other vernal pools throughout the state. When the watery perimeter of the pool contracts during the lengthening and warming days of spring, successive waves of annual wildflowers bloom along the drying margin. By July or August, all water is gone, and nothing remains but a desiccated depression.

Continue east on the Vernal Pool Trail, and descend from Mesa de Colorado to the two adobe buildings of the former Santa Rosa Ranch, 3.3 miles from the start.

Constructed around 1845, these are Riverside County's oldest standing structures.

After a look at the adobes and a refreshing pause in the shade, make a beeline north on the Lomas Trail. You'll jog briefly right on Monument Road, then go left to stay on the Lomas Trail. At the junction with Tenaja Truck Trail ahead, go straight across toward the looping Oak Tree Trail. The left (streamside) branch is better—assuming the creek is flowing. Both alternatives give you a close-up look at some of the finest Engelmann-oak woodland anywhere. The Engelmann oak tree, with its distinctive gray-green leaves, is endemic to a narrow strip of coastal foothills stretching from Southern California into northern Baja California. It's becoming one of the rarer of the state's oak species, primarily because its native range is squarely in the path of current and future suburban and rural development.

At the far end of the Oak Tree Trail loop, you come to the Trans Preserve Trail. Use it to reach the Coyote Trail, where a turn to the right and a retracing of earlier steps takes you a final half mile to your starting point.

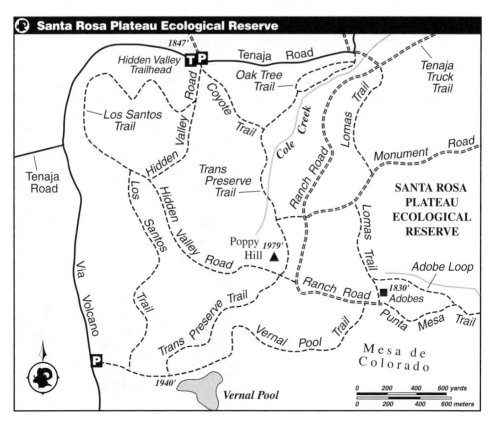

HIKE 64

Dripping Springs Trail

Location	Agua Tibia Wilderness
Highlights	Spring wildflowers; valley and mountain views
Distance	14.0 miles round trip (to head of Castro Canyon)
Total Elevation Gain/Loss	3100'/3100'
Hiking Time	8 hours (round trip)
Recomended Map	USGS 7.5-min *Vail Lake*
Best Times	November through May
Agency	CNF/PD
Difficulty	★★★★

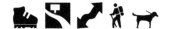

The 18,000-acre Agua Tibia Wilderness lies northwest of Palomar Mountain, straddling the San Diego-Riverside county line in Cleveland National Forest. Agua Tibia Mountain, one of the three distinct mountain blocks of the Palomar range, is the centerpiece of the wilderness that bears its name. Sparse groves of Coulter pine, bigcone Douglas-fir, incensecedar, live oak, and black oak cover the highest elevations, while the lower slopes are scrub-covered and fluted by many steep canyons holding intermittent streams. The wilderness was named after one of these streams, Agua Tibia ("tepid water") Creek.

The Dripping Springs Trail, which is the primary route into the wilderness area, originates at Dripping Springs Campground. With only minimal interruptions, the trail ascends from the 1620-foot elevation of the campground to a 4400-foot crest near the high point of Agua Tibia Mountain, passing through belts of chamise chaparral, manzanita and ribbonwood chaparral, and finally oak/pine forest. In March or April of an average or better rain year, the blooming of annual wildflowers along the lower trail can be stupendous. The trail's upper part offers ever-widening, pseudo-aerial views to the north, where the distant

Transverse Ranges rise out of valley mists as if they were the rim of the world.

The Vail Fire of 1989 burned nearly all of the area traversed by the Dripping Springs Trail to a crisp. In 2000 the Pechanga Fire swept across the uppermost part of the trail, singeing many of the

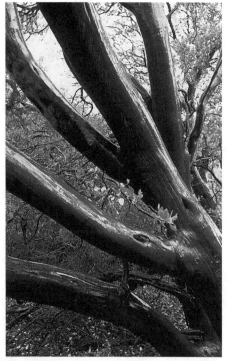

Manzanita in the rain

places the earlier fire had missed. After those fires, considerable efforts were devoted to clearing the Agua Tibia trails of new growth and fallen trees. Be aware that just one or two future years of heavy rain or inattention by trail crews could render the Dripping Springs Trail nearly impassable, or certainly make it uncomfortably scratchy for anyone not wearing long pants. That was the case during most of the 1990s when most of the trail mileage in Agua Tibia became severely overgrown. Another thing to remember: Water tends to disappear quickly into the porous, decomposed granite soil, and flowing water tends to dry up quickly in the ravines. Bring all the drinking water you'll need.

To Reach the Trailhead: From I-15 in Temecula, drive 10 miles east on Highway 79 to Dripping Springs Campground, on the right (south) side of the road. The campground lies just behind the Dripping Springs Fire Station. If the campground is closed, you can park outside the gate and walk 0.4 mile past the campsites to reach the "inner" trailhead, where you sign in at a register before entering the national-forest wilderness area that lies just ahead. You'll need a National Forest Adventure Pass for parking either inside or outside the campground.

Description: The trail mileages given below are keyed to the inner trailhead. From the campground, the Dripping Springs Trail immediately fords Arroyo Seco Creek, and then begins a switchbacking ascent through sage scrub and chaparral vegetation, liberally sprinkled with annual wildflowers in early spring. After only 0.1 mile, there's a trail junction. The Wild Horse Trail, on the left, gains elevation relatively slowly, sticking to the slopes overlooking Agua Tibia Creek. Your way stays right, up the Dripping Springs route that is sure to give you a good cardiovascular workout.

After a mile, the trail gains the top of a nearly flat ridge and then continues

south toward a series of 10 ascending switchbacks that cross an old firebreak (stay on the zigzagging trail and don't make short cuts). Vail Lake and Southern California's highest mountains—Old Baldy, San Gorgonio and San Jacinto—come into view. On a clear winter day, the snow-covered summits standing bold against the blue sky are a memorable sight.

At about 3.5 miles (3100 feet elevation), the Dripping Springs Trail crosses the head of a small creek and continues upward amid new growths of manzanita and ribbonwood. At about 4 miles (3300 feet) you'll pass what remains of the truly giant specimens of manzanita and ribbonwood that stood here until the 1989 fire. These century-old shrubs, up to 20 feet high, represented the equivalent of a "climax forest" consisting entirely of chaparral. The nearly complete loss of this mature patch of vegetation was unfortunate, but it must be remembered that without the effect of fire-suppression measures enacted over the past century, the natural cycle of growth and incineration by natural causes (every decade or two) would probably have never allowed so mature a stand of chaparral to develop in the first place.

The bleached skeletons of the giant shrubs sometimes fall across the trail along this stretch, blocking it until someone can clear the debris. Be aware also of roots stretching across the trail that might act like trip wires.

At about 4.5 miles, the trail descends a little and crosses an area of poor soil. A view opens up to the southeast and south. The white dome of the Hale Telescope at Palomar Observatory gleams on a ridge about 9 miles southeast. You can now see the pine- and oak-fringed summit ridge of Agua Tibia Mountain ahead.

Soon you follow sharp switchbacks again, with the scenery changing from low chaparral to scattered, singed oak and pine trees. At the trail's end, 6.8 miles, you join the Magee-Palomar Trail, an abandoned fire road along the Agua Tibia crest which is maintained today as a foot trail. Flat sites for trail camping exist in abundance in the area.

Much rambling could be done around here; at the very least, you should walk 0.2 mile south down the Magee-Palomar Trail

to a point overlooking Castro Canyon. There, on most clear winter days, a clear panorama of north San Diego County spreads before you, including a conspicuous, undulating, linear feature—I-15. On the far horizon to the west and south you can often see the Pacific Ocean and the mountains of Baja California.

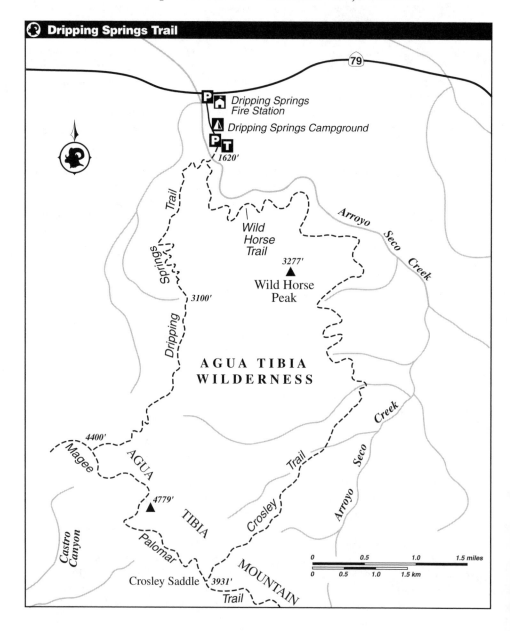

Dripping Springs Trail

HIKE 65

La Jolla Shores to Torrey Pines Beach

Location	La Jolla
Highlights	Remote beach backed by sheer cliffs; body surfing
Distance	5.0 miles
Total Elevation Gain/Loss	sea level
Hiking Time	2 ½ hours
Optional Maps	USGS 7.5-min *La Jolla, Del Mar*
Best Times	All year
Agency	TPSR
Difficulty	★★

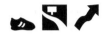

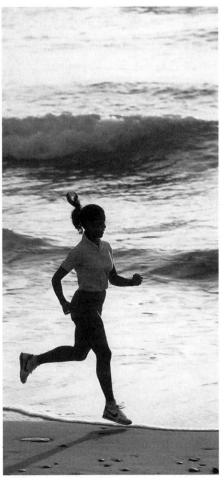

Jogging on Torrey Pines Beach

There are only a few places along the Southern California coastline where a person can hike for miles in a single direction and not catch sight of a highway, railroad tracks, powerlines, houses, or other signs of civilization. The Torrey Pines beaches are one such place. Here, for 3 or 4 miles, cliffs front the shoreline and cut off the sights and sounds of the world beyond.

Plan to do this beach walk at low tide. High tides—especially in winter—could force you to walk on cobbles at the base of the cliffs or oblige you to wade in the surf. Beach sand is often carried away by the scouring action of the winter waves, but is usually replenished by currents as summer approaches.

To Reach the Trailhead: As you approach La Jolla from the east on La Jolla Parkway (formerly Ardath Road), turn right on La Jolla Shores Drive. Drive 0.3 to 0.6 mile north and turn left on any street, all of which lead two or three blocks to La Jolla Shores Beach and the grassy park alongside it known as Kellogg Park. If you're making this a one-way trip, leave a second car along North Torrey Pines Road (the Old Coast Highway 101), next to Torrey Pines State Beach, or in the adjacent Torrey Pines State Reserve. It may be easiest to have someone drop you off at the start and later pick you up at the end. Another option is to use local buses to get from the finish back to the start: At Torrey Pines State Beach you can take a North County Transit bus south to UCSD, from where a transfer to a Route 34 San Diego city bus takes you to Kellogg Park.

Description: Start your hike at La Jolla Shores Beach by walking north under Scripps Pier and on past the rocky tidepool area. Once beyond the last of the cobbles and wave-rounded boulders, you can slip off your shoes and enjoy the feel of the fine, clean sand underfoot.

Beyond the tide pools, you may notice that some people have doffed more than just shoes. You're now on Torrey Pines City Beach, also known as Black's Beach, San Diego's unofficial nude-bathing spot. The city rescinded a "clothing optional" policy for this beach in the late '70s, but old traditions have never died.

About a half mile past the tidepools, you'll see a paved road (closed to car traffic) going up through a small canyon. This is a good, safe way to reach (or exit from) the beach. There's a limited amount of 2-hour parking at the top along La Jolla Farms Road.

A bit farther ahead, where most Black's Beach users congregate, two precipitous trails ascend about 300 feet to the Glider Port, where hang-gliders launch their craft. Look up to see antlike beachgoers lugging their gear up or down the zigzagging paths, and hang-gliders soaring overhead. The southern of the two trails, improved and widened, is the safer one. There's plenty of free, all-day parking at the top if you want to start or end your beach walk there.

Lifeguards patrol some areas of Black's Beach during busy periods, so you can feel fairly safe about jumping into the water, which may reach a temperature warmer than 70°F in July through September. Elsewhere you swim at your own risk—watch out for rip currents.

At about 4 miles from Kellogg Park, you reach Flat Rock, where a protruding sandstone wall blocks easy passage. Follow the narrow path cut into the wall. From a low shelf on the far side, the Beach Trail begins its ascent to Torrey Pines State Reserve's visitor center.

In the fifth and last mile, the narrow beach is squeezed between sculpted sedimentary cliffs on one side and crashing surf on the other. These are the tallest cliffs in western San Diego County. A close look at the faces reveals a slice of geologic history: the greenish siltstone on the bottom, called the Del Mar Formation, is older than the buff or rust-colored Torrey Sandstone above it. Higher still is a thin cap of reddish sandstone, not easily seen from the beach—the Linda Vista Formation.

In the end, the beach widens, the cliffs fall back, and you arrive at Torrey Pines State Reserve's entrance along North Torrey Pines Road.

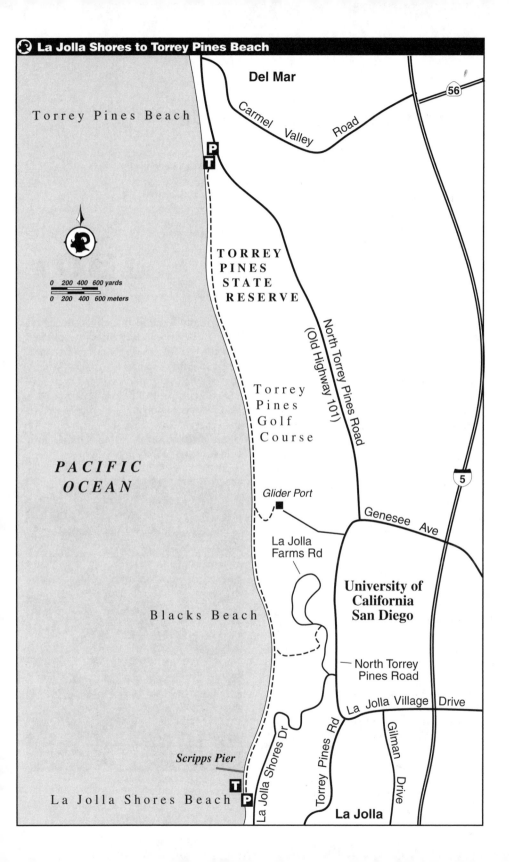

Del Mar

56

Torrey Pines Beach

P
T

Carmel Valley Road

TORREY PINES STATE RESERVE

North Torrey Pines Road
(Old Highway 101)

Torrey Pines Golf Course

0   200 400 600 yards
0   200 400 600 meters

PACIFIC OCEAN

Glider Port

Genesee Ave

5

La Jolla Farms Rd

University of California San Diego

Blacks Beach

North Torrey Pines Road

La Jolla Village Drive

La Jolla Shores Dr

Torrey Pines Rd

Gilman Drive

Scripps Pier

T
P

La Jolla Shores Beach

La Jolla

HIKE 66

Torrey Pines State Reserve

Location	Del Mar
Highlights	Rare vegetation, wildflowers, ocean views
Distance	short loops; up to 4 miles total distance
Total Elevation Gain/Loss	up to 600'
Hiking Time	up to 2 hours
Optional Map	USGS 7.5-min *Del Mar*
Best Times	All year
Agency	TPSR
Difficulty	★ to ★★

The rare and beautiful Torrey pines atop the coastal bluffs south of Del Mar are as much a symbol of the Golden State as are the famed Monterey cypress trees native to central California's coast. Torrey pines grow naturally in only two places on Earth: in and around Torrey Pines State Reserve and on Santa Rosa Island, off Santa Barbara. Of the estimated 10,000 native Torrey pines now living, about one-third grow within the reserve. A combination of drought and bark-beetle infestation killed about 15 percent of the reserve's Torrey pines during the late 1980s, but new seedlings planted in their place are thriving today.

Torrey Pines State Reserve would be botanically remarkable even without its pines. Three major plant communities can be found on the reserve's 1750 acres: the sage-scrub, chaparral, and salt-marsh plant communities. More than 330 plant species have been identified within the reserve so far. That number is approximately 20 percent of all the known plants native to San Diego County. This is especially noteworthy because San Diego County is widely regarded as being the most geographically and botanically diverse county in the continental United States.

If you're interested in identifying plants and wildflowers typical of coastal and inland Southern California, come here in the spring. Excellent interpretive facilities at the reserve's museum make plant identification an easy task. Besides the exhibits, you can browse through several notebooks full of captioned photographs of common and rare plants within the reserve. You can also visit the native plant gardens surrounding the museum building and at the Parry Grove trailhead.

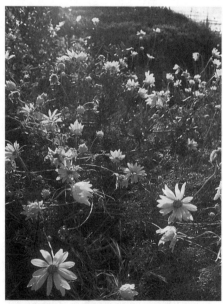

Sea Dahlia in bloom, Torrey Pines State Reserve

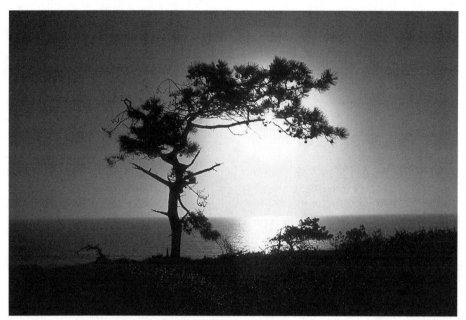

Wind-battered Torrey pine near Razor Point

A network of trails over the eroded bluffs will take you nearly everywhere in the reserve, except into most canyon bottoms. It's important that you stick to these trails and eschew shortcuts and cross-country travel. The thin soils are easily eroded without the protection of healthy vegetation. As you'll plainly see, there are already enough instances of erosion here, due to both natural and human causes.

To Reach the Trailhead: Exit I-5 at Carmel Valley Road, and drive west 1.5 mile to the Old Coast Highway 101 (which is named Camino del Mar to the north, and North Torrey Pines Road to the south). Turn left, drive 1 mile to the Torrey Pines State Reserve entrance on the right, pay the day-use fee for the reserve. Past the entrance a paved road goes up to a parking lot adjacent to the reserve office and museum. From there, you can walk to the beginning of any of the trails in 10 minutes or less. If that lot is full, you may be able to park in turnouts along the entrance road, in the beach parking lot at the reserve entrance, or along the shoul-

der of North Torrey Pines Road. The reserve has a finite carrying capacity. Access may be restricted on busy weekends, so get there early if you can.

Description: After a stop at the museum for a bit of educational browsing, you might first explore nearby High Point, where your gaze encompasses a steep, off-limits section of the reserve known as East Grove. There, young Torrey pines are establishing a foothold on the bluffs and canyons in the aftermath of past wildfires.

Next, you might head south on the concrete roadbed of the "old" old coast highway (closed to car traffic) and pick up the Broken Hill Trail. The two east branches of this trail wind through thick chamise chaparral and connect with a spur trail leading to Broken Hill Overlook. You'll be able to step out (very carefully) onto a precipitous fin of sandstone and peer over to see what, except for a few Torrey pine trees here and there, looks like desert badlands. A third (west) branch of the Broken Hill Trail winds down a slope festooned with wildflowers and joins the Beach Trail at a point just above where the latter drops sharply to the beach.

The popular Beach Trail originates at the parking lot near the museum and intersects with trails to Yucca Point and Razor Point. Fenced viewpoints along both of these trails offer views straight down to the sandy beach and surf.

The Parry Grove and Guy Fleming loop trails wind among Torrey pine groves hit hard by the late '80s drought. The Guy Fleming Trail is mostly flat, while the Parry Grove Trail starts with a steep descent on stair steps. In spring, the sunny slopes along the Guy Fleming Trail come alive with phantasmagoric wildflower displays. Fluttering in the sea breeze, the flowers put on quite a show as several vivid shades of color dynami-

cally intermix with the more muted tones of earth, sea, and sky.

The Torrey Pines trails can be enjoyed the year round, but they're open only during daylight hours. Ranger-led walks are featured on weekends. You can't picnic in the reserve, but after you do your hiking, you can use the tables or the beach down near the entrance. Bring along binoculars: the soaring ravens and the red-tailed and sparrow hawks are interesting to watch, as are the hang-gliding humans you'll sometimes see.

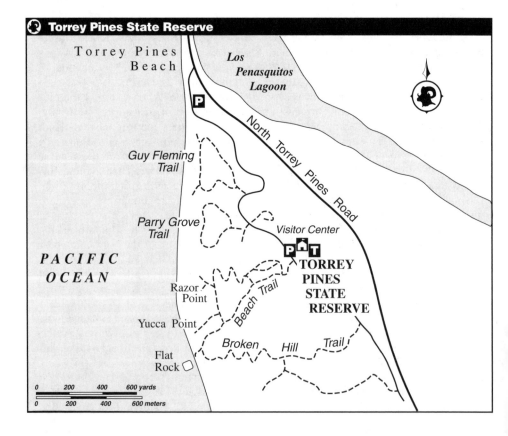

HIKE 67

Los Penasquitos Canyon

Location	Northern San Diego
Highlights	Oak-shaded coastal canyon; waterfall
Distance	6.2 miles round trip
Total Elevation Gain/Loss	300'/300'
Hiking Time	3 hours (round trip)
Optional Map	USGS 7.5-min *Del Mar*
Best Times	All year
Agency	LPCP
Difficulty	★★

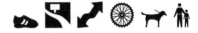

Crickets sing, cicadas buzz, and bullfrogs groan. A sparrow hawk alights upon a sycamore limb, then launches with outstretched wings to catch a puff of sea breeze moving up the canyon. A cottontail rabbit bounds across the trail, and stops to take your measure with a sidelong stare. Los Penasquitos Creek slips silently through placid pools and darts noisily down multiple paths in the constriction known as "the falls."

Despite the noose of suburban development tightening around it, Los Penasquitos Canyon Preserve still retains its gentle, unselfconscious beauty. The preserve's 3000 acres of San Diego city- and county-owned open-space stretch for almost 7 miles between I-5 and I-15, encompassing much of Los Penasquitos Creek and one of its tributaries—Lopez Canyon.

Visitor facilities at the preserve include parking/equestrian staging areas off Black Mountain Road on the east side, and next to Sorrento Valley Boulevard on the west side. Near the east entry stands the Johnson-Taylor ranch house, now the preserve's headquarters, dating from 1862. In 1991, archaeologists announced the discovery that part of the ranch house is a surviving remnant of a house built in 1824 for Captain Francisco Maria Ruiz. Ruiz was commandant of the Presidio of San Diego, and the recipient of the county's first Spanish land grant. The crumbling remnants of another adobe structure, also owned by Ruiz, stand under a protective roof at the west entrance to the preserve.

Farther afield, hikers, joggers, and equestrians have the run of the preserve. Take along a picnic lunch and a blanket. There are many fine places—sunny mead-

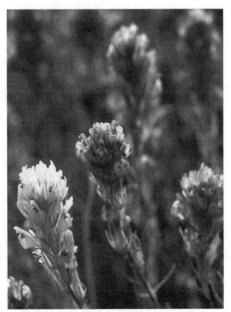

Owl's clover, Los Penasquitos Canyon

ows, oak-shaded flats, and the sycamore-fringed streamside—to stop for an hour's relaxation. For starters, you can try the following, nearly level hike to the falls and back.

To Reach the Trailhead: Exit I-15 at Mercy Road/Scripps Poway Parkway, and go west on Mercy Road 1 mile downhill to a traffic light at a T-intersection with Black Mountain Road. The main entrance to Los Penasquitos Canyon Preserve is straight across this intersection. Drive in, pay a small day-use fee, and park in the large parking lot.

Description: On foot (or on bike wheels—the route sometimes swarms with mountain bikers), head west on a dirt road. In the first mile the road hugs Los Penasquitos Canyon's south wall, a steep, chaparral-covered hillside (Penasquitos means "little cliffs").

As you pass near the Johnson-Taylor ranch (screened from view by willows and dense vegetation along the creek), you'll notice several non-native plants—eucalyptus, fan palms, feather-duster palms, and fennel, for example—introduced into this area over the past century. Efforts continue to remove these exotic species. Next, you enter a long and beautiful canopy of intertwined live oaks, accompanied by a lush understory of mostly poison oak.

Mile posts along the roadside help you gauge your progress. At mile 2 the trail winds out of the dense cover of oaks and continues through grassland dotted with a few small elderberry trees. Wildflowers such as wild radish, mustard, California poppies, bush mallow, blue-eyed grass, and violets put on quite a show here in March and April. Look, too, for the fuchsia-flowered gooseberry, quite unmistakable when in bloom.

At the 3-mile marker the road starts winding up onto a chaparral slope in order to detour a narrow, rocky section of the canyon. At a wide spot in the road, where there are bike racks, take a path descending on the right toward a narrow, rocky constriction along the canyon bottom. During winter and early spring, water in decent quantity tumbles through here. Polished rock 10 feet up on either side and deep, circular potholes testify to its sometimes violent flow. The outcroppings of greenish-gray rock have been identified as Santiago Peak volcanics—the same hardened metavolcanic rock found farther north at Santiago Peak in the Santa Ana Mountains and farther south into Baja California.

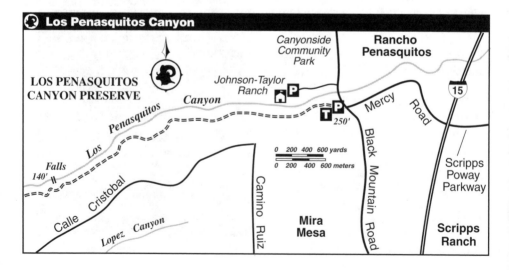

HIKE 68

Bernardo Mountain

Location	Escondido
Highlights	Wildflower-dotted hillsides; lake views
Distance	7.2 miles round trip
Total Elevation Gain/Loss	1000'/1000'
Hiking Time	3 hours (round trip)
Optional Map	USGS 7.5-min *Escondido*
Best Times	All year
Agency	SDRP
Difficulty	★★★

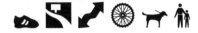

Imagine a hiking, biking, and equestrian trail extending from the coast at Del Mar to the crest of the mountains in mid-San Diego County. Today, certain sections of this 55-mile-long route, known as the Coast to Crest Trail, are already open. These and other future sections of the trail will define the main axis of the San Dieguito River Park, now taking shape along the watersheds of the San Dieguito River and its main tributary, Santa Ysabel Creek. Many pieces of the proposed park are in place today and open to the public, but fleshing out the entire 60,000 acres of parkland promises to involve much wrangling with landowners and long-term efforts by interested citizens and various local governments.

On this hike you'll travel one of the more accessible and scenic segments of the Coast to Crest Trail, overlooking scenic Lake Hodges, and you'll climb to the summit of Bernardo Mountain, which was purchased in 2002 for inclusion in the San Dieguito River Park.

To Reach the Trailhead: Exit I-15 at Via Rancho Parkway and go east to the first southbound street on the right, Sunset Drive. Drive to the end of Sunset Drive and park (no charge).

Description: From Sunset Drive, continue south on the Coast to Crest Trail, initially a concrete pathway parallel to the freeway. After about 0.4 mile, the pathway turns sharply right and passes under the I-15 bridge that goes over the east arm of Lake Hodges. Depending on the amount of rainfall over the past year or two, the lake (a San Diego city reservoir) could be

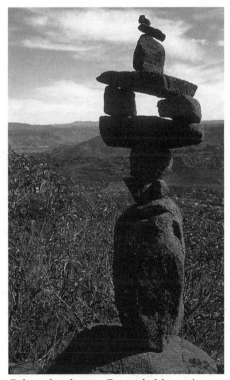

Balanced rocks atop Bernardo Mountain

brimming with water at this spot—or be completely dry, as it has been in the early years of this decade. A foot/bicycle bridge going across the water, parallel to the freeway on the west side, is slated for imminent construction.

After swinging north on the far side (west side) of the freeway, the Coast to Crest Trail joins for a short time the crumbling pavement of the long-abandoned Highway 395, the former inland highway running north from San Diego into Riverside County and beyond. Soon, however, the pavement disappears and you're on a dirt trail following the shoreline west. At 1.5 miles from the start, you cross Felicita Creek, a small perennial brook deeply shaded by oaks, sycamores, palms, and other water-loving vegetation.

You rise out of the creek and ascend moderately, wrapping around the broad flank of Bernardo Mountain. The sunny slope on the right hosts an eye-popping assortment of wildflowers March through May. On the left, look for snow-white egrets parasailing over the wind-rippled surface of the lake. Overhead, hawks and ravens can often be seen patrolling the afternoon skies, riding on thermals. Ospreys and golden eagles have been seen in this area as well—not to mention small and circumspect California gnatcatchers, which are classified as an endangered species.

At 1.7 miles, a few minutes past the creek crossing, make a very sharp right turn on the path heading north. You ascend slowly, with the oaks and sycamores of Felicita Creek just below you on the right and Bernardo Mountain rising on the left. By about 2.5 miles, you've swung around to the north side of the mountain, where the chaparral vegetation thickens to junglelike proportions and the ascent quickens. Stay left (uphill) at the next two trail intersections, always heading upward.

You continue either rising or contouring in a zigzag pattern, passing a large water tank at 3.2 miles, and finally reaching the rocky summit at 3.6 miles. From this lofty vantage point you can clearly see the patchwork of urban/suburban/wildland that inland north San Diego County has become. The white noise of traffic on I-15 wafts upward to you—but peering in certain other directions you see little apparent human impact on the landscape. Westward, down the valley below Lake Hodges, a slice of Pacific Ocean is visible on clear days.

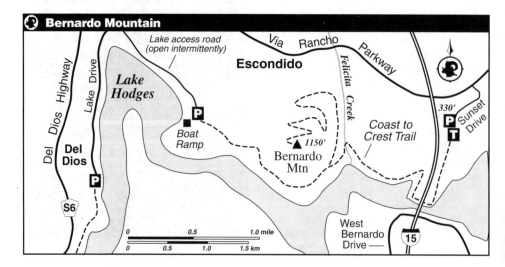

HIKE 69

Cowles Mountain

Location	Mission Trails Regional Park
Highlight	Best view of urban San Diego County
Distance	3.0 miles round trip
Total Elevation Gain/Loss	950'/950'
Hiking Time	2 hours (round trip)
Optional Map	USGS 7.5-min *La Mesa*
Best Times	All year
Agency	MTRP
Difficulty	★★

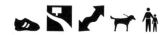

Touted as one of the largest urban parks in the country, Mission Trails Regional Park, in San Diego's San Carlos district, preserves some of the last remaining open space close to the heart of this sprawling city. Cowles Mountain, centerpiece of the regional park, stands 1591 feet above sea level, and is recognized as the highest point within San Diego's city limits. Hundreds of people walk the main south trail to its summit daily. Several newer trails have been laid out on the east and north slopes of the mountain in recent years, so now hikers can choose among several summit routes. We describe the ever-popular south route, which consistently offers vistas stretching from the Pacific Ocean to Mexico.

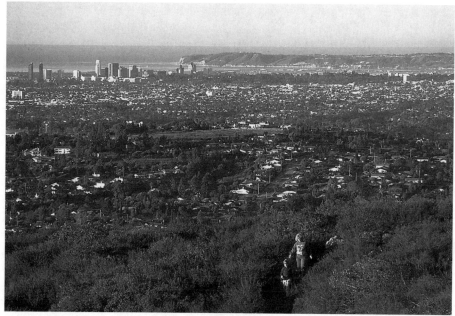

Cowles Mountain vista of downtown San Diego and Point Loma

To Reach the Trailhead: Exit I-8 at College Avenue, go north for 1 mile, and turn right (east) on Navajo Road. Continue 2 miles to the Cowles Mountain trailhead (parking lot, restrooms) on the northeast corner of Navajo Road and Golfcrest Drive..

Description: From the trailhead you ascend steadily, zigzagging almost constantly up through low-growing chaparral punctuated by outcrops of granitic rock. The trail was cut into decomposed granite, so it is quite susceptible to erosion. Don't shortcut the switchbacks, tempting as this may be, as this tramples plants and tends to destabilize the trail.

Nearly 1 mile up, a spur trail branches right toward a flat spot on the mountain's south shoulder. This, the site of ancient winter-solstice ceremonies by the ancestral Kumeyaay Indians, has become a popular place to visit at dawn on or near the solstice (December 21). If viewed from the right spot, the sun's disk, just peeping over the mountains to the east, gets momentarily split into two brilliant points of light by a large outcrop atop a distant ridge.

Just beyond the spur trail, another trail branches right and eventually descends the east slope. Stay left and continue up the slope on the series of long switchback segments leading to the rocky summit of the mountain. A cluster of antennas obstructs the northward view somewhat, but otherwise the panorama is complete. With binoculars and with the help of two large interpretive panels that identify nearby and distant landmarks, you could spend a lot of time getting to know the region. In the rift between the mesas to the west, there's a good view of Mission Valley and the tangle of freeways that pass over and through it. Southwest, the towers of downtown San Diego stand against Point Loma, Coronado, and sparkling San Diego Bay. Lake Murray shimmers to the south. The chain of Santee Lakes contrasts darkly with pale hills to the north. In all directions you look out over the abodes of

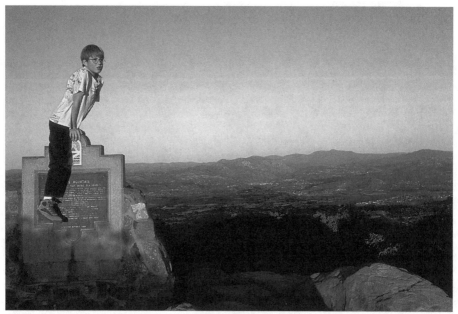

Cowles Mountain summit

the nearly five million people now living in the combined metropolis of San Diego and Tijuana.

On the clearest days, the higher peaks of San Diego County stand in bold relief against the sky. Southward into Baja, you should spot the flat-topped "Table Mountain" behind Tijuana, and the Coronado Islands offshore. Try looking for the dusky profiles of Santa Catalina and San Clemente islands, to the northwest and west respectively.

Here's a suggestion for romantics and adventurers who don't mind descending the trail by flashlight: Catch the sunset from Cowles' summit when the moon is full. After the sun slides into the Pacific, turn around and enjoy the moonrise over the El Cajon valley!

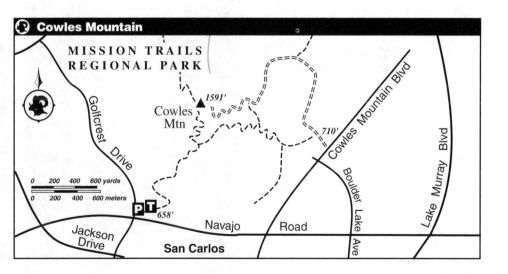

HIKE 70

Blue Sky Ecological Reserve

Location	Poway
Highlights	Riparian and oak woodland; spring wildflowers
Distance	5.0 miles round trip
Total Elevation Gain/Loss	800'/800'
Hiking Time	2 ½ hours (round trip)
Optional Map	USGS 7.5-min *Escondido*
Best Times	All year
Agency	BSER
Difficulty	★★

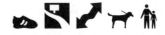

The 700-acre Blue Sky Ecological Reserve near Poway protects one of the finer examples of riparian (streamside) vegetation in Southern California. As one of the most popular of the 119 California Department of Fish and Game wildlife reserves in the state, much attention here is focused on nature education as well as habitat preservation. Motorized vehicles and mountain bikes are banned—so you'll be assured of peace and quiet, and more frequent wildlife sightings, as you stroll along.

To Reach the Trailhead: Exit I-15 at Rancho Bernardo Road, and drive east through Rancho Bernardo and Poway (where the road changes its name to Espola Road). At 3 miles east, the road bends 90° to the right. Just after that bend look for the Blue Sky reserve entrance/trailhead on the left. If you are coming from the south on Espola Road, the Blue Sky turnoff is 0.6 mile north of Lake Poway Road.

Description: On foot, follow the unpaved Green Valley Truck Trail along the south bank of a creek. Traffic noise disappears, and frogs entertain you with their guttural serenades. Live oaks spread their limbs overhead, casting pools of shade, while willows, sycamores, and lush thickets of poison oak cluster along the creek itself. On the left, about one-quarter mile

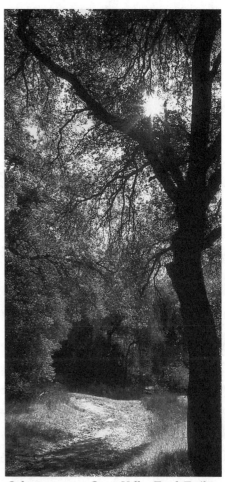

Oak canopy over Green Valley Truck Trail

out, a wide side trail diverges toward the creek itself. There you can spot tadpoles, frogs, and perhaps other amphibious creatures. A narrower path takes you back to the truck trail.

After a wet winter, usually by March, the creekside landscape turns an almost unbelievably bright shade of green. Mosses, ferns, annual grasses, and fresh new shrub growth coats everything, even the rocks. Wildflowers appear in great numbers by about April, and start to fade by June, after the grasses have bleached to a straw-yellow color. More than 100 kinds of wildflowers have been identified here in a single year.

At 1.0 mile, a trail branching right (south) heads uphill to join the trail system of the Lake Poway Recreation Area. About 0.2 mile farther on the main road, where powerlines pass overhead, there's a major split. The left branch (Green Valley Truck Trail) fords the creek and starts climbing a dry south slope toward the Ramona Reservoir dam. In the next 1.3 miles of steady ascent, you gain about 700 feet of elevation and enjoy an ever-expanding view of Poway, Rancho Bernardo, and much of the rest of inland north San Diego County's rapidly urbanizing region.

Once you reach the dam you can turn around and return on the same route in much less time.

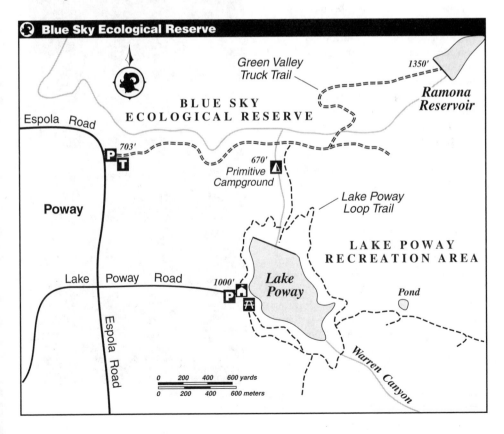

HIKE 71

Woodson Mountain

Location	Poway-Ramona
Highlights	Giant boulders; superb views
Distance	5.5 miles
Total Elevation Gain/Loss	1500'/1500'
Hiking Time	3 hours
Optional Map	USGS 7.5-min *San Pasqual*
Best Times	October through June
Agency	LPRA
Difficulty	★★

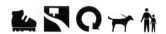

Indians called it "Mountain of Moon-lit Rocks," an appropriate name for a landmark visible, even at night, over great distances. Early white settlers dubbed it "Cobbleback Peak," a name utterly descriptive of its rugged, boulder-strewn slopes. For the past 100 years, however, it has appeared on maps simply as "Woodson Mountain," in honor of a Dr. Woodson who homesteaded some property nearby well over a century ago.

The light-colored bedrock of Woodson Mountain and several of its neighboring peaks in the Poway/Ramona area is a type geologists call "Woodson Mountain granodiorite." When exposed at the surface, it weathers into huge spherical or ellipsoidal boulders with smooth surfaces. The largest boulders have a tendency to cleave apart along remarkably flat planes, forming "chimneys" from several inches to several feet wide. Sometimes, one half of a split boulder will roll away, leaving a vertical and almost seamless face behind. It's no wonder that Woodson Mountain (or "Mt. Woodson," as it is popularly called) is regarded as one of the finest places to practice the craft of bouldering in Southern California.

This looping route up and over Woodson's summit takes advantage of the newer Fry-Koegel Trail along the mountain's bouldery north slope. Hikers have

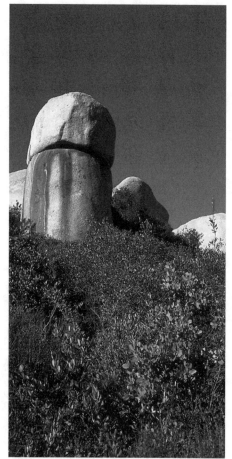

Granodiorite boulders, east slope of Woodson Mountain

long had the opportunity of reaching the summit by either of two major routes, but there was never any easy way to avoid re-tracing steps.

To Reach the Trailhead: From the intersection of Poway Road and Highway 67, in eastern Poway, drive north on Highway 67 to a large turnout on the right (east) side of the road, opposite the California Division of Forestry fire station. (Some parking space is also available on the narrower west shoulder of the highway as well.)

Description: After parking, carefully cross the four lanes of the highway (there's no crosswalk, though pedestrians scoot across here frequently), and follow a well-beaten path south past the fire station to where it hooks up with a paved service road (closed to vehicular travel) curling up the mountain's east slope. The road underfoot is at times very steep, but offers good traction.

On most weekends, the sounds of nature along the road will be accompanied by the clink of aluminum hardware, plus the shouts of "On belay!" and other phrases in climbers' parlance. Even if you don't see climbers, chalk marks (from gymnast's chalk) on the larger boulders mark their favorite routes. Near the top of the mountain, the road passes narrowly between immense, egg-shaped boulders and split-boulder faces 20 to 30 feet high.

When you reach the top of the mountain, at 1.7 miles, you'll be amid a forest of radio antennas rising from the outsized boulders. Walk west, on dirt now, along the narrow summit ridge to reach a vantage point overlooking Poway, north San Diego County's coastal region, and the great blue expanse of the Pacific Ocean. Santa Catalina and San Clemente islands are visible on the clearest days. Nearby you'll spot an amazing cantilevered "potato-chip" flake of rock, the result of exfoliation and weathering. If you're weary, this is a good spot to turn back and return the way you came.

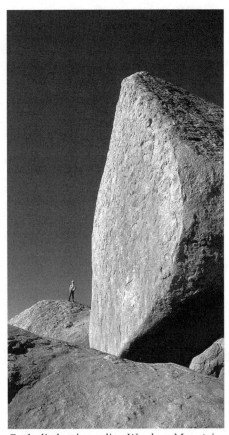

Rock climbers' paradise, Woodson Mountain

Otherwise, on ahead, you quickly pick up a rough trail which tilts downward, steeply at times, along Woodson's boulder-punctuated west ridge. After about 0.5 mile, there's a fork. Ignore the left branch, which descends toward the Mt. Woodson Trail and Lake Poway, and continue west, down-ridge, on the Fry-Koegel Trail.

After a few minutes, the trail switches back and starts an oblique dive down through wildly tangled, mature chaparral, bound for the Mt. Woodson Estates subdivision at the north base of the mountain. Near the bottom, the trail meanders through spooky clusters of coast live oaks. Watch out for copious growths of poison oak through here.

Back in the open air again, the trail executes a rather annoying switchbacking detour around a block of new houses. Then it's a straight shot to Archie Moore Road, near Highway 67. A few minutes' walk along the highway shoulder from there takes you back to your car.

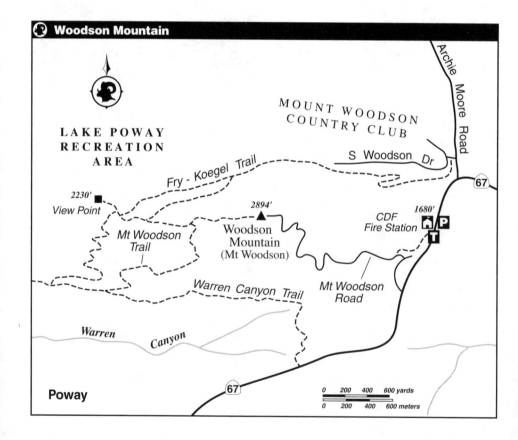

HIKE 72

Iron Mountain

Location	Near Poway
Highlights	Panoramic views
Distance	6.4 miles round trip
Total Elevation Gain/Loss	1200′/1200′
Hiking Time	3 ½ hours (round trip)
Optional Map	USGS 7.5-min *San Vicente Reservoir*
Best Times	October through June
Agency	LPRA
Difficulty	★★

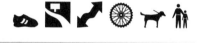

North San Diego County's Iron Mountain thrusts its conical summit nearly 2700 feet above sea level, frequently well above the low-lying coastal haze. On many a crystalline winter day, the summit offers a sweeping, 360° panorama from glistening ocean to blue mountains and back to the ocean again. Access to the summit—by foot, horse, or mountain bike—is now afforded by a key link in the City of Poway's ever-expanding multi-use trails system.

To Reach the Trailhead: The popular Iron Mountain trailhead is located just south of the intersection of Highway 67 and Poway Road—5 miles east of central Poway by way of Poway Road, and 9 miles north of Lakeside by way of Highway 67. A secondary trailhead at Ellie Lane, 0.7 mile north on Highway 67 from the main trailhead, can be used instead if you opt for the extended route noted at the end of this hike description.

Description: From the main trailhead, the shortest way up the mountain (just over 3 miles one-way) takes you along signed pathways. Thick stands of chaparral stood along these trails until 1995, when a wildfire swept east from Highway 67 and topped Iron Mountain's summit, burning to a crisp everything in its path. The mountain was swept by flames yet again in October 2003 by the 300,000-acre Cedar Fire (the largest blaze in contem-

porary California history). The summit trail remains in excellent shape, however, and the coming years will see the return of the vegetation and provide interesting lessons in fire ecology.

At 1.0 mile east of Highway 67, just before the trail dips to cross a ravine, an obscure side trail goes north almost straight up a hill. If you care to make the

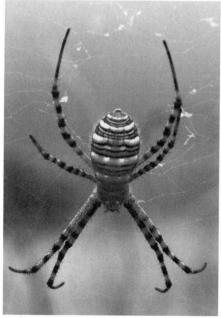

Early-morning spider, Iron Mountain Trail

short, strenuous side trip, you'll find a small pit where iron ore was once mined in small quantities. Dark, dense chunks of the ore lie strewn about—bring along a magnet to confirm their identity.

Once across the ravine, you commence a steeper ascent. At 1.5 miles you reach, in a saddle, a trail junction, where you turn right to head for Iron Mountain's summit, 1.7 meandering trail miles away. Numerous switchbacks on the trail's final half mile take you back and forth across the ever-narrowing summit cone. On the summit you'll find a massive, pier-mounted telescope (no coins required) thoughtfully provided for the purpose of scanning the near and far horizons.

Return the easy way by simply reversing your steps, or you can opt for a more challenging traverse over hill and dale to the north. The northern loop,

which passes Table Rock and two old cattle ponds, adds three additional miles to the round trip and involves several severe up and down pitches. You'll end up at the Ellie Lane trailhead, 0.7 mile north of the main trailhead.

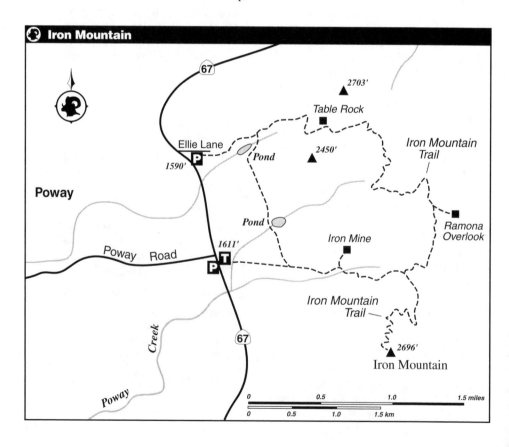

HIKE 73

El Capitan Open Space Preserve

Location	Near Lakeside
Highlights	Frequent vistas of coastal lowlands and ocean
Distance	11.0 miles round trip (to saddle)
Total Elevation Gain/Loss	4000'/4000'
Hiking Time	6 hours (round trip)
Optional Maps	USGS 7.5-min *San Vicente Reservoir, El Cajon Mtn.*
Best Times	November through April
Agency	SDCP
Difficulty	★★★★

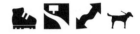

As you walk along the granite-ribbed ridgeline, down the middle of the El Capitan Open Space Preserve, a binational panorama of ocean, islands, and innumerable mountain peaks lies in view. The broad San Diego River valley below curves beneath the sheer south face of El Cajon Mountain—the landmark informally known as "El Capitan."

The 2800-acre preserve was pieced together out of former Bureau of Land Management (BLM) lands adjacent to the Cleveland National Forest. If you have the determination to tackle some really severe uphills and downhills, and get the benefit of a serious cardiovascular workout, try following the main route into the preserve—an old, sometimes precariously steep road bulldozed by miners years ago. It twists and turns over a scrubby, boulder-punctuated landscape that in spring comes alive with a blue frosting of ceanothus (wild lilac) blossoms. Parts of this mining road are gradually being bypassed or improved and incorporated into the fledgling Trans-County Trail—a major multi-use pathway that will stretch east-west across San Diego County from Del Mar on the coast to Borrego Springs in the desert.

The statistics in the capsulized summary above do not include additional miles and time spent on three possible

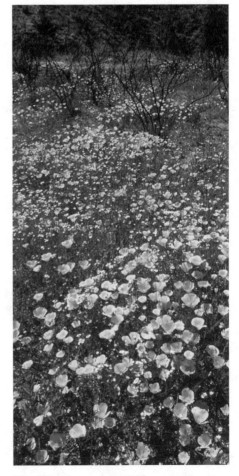

Fire-following spring wildflowers

side trips, mentioned below. Even the main route, however, is surprisingly difficult, due to both the ups and downs, and a lack of abundant shade. Many hikers underestimate the amount of drinking water they will need. Bring more than you think you should. [El Capitan Open Space Preserve will likely be the last county-operated recreational facility to reopen after 2003's devastating Cedar Fire. As of this writing, no opening date has been announced.]

To Reach the Trailhead: To reach the trailhead from the town of Lakeside (northeast of San Diego), turn east on Mapleview Street where the freeway portion of Highway 67 ends. After 0.3 mile on Mapleview, turn left (north) on Ashwood Street. Ashwood soon becomes Wildcat Canyon Road, Proceed north on the combined Ashwood/Wildcat Canyon road 4.2

miles to a signed parking lot and trailhead for the El Capitan preserve on the right. (You can use the green mile markers by the roadside as your guide; slow down after mile marker 4.0.)

Description: From the lot, walk east 0.4 mile on the entry road to the private Blue Sky Ranch, past that ranch, to where the trail starts a steep, zigzag ascent up a cool, north-facing slope. You soon hook up with the old mining road, and the going gets easier for a while. [NOTE: These directions will change once a planned bypass trail is completed between the trailhead and the old mining road.]

As you reach a small summit (about 1.2 miles from the start) and start descending on the old mining road, the round top and sheer south brow of El Cajon Mountain (El Capitan) becomes visible in the middle distance. A very steep

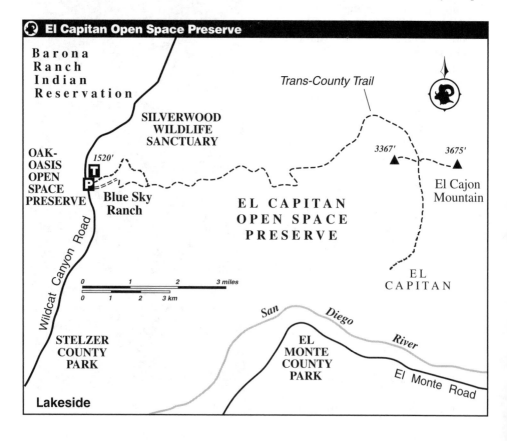

uphill pitch, commencing at about 3 miles, will surely reduce you to painfully slow uphill scrambling, if only for a few minutes. At just under 4 miles, you reach another significant summit. From this spot, a short side path leads north to some abandoned mines—shallow tunnels cut into a chalky hillside.

Like Sisyphus, your elevation gain is tragically interrupted just ahead. You sink 300 feet in less than a half mile on a slippery, decomposing granite surface, before once again resuming uphill progress. At 4.7 miles there's a rock-lined spring on the left, brimming with iron-rich, non-potable water, or possibly dry. At 5.5 miles, the road arrives on a saddle between El Cajon Mountain's summit on the left (east) and a smaller 3367-foot peak on the right (west). You'll be retracing your steps from this point to get back to your car. Ahead, though, you have three choices for further exploration.

By turning right (west) and walking 0.2 mile, you reach a 3367-foot summit, with evident remnants of a radio antenna installation. This rocky peaklet offers a nice panoramic view west and south.

By turning left (east) you can follow a narrow path threading 0.5 mile through thick chaparral and around jumbo-sized granitic boulders to El Cajon Mountain's summit. (The route is slated to be improved and incorporated into the Trans-County Trail.) Although the summit is rounded and clogged with boulders, the view from there is panoramic in all directions.

The third, most difficult alternative is a 1.4-mile-long trek straight ahead (south) from the saddle, using a severely eroded and partially overgrown roadbed. This route takes you to the sheer brow of El Capitan. Walk out to the edge, beyond the end of the old roadbed, and descend over boulders 50 or 100 yards for a pseudo-aerial view of the San Diego River Valley and El Capitan Reservoir, complete with toy-like boats floating on its blue surface.

HIKE 74

Doane Valley

Location	Palomar Mountain State Park
Highlight	Verdant meadows, bubbling streams
Distance	2.5 miles
Total Elevation Gain/Loss	300'/300'
Hiking Time	1 ½ hours
Optional Map	USGS 7.5-min *Boucher Hill*
Best Times	All year
Agency	PSP
Difficulty	★★

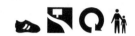

This is a hike for inspiration. Here, at Palomar Mountain State Park, you'll find some of Southern California's finest montane scenery, complete with trickling streams, mixed forests of pine, cedar and oak, and rolling meadows. The long, stomach-churning drive up the mountain's slopes is well worth the trouble once you get out of the car and start breathing in Palomar's sweet, tangy air.

To Reach the Trailhead: Palomar Mountain State Park lies in far-north San Diego County, about 20 miles east of I-15 by way of State Highway 76, County Highway S6 (South Grade Road), and County Highway S7 (East Grade Road). From most parts of San Diego County, it's fastest to use Highway S6 (Valley Center Road) to reach Highway 76 near the foot of Palomar Mountain. Day-use and camp-

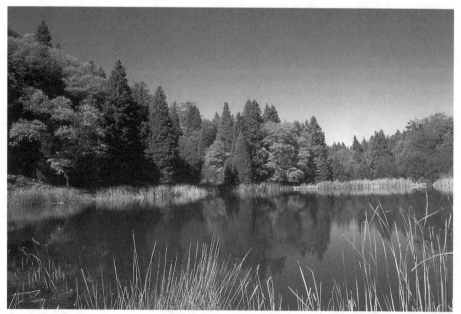

Doane Pond

ing fees are payable at the state park entrance, at the west end of East Grade Road. Continue driving past that entrance until you reach the Doane Pond parking lot, which is the starting point for the Doane Valley Nature Trail.

Description: You begin your hike by following the Doane Valley Nature Trail downstream along Doane Creek. Along the bank grow boxelder trees, creek dogwood, wild strawberry, mountain currant, and Sierra gooseberry. You pass a massive incense-cedar tree towering more than 100 feet high. If you weren't informed of its true identity, you might think it was a giant (sequoia) redwood.

After 0.3 mile, the nature trail curves and climbs around a hill to connect with Doane Valley Campground. At a trail junction here, bear left on the Weir Trail, following Doane Creek through stately groves of white fir and incense-cedar. Walk all the way down to the weir at the end of the trail, and admire the stone-and-mortar structure above it. This small dam and gauging station were used in the late 1920s to test the hydroelectric potential of the stream. The tests proved there was not enough flow to justify construction of a power plant. Today, the silted-in dam holds barely enough water to soak your feet in.

Some fishermen and hikers are familiar with the rugged and beautiful stretch of Pauma Creek below the weir. It's legal to scramble down the creek to the park boundary, only 0.2 mile away. Beyond that point access is forbidden. The creek flows through the Pala Indian Reservation and eventually joins the San Luis Rey River in Pauma Valley. During high water, even the less-rugged stretch within the park can be quite treacherous. Some years ago, park rangers were surprised to discover banana slugs (like those in California's central and northern coast ranges) in this drainage.

From the weir, backtrack 0.2 mile and take the Lower Doane Trail left across the

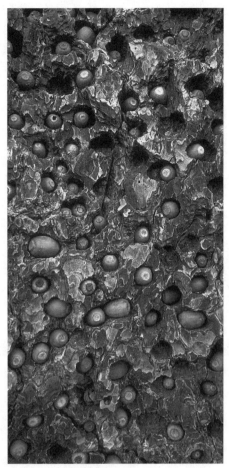

Acorn cache in pine

valley to the French Valley Trail. Go left (north), passing into Lower French Valley. The setting is idyllic: rolling grasslands dotted with statuesque ponderosa pines, surrounded by hillsides clothed in oaks and tall conifers.

Several of the pines are riddled with holes—some plugged with acorns. This is the handiwork of the acorn woodpecker, who uses the holes to store acorns filled with larvae. The birds retrieve these acorns and the grubs in leaner times. Listen for the repetitive, guttural call of this bird, and observe the distinctive red patch on its head and the white wing patch when in flight.

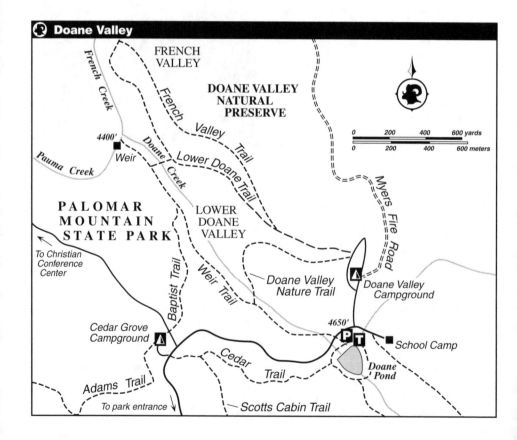

Hike as far as the bank of French Creek, then head back toward your starting point along the upper part of the French Valley Trail. You'll join Lower Doane Trail and pass through Doane Valley Campground before arriving at the Doane Pond parking lot.

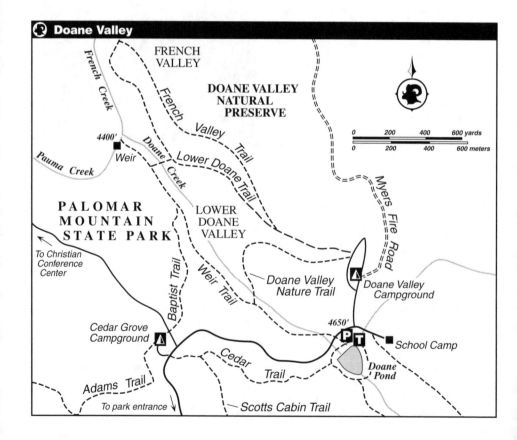

HIKE 75

Barker Valley

Location	Palomar Mountain
Highlights	Remote valley; spectacular cascades
Distance	6.2 miles round trip (to foot of trail)
Total Elevation Gain/Loss	1000'/1000'
Hiking Time	4 hours (round trip)
Optional Map	USGS 7.5-min *Palomar Observatory*
Best Times	October through July
Agency	CNF/PD
Difficulty	★★★

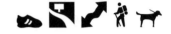

Tucked into a dry and isolated corner of Cleveland National Forest, the oak-rimmed oasis of Barker Valley is a real surprise. The perennial west fork of the San Luis Rey River gurgles through the narrow valley floor, sustaining a growth of willows and sycamores along its banks. Centuries-old live oaks cast inviting pools of shade across grassy meadows that in late spring metamorphose from green to gold under the relentless rays of the sun.

Getting there requires some serious driving and hiking—first on an 8-mile stretch of bone-shaking truck trail that will surely loosen a nut or two on your vehicle, then on a gently descending, sun-exposed, 3-mile hiking trail. Get an early start if you're heading down for a picnic, so as to avoid some of the midday heat. (Check with the Forest Service to see if the road is open; storms can render it temporarily unusable.) Barker Valley is a popular destination for backpacking. No campfires are allowed, and you'll need a remote camping permit from the Forest Service for an overnight stay.

To Reach the Trailhead: To reach the trailhead, turn west from Highway 79 onto Palomar Divide Road (Forest Road 9S07), 6.5 miles northwest of Warner Springs. Continue on the winding, unpaved road 7.8 miles to the Barker Valley

Spur trailhead on the left side. Park off of the roadway.

Description: From your car, head down the trail (an old roadbed), which gradually descends along a chaparral-covered slope. The uneven growth is a consequence of various fires—some prescribed (to rid the hills of half-dead, mature shrubbery), others unintentional. For a while you pass through a grown-in section, unburned for perhaps several decades, choked with an attractive and colorful mix of manzanita, chamise, mountain mahogany, silk-tassel bush, ceanothus, and ribbonwood. The latter, almost the dominant shrub, spreads feathery plumes of light green foliage across the slopes. Notice its perpetually peeling, ribbonlike bark.

Keep an eye out for hawks and ravens soaring overhead. During the winter bald eagles are sometimes seen here, not far from where they roost on old snags near the shore of Lake Henshaw. Also keep a sharp eye on the ground for horned lizards. When not scurrying about, they're practically invisible against the decomposed granite soil.

After 1.7 miles of gradual descent, the old road bends sharply left. Continue around the U-curve, and within 0.1 mile veer to the right on a newer trail. You lazily zigzag down a dry slope and emerge on the floor of oak-rimmed Barker Valley. If you're looking for a campsite, they're abundant here. Just remember to select one at least 100 feet away from the nearest water—in this case, the West Fork San Luis Rey River. Barker Valley is notorious for cold air drainage at night. I once had the interesting experience of sweating out an 85°F July day, and awakening next morning to find frost along the stream.

By poking around the valley a bit, you may find evidence of former homesteads (various rusty pieces of metal and square nails), and evidence of early Indian use as well. Bedrock mortars (holes for grinding acorns) have been worn into some of the larger slab rocks. Keep in mind that all features are protected; there's no collecting allowed.

Many hikers come to Barker Valley in search of the rugged set of falls and pools a mile or so downstream from the foot of the Barker Valley Spur Trail. These lie just below an old stone weir and gauging station. By following rough paths traversing the steep, brushy, north canyon wall, it's possible to reach hidden swimming holes worn in the water-polished rock. Wild trout can be found in the pools below the first falls (a license is needed for fishing). Don't attempt to explore this area unless you have the right footgear, and you're adept at scrambling across steep terrain and potentially slippery, water-polished rock. An ill-timed slip in a couple of places could result in a deadly, 50-foot plunge down a cascade.

When it's time to return, go back the same way, uphill this time. The consistently gradual trail is not at all challenging, but it may prove difficult after many hours of exposure to the warm sun.

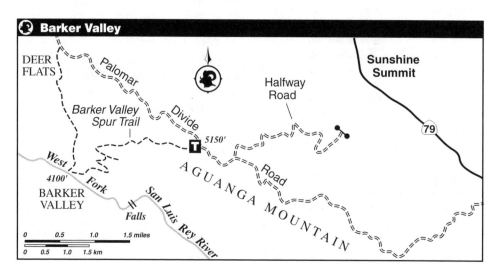

HIKE 76

Love Valley

Location	Palomar Mountain
Highlights	Secluded meadows and ponds
Distance	2.0 miles round trip
Total Elevation Gain/Loss	300'/300'
Hiking Time	1 ½ hours (round trip)
Optional Map	USGS 7.5-min *Palomar Observatory*
Best Times	November through June
Agency	CNF/PD
Difficulty	★

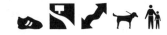

After a wet winter, shallow ponds in Love Valley hold the shimmering, upside-down image of a classic California landscape: a weathered barn nestled at the far end of an Ireland-colored meadow, rounded foothills studded with oaks, and white cumulus clouds billowing over the dark, conifer-draped Palomar crest. By May or June, the shallow ponds in the valley bottom shrink and disappear, leaving in their wake a brilliant display of yellow tidy tips and assorted other wildflowers. This little-known, day-use destination near the foot of Palomar Mountain is great for a picnic of the sit-on-a-blanket type.

To Reach the Trailhead: First, drive to Lake Henshaw, 30 miles east of I-15 by way of Highway 76, or 4.5 miles west of Highway 79 by way of Highway 76. Just west of the little resort community of Lake

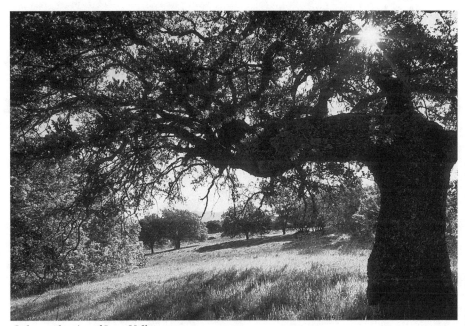

Oaks on the rim of Love Valley

Henshaw near the Lake Henshaw dam, turn north on East Grade Road. Proceed 3.3 miles uphill on East Grade Road and find the marked parking turnout for Love Valley on the left side of the road. Using the mile markers on East Grade Road, the turnout is between mile markers 3.0 and 3.5.

Description: From your car parked at the turnout, walk around the locked vehicle gate, and follow a wide, dirt path over a low rise and then gently downhill.

As you descend, watch for three kinds of oak trees—black, coast, and Engelmann oaks. The Engelmann variety, characterized by gray-green leaves, is noted for its limited and shrinking habitat. The 3600-foot elevation here is a bit too low for the pines, cedars and firs that are so common a little higher on Palomar Mountain.

Presently, Lake Henshaw comes into view, tucked into a corner of the large Valle de San Jose, a down-dropped basin along the Elsinore Fault. The fault, which runs right along the base of Palomar Mountain to the south, is responsible for your elevated position here.

When you reach the edge of Love Valley at 0.8 mile, you can walk straight to the old barn (which, upon closer inspection, is made of unromantic and rusty cor-

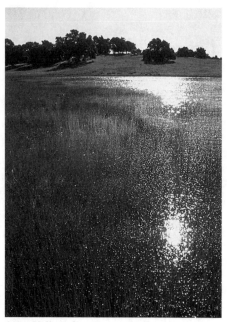

Love Valley after a wet winter

rugated metal), or you can veer left toward the two ephemeral ponds on the valley floor. Choose your picnic site so as to trample as little vegetation as possible. There are no trash barrels or other facilities in Love Valley, so remember to pack out whatever you packed in and did not consume.

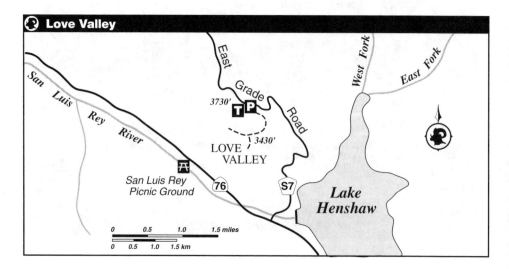

HIKE 77

Agua Caliente Creek

Location	Near Warner Springs
Highlights	Beautiful mountain stream
Distance	8.0 miles round trip
Total Elevation Gain/Loss	900'/900'
Hiking Time	4 hours (round trip)
Optional Maps	USGS 7.5-min *Warner Springs, Hot Springs Mtn.*
Best Times	November through May
Agency	CNF/PD
Difficulty	★★★

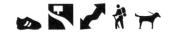

Until the early 1970s, the middle reaches of Agua Caliente Creek seldom saw the intrusion of humans. After the Pacific Crest Trail was routed through, it became a favorite resting spot for hikers heading north or south. This is one of only four places in San Diego County where the PCT dips to cross a fairly dependable stream, and the only place where the trail closely follows water for a fair distance. The stream—if not perennial every year—is at least alive from the first rains of fall into early summer.

To Reach the Trailhead: From I-15 at Temecula, drive east on Highway 79 for 37 miles to reach the resort community of Warner Springs. From the San Diego area, use Highway 78 or Highways 67 and 78 to reach Santa Ysabel, and then proceed north on Highway 79 for 14 miles to Warner Springs. Just west of Warner Springs (toward Temecula), there's a turnout for parking at mile 36.7 on Highway 79. Note the dirt road slanting over to where the PCT crosses under the highway.

Description: Join the PCT at the Agua Caliente Creek bridge at mile 36.6 on Highway 79. Proceed upstream along the cottonwood-shaded creek, first on the left (north) bank, then on the right. In this first mile, the trail goes through Warner Ranch resort property on an easement. Near the

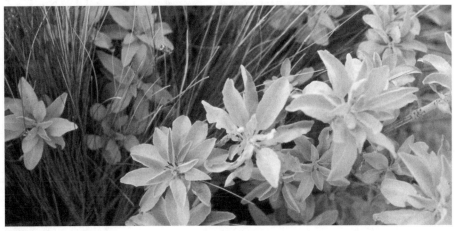

White sage

Cleveland National Forest boundary, about 1 mile out, water flows or trickles from a canyon mouth (trail camping, with permit, is allowed on the lands beyond this point). The trail detours this canyon by swinging to the east and climbing moderately onto gentle, ribbonwood-clothed slopes. After almost 2 miles of somewhat tedious twisting and turning in the chaparral you join the creek again at the 3200-foot contour. ("Unofficial" paths worn in by local equestrians intersecting the PCT may confuse navigation through here a bit.)

Gorgeous scenery begins when you reach the creek. In the next mile the trail (or at least remnants of the trail, since it is easily subject to washouts) crosses the stream several times and passes a number of appealing small campsites well up on the bank. Live oaks, sycamores, willows,

and alders line the creek. The canyon walls soar several hundred feet on either side—clad in dense chaparral on the southeast side, dotted with sage and yucca on the northwest.

After a final crossing of the creek, the trail doubles back and begins a switch-backing (and not very scenic) ascent northwest toward Indian Flats Road. This is a good place to turn around and return the same way.

If you want to explore farther upstream along Agua Caliente Creek from where the trail ascends out of the canyon, you can do it by boulder hopping and wading. Ahead, there's some serious scrambling around small waterfalls, and personal battles with the ever-present alder branches. Los Coyotes Indian Reservation property, requiring permission for entry, lies about a mile ahead.

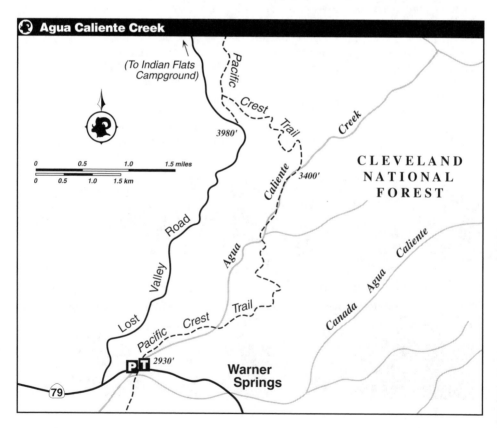

HIKE 78

Hot Springs Mountain

Location	Near Warner Springs
Highlight	Summit is San Diego County's high point
Distance	5.6 miles round trip
Total Elevation Gain/Lost	1250'/1250'
Hiking Time	3 ½ hours (round trip)
Optional Map	USGS 7.5-min *Hot Springs Mtn.*
Best Times	March through November
Agency	LCIR
Difficulty	★★★

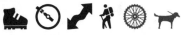

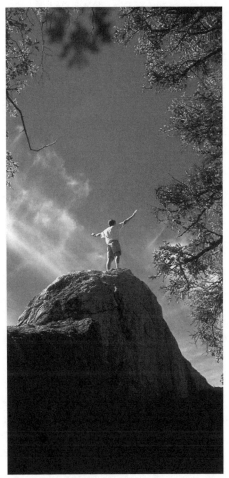

True summit of Hot Springs Mountain

Some of the loftiest—and least visited—mountain country in San Diego County surrounds the resort community of Warner Springs. Hot Springs Mountain, on the Los Coyotes Indian Reservation to the east, is recognized as the county's highest point. At 6533 feet, it beats the better-known, 6512-foot Cuyamaca Peak to the south by a whisker.

Hikers and backpackers are in on a little secret when they discover the Los Coyotes Indian Reservation. This is the largest (25,000 acres) of the 18 reservations in San Diego County, yet one of the least populated. Visitors can make use of developed camping facilities there, as well as explore the undeveloped parts on a network of graded dirt roads, 4-wheel-drive roads, and trails. Motorcycles are prohibited on the reservation and the vehicle traffic is light on the roads, so you're quite likely to find this a pleasant place to go hiking. With its network of roads and trails that seem to go everywhere, the reservation has also become popular among mountain bikers. Los Coyotes is open year-round on the weekends and holidays, weather and road conditions permitting, and visits may be possible on weekdays.

NOTE: At times the Los Coyotes Indian Reservation is closed to all public entry. Please call the reservation at (760) 782-0711 before you try a visit.

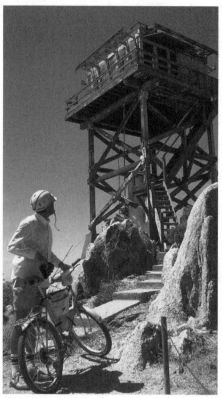

Old lookout tower

To Reach the Trailhead: From I-15 at Temecula, drive east on Highway 79 for 37 miles to reach the resort community of Warner Springs. From the San Diego area, use Highway 78 or Highways 67 and 78 to reach Santa Ysabel, and then proceed north on Highway 79 for 14 miles to Warner Springs. Turn east on Camino San Ignacio from Highway 79 (mile 35.0) at Warner Springs. After 0.6 mile, bear right on Los Tules Road and continue 4.5 miles to the reservation entrance gate. There you pay a $10 fee for entry and pick up a sketch map of the roads and trails. When road and weather conditions allow, it is possible to drive nearly all the way to the Hot Springs summit by way of the semi-maintained Lookout Road, which starts just beyond the entrance gate.

More rewarding from a hiker's point of view, though, is the moderately stren-uous trek we describe here, starting from Nelson's Camp, northeast of the summit and several miles by car into the reservation. So, for that approach drive up the main reservation road, past the campground, to an intersection in a valley 6.1 miles past the entrance gate. Turn left (west) and drive up the valley on a sandy road to reach a saddle above the valley, 2.2 miles farther. Just beyond this saddle, on the left (west) side of the road, you'll find Nelson's Camp amid a pleasant grove of live oak, pine and cedar trees. Park here.

Description: Begin hiking southwest up along a small stream, following what the reservation trail map calls "dangerous trail"—an old jeep track sometimes used by daring 4-wheel drivers who risk and probably relish getting stuck at the top, very steep section. You gain about 500 feet in just over a mile on that road, joining Lookout Road on the crest. Turn right (west) on Lookout Road and climb another 1.6 miles along the ridgeline to a roadend near the top of the mountain. Along this pleasant stretch you'll pass through groves of black oak, Coulter pine and white fir, and across sunny meadows dotted in late spring with wildflowers. In late October, the black oaks shimmer with yellow leaves, and gusts of wind unleash a pitter-patter of acorns.

Just west of the roadend stands a rickety old fire lookout tower, disused since 1976, with rotting and broken wooden steps. A better view awaits you just east, on a flat concrete platform topping a large boulder. This is the true summit of Hot Springs Mountain. A bit of hand-and-toe climbing is required to gain the last 20 feet of elevation. As seen from the flat platform, steep canyons yawn to the west and north, and the Salton Sea often shimmers like a mirage on the eastern horizon. On sunny days, soaring enthusiasts riding the thermals quietly buzz the summit using their lean-looking aircraft.

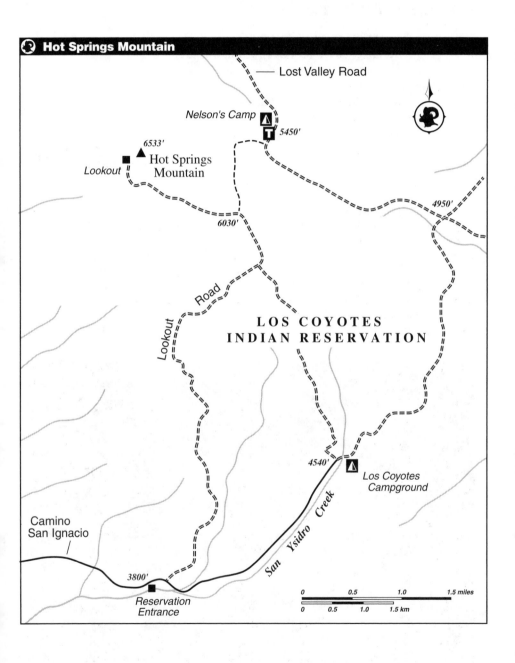

Hot Springs Mountain

Lost Valley Road

Nelson's Camp — 5450'

6533'
Lookout — Hot Springs
Mountain

6030'

4950'

Road

Lookout

**LOS COYOTES
INDIAN RESERVATION**

4540'   Los Coyotes
Campground

San Ysidro Creek

Camino
San Ignacio

3800'
Reservation
Entrance

| 0 | 0.5 | 1.0 | 1.5 miles |
| 0 | 0.5 | 1.0 | 1.5 km |

Cedar Creek Falls

Location	West of Julian
Highlights	Beautiful cascade and "punchbowl"
Distance	4.5 miles round trip
Total Elevation Gain/Loss	1200'/1200'
Hiking Time	2 ½ hours (round trip)
Optional Maps	USGS 7.5-min *Santa Ysabel, Tule Springs*
Best Times	November through June
Agency	CNF/PD
Difficulty	★★

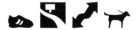

The San Diego River and its upper tributaries drain the pastoral valleys and forested hillsides around Julian, and the rugged western slopes of the Cuyamaca Mountains. The water flows generally southwest through V-shaped canyons, and eventually reaches El Capitan Reservoir, not far from San Diego's eastern suburbs. Quite frequently the water encounters resistant layers in the underlying igneous and metamorphic rocks. In several places it tumbles over cataracts up to a hundred feet high. The grinding of stones trapped in pockets below these falls has created deep pools, or "punchbowls." Cedar Creek Falls, along with its punchbowl, is one of the more attractive and accessible of these wonders.

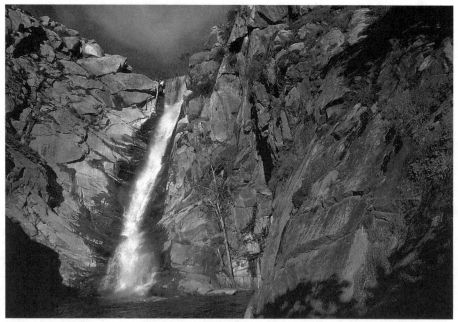

Cedar Creek Falls

Before the construction of El Capitan Dam in the early 1930s, the falls were a popular destination for Sunday outings, and could be reached relatively easily on an auto road up the San Diego River valley from Lakeside. Now, the drive to the Cedar Creek Falls trailhead, which takes San Diegans nearly as far as Julian, is far more circuitous—but very scenic nonetheless.

To Reach the Trailhead: From the town of Julian, on Highway 78 drive west 1 mile and turn south on Pine Hills Road. After 1.5 miles, bear right on Eagle Peak Road. After 1.4 more miles, Eagle Peak Road veers right (Boulder Creek Road goes left). Now you and your vehicle face 8.2 miles of progressively poorer road, parts of which become slippery and muddy in wet weather. In the end, you'll come to an intersection of roads (called "Saddleback"

on detailed maps of the area) and a sign denoting the abandoned road ahead as the Cedar Creek Falls hiking and equestrian trail. Park here so as not to block the intersection

Description: As you head downhill on foot, look up the canyon in the north to see Mildred Falls, arguably San Diego County's highest at more than 100 feet. Unfortunately, it's often little more than a dark stain on an orange-tinted cliff. In flood, however, it is truly an awesome sight.

The old road winds farther west, offering a splendid view of the upper San Diego River canyon, then turns south for a long descent to the river bed. At 1.4 miles, take the spur road that goes left (southeast) over a low saddle into the Cedar Creek drainage. Descend to the bank of the creek and continue following

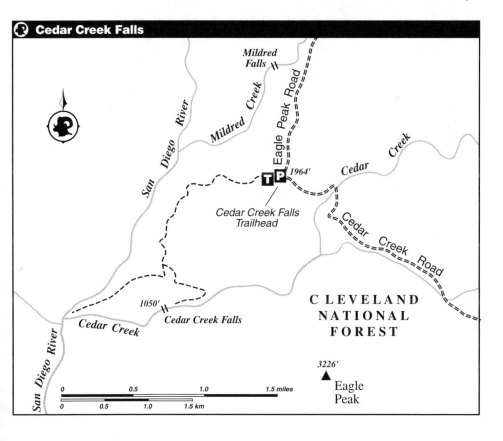

the old road and trail down to the shallow, reflecting pool at the brink of the falls. Be extremely cautious here, as the rock is very slippery. Several fatalities and serious injuries have occurred at the falls as a result of people slipping or unsafely diving into the pool.

From a ridge on the right side, it's possible to admire the 90-foot-high cascade and the cottonwood-framed punchbowl at the bottom—some 50 feet across and 20 feet deep. After heavy rains, water thunders over the precipice, but by late summer the falls merely whisper. Many people obviously make the steep traverse down to the pool at the bottom, though the Forest Service advises against it.

There are other routes to the falls via the mouth of Cedar Creek canyon, but they necessitate crossing property owned by the Helix Water District (land below the 995-foot contour in the San Diego River drainage.) The Forest Service says that permission must be obtained from the landowner to cross this land.

When you've had your fill of the almost overwhelming natural beauty, return to your starting point the same way. If the spirit moves you, you can try this more adventurous, difficult route on the return: From the top of the falls, walk east along the north bank of Cedar Creek about 0.5 mile until the canyon walls close in. There you'll be forced into the creekbed. After about two hours (about 1.2 miles) of boulder-hopping, bushwhacking, and wading through a beautiful and isolated stretch of canyon, Cedar Creek Road will lie above you on the left. Climb north up the slope to that road and follow it a short distance up to your starting point.

HIKE 80

Volcan Mountain

Location	Near Julian
Highlights	Pastoral mountain landscapes
Distance	3.0 miles
Total Elevation Gain/Loss	900'/900'
Hiking Time	2 hours (round trip)
Optional Map	USGS 7.5-min *Julian*
Best Times	October through June
Agency	SDCP
Difficulty	★★

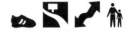

Rising boldly above the apple orchards outside Julian, Volcan Mountain's oak- and pine-dotted slopes are swept by some of the freshest breezes found anywhere. Soughing through the trees like waves spending themselves against a sandy beach, these gusts bear the astringent dryness of the nearby desert as well as the volatile scents of pine needles and sun-baked grass.

Named by early Spanish or Mexican travelers for its dubious resemblance to a volcano, Volcan Mountain (called the "Volcan Mountains" on topographic maps) is really a fault-block mountain, like many others in the Peninsular Ranges. Two faults—the Elsinore and the Earthquake Valley faults—bracket the mountain on the southwest and northeast sides respectively.

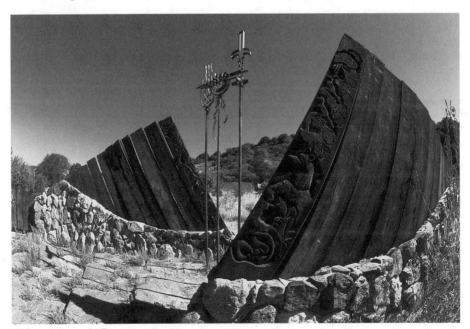

Volcan Mountain Preserve entrance

Off-limits to public use for the past century, Volcan Mountain is gradually falling into the public domain today. As funding becomes available, privately owned land on the mountain is being purchased piecemeal by San Diego County and by the San Dieguito River Park joint powers authority. One such parcel has already become an unsung crown jewel in the county parks system—Volcan Mountain Wilderness Preserve.

To Reach the Trailhead: From the center of Julian (50 miles northeast of San Diego), drive 2.3 miles north on Farmer Road to Wynola Road. Jog right briefly, and then go left on the continuation of Farmer Road. Just ahead, on the right, an obscure wooden sign announces the preserve. Park alongside Farmer Road.

Description: From your parked car, walk east on a dirt access road. After 0.2 mile, you come upon a carved entry structure and stonework designed by noted Julian artist James Hubbell. There's also a small, open-air "kiva" with a compass rose imbedded in the floor, used during interpretive programs. The Elsinore Fault, a major splinter of the San Andreas, passes almost directly under this spot.

Just beyond this formal entrance, your wide path leads sharply up a hill over-looking an apple orchard. You soon swing sharply right and continue climbing in earnest along a rounded ridgeline leading toward the Volcan Mountain crest. Along the ridge, wind-rippled expanses of grassland alternate with dense copses of live oak and black oak. The rust-red bark of the many manzanita shrubs along the way perpetually peels, revealing a green undercoat. Look for the *manzanitas* ("little apples" in Spanish)—the ripe, reddish brown berries that look and taste a bit like the apples hanging from the trees down in the valley below. As you climb higher, the view expands to include parts of Julian, the dusky Cuyamaca Mountains to the south, and—on the clearest days— the blue arc of the Pacific Ocean in the west and southwest.

A locked gate at 1.5 miles (and 900 feet higher than where you started) blocks further progress up the dirt road. At some future date, when the property above opens to the public, you will be able to continue walking toward Volcan peak (elevation 5353 feet) on the summit ridge.

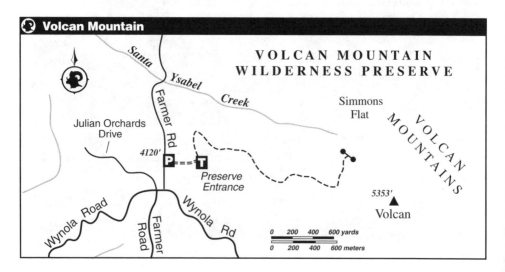

HIKE 81

Cuyamaca Peak

Location	Cuyamaca Rancho State Park
Highlights	Panoramic views; lessons in fire ecology
Distance	5.5 miles round trip
Total Elevation Gain/Loss	1650'/1650'
Hiking Time	3 hours (round trip)
Optional Map	USGS 7.5-min *Cuyamaca Peak*
Best Times	All year
Agency	CRSP
Difficulty	★★★

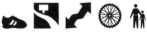

Cuyamaca Peak, San Diego County's second highest summit, lies only a few miles from the county's geographical center. Its unique position and height make it the best land-based vantage point for studying the topography of the southernmost section of California. The 2003 Cedar Fire actually improved the view from the top by effectively removing most of the trees that used to block the panoramic view.

The one-lane, paved Lookout Road ("Cuyamaca Peak Fire Road" on some maps) is closed to public vehicles, but provides a straightforward passage to the top of the peak for self-propelled travelers: hikers, runners, cyclists, and (rarely) cross-country skiers.

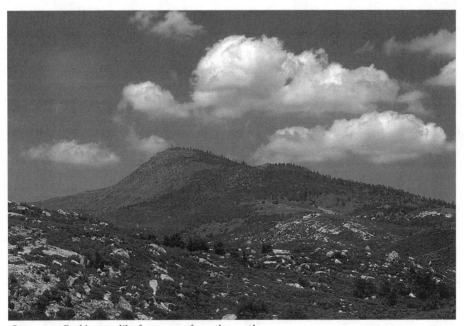

Cuyamaca Peak's wavelike form, seen from the south

To Reach the Trailhead: You'll begin this hike at Paso Picacho Campground/Picnic Area on Highway 79, about 12 miles north of I-8 near Descanso and about 11 miles south of Julian. Day-use parking is available here for a fee, next to the picnic sites. You can start hiking where the Lookout Road meets the highway just south of Paso Picacho's entrance, or you may access that same road by walking through Paso Picacho's southernmost campsites.

Description: Once you are walking on the Lookout Road, you will find the initial uphill grade to be only moderately steep and, of late, only slightly shaded. The dense pine, fir, cedar, and oak forest that grew on these Cuyamaca slopes before October 2003 was hard-hit by the fire. Many of the oaks will survive, though the future of the coniferous trees here is in

doubt. If a long-term drought is in store for the region, the landscape may be transformed into chaparral and oak woods. If the climate turns wet, the mixed coniferous-oak forest will regenerate in a few decades.

After you cross the California Riding and Hiking Trail, which is called Fern Flat Fire Road to the south and Azalea Spring Fire Road to the north (1.2 miles), the paved road gets seriously steep, and remains so for most of the remainder of the climb. The widening vista to the north and east includes Cuyamaca Reservoir and several desert mountain ranges. Notice how the aptly named Stonewall Peak to the east (just across Highway 79) appears to shrink in stature as you continue your climb. In the final steep stretch, you go climb past timber snags and suddenly arrive at the antenna-cluttered summit of

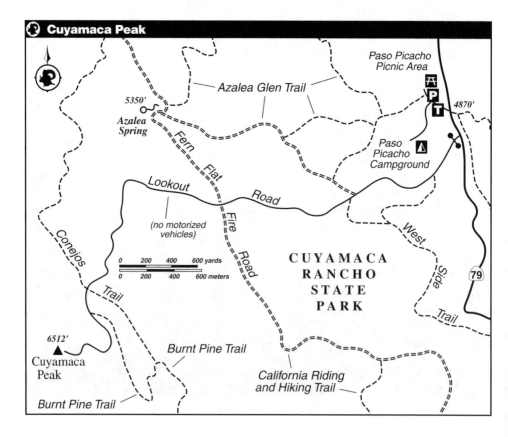

the peak. A fire-lookout structure stood here until the late 1980s, when it was removed for lack of use.

During a Santa Ana condition in fall or winter, and after the passage of major winter storms, Cuyamaca Peak becomes a grandstand seat for views stretching into at least five counties and one foreign state. To name some of the features visible within San Diego County: the Palomar Mountains (look for the tiny white speck on the summit ridge—the Hale Telescope dome) northwest more than 30 miles away; Hot Springs Mountain, 26 miles almost due north over the summit of nearby Middle Peak; Granite Mountain, 11 miles to the northeast; the south end of the Santa Rosa Mountains, 40 miles northeast; and Whale Peak and the Vallecito Mountains, 18 miles east-northeast.

Close in, just 10 or so miles to the southeast, are the wooded Laguna Mountains. South and southwest along the international border are Tecate Peak and Otay Mountain, 25–30 miles away. The Pacific Ocean gleams in the west, with Point Loma, the Silver Strand, San Diego Bay, and Mission Bay visible at distances of about 35–40 miles. Along an arc from west to southwest, you'll spot coastal peaks like Black Mountain, Soledad Mountain, Fortuna Mountain, Cowles Mountain, Mt. Helix, and San Miguel Mountain. Along a west-to-south arc, but closer in, you'll see El Cajon Mountain, Viejas Mountain, Lyons Peak, and Corte Madera Mountain.

You'll enhance the pleasure of your resting time on the peak if you bring along a map of regional features and binoculars.

HIKE 82

Stonewall Peak

Location	Cuyamaca Rancho State Park
Highlights	Outstanding views from summit block
Distance	4.5 miles round trip
Total Elevation Gain/Loss	850'/850'
Hiking Time	2 ½ hours (round trip)
Optional Map	USGS 7.5-min *Cuyamaca Peak*
Best Times	All year
Agency	CRSP
Difficulty	★★

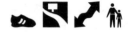

Stonewall Peak's angular summit of white granitic rock is a conspicuous landmark throughout Cuyamaca Rancho State Park. Although Stonewall stands some 800 feet lower than nearby Cuyamaca Peak, its unique position and steep, south exposure provides a more inclusive view of the park area itself.

To Reach the Trailhead: You'll begin this hike at Paso Picacho Campground/Picnic Area on Highway 79, about 12 miles north of I-8 near Descanso and about 11 miles south of Julian. Day-use parking is available here for a fee, next to the picnic sites.

Description: Beginning across the highway from the entrance to Paso Picacho,, the trail climbs steadily and moderately on a set of well-graded switchback segments up the west slope of Stonewall Peak. For many years to come, the trail will probably offer a fairly unobstructed view, since the majority of trees that grew here prior to the 2003 Cedar Fire did not survive.

About halfway up the trail, you can gaze down on Cuyamaca Reservoir to the north, its water level and areal extent varying according to the season and the year's precipitation. When it is full, water covers nearly 1000 acres.

When you reach the top of the switchbacks, turn right and continue south to-

ward the summit of the peak. (The trail to the left descends sharply to Los Caballos equestrian camp. It could be used as an alternate longer, looping route on your way back.) Soon you arrive at the base of the granite cap that crowns the peak. The trail veers right onto that rock, and goes up some rough steps (with guardrail) to

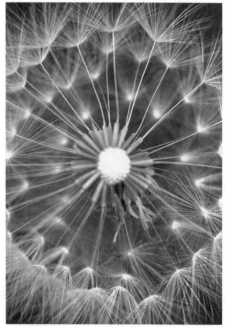

Dandelion

the top. Small children may need assistance on this last airy segment.

The main Cuyamaca massif stands taller in the west, blocking views of the coastline, but the foreground panorama of the park's rolling topography is impressive enough. Patches of meadow along the streamcourses and the bald grassland areas below change color with the seasons: green in spring, yellow in summer, brown or gray in fall, and occasionally white with fallen snow in winter. The recovering forests in view below will probably appear different from year to year as they evolve toward a mature stage.

Swallows or swifts may buzz the Stonewall summit like miniature fighter jets, and larger birds—ravens, hawks, and even bald eagles may cruise by. Eagles, along with egrets, herons, and ospreys, are sometimes attracted to the shoreline of nearby Cuyamaca Reservoir, especially in winter.

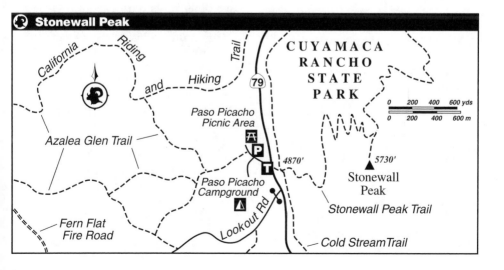

HIKE 83

Sweetwater River

Location	Cuyamaca Rancho State Park
Highlight	Riparian and oak woodland; sparkling mountain stream
Distance	3.8 miles round trip
Total Elevation Gain/Loss	400'/400'
Hiking Time	1 ½ hours (round trip)
Optional Maps	USGS 7.5-min *Descanso, Cuyamaca Peak*
Best Times	October through June
Agency	CRSP
Difficulty	★★

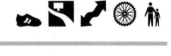

Fed by countless ravines and rivulets on the slopes of the Cuyamaca Mountains, the Sweetwater River eventually becomes a watercourse worthy of the name "river"—at least in the rain or snow season. In the south end of Cuyamaca Rancho State Park, the sweet, bubbling liquid slides placidly down a pleasant little gorge lined by alders, willows, and live oaks. The Merigan Fire Road—a wide, oak-shaded path for hikers, horses and mountain bikers—clings to the high bank of the river for more than a mile, offering the self-propelled traveler vistas of cool, sparkling water tumbling over a gravelly canyon floor. The 2003 Cedar Fire swept most of the area covered along this hike, but it won't be very many years before the chaparral, oak, and riparian habitats fully recover.

To Reach the Trailhead: To reach the starting point from I-8 near Descanso, drive north 2.7 miles on Highway 79 and turn left (north) toward Cuyamaca Rancho State Park, staying on 79. After another 0.2 mile, turn left on Viejas Boulevard. Continue 1.1 miles to a trailhead parking lot next to a ranger residence on the right.

Description: From the lot, walk past a vehicle gate. The fire road beyond takes you across a sunny meadow, then up onto a brushy slope toward a saddle. In spring-

time, the air rising along the slopes bears both the tangy fragrance of new growth in the chaparral and the humid scent of riparian vegetation along the river just ahead.

Just beyond the saddle, the first of two short spur trails branches left and downward toward the river bottom. The second spur trail, 0.4 mile farther, leads to an artificial waterfall—a silted-in diversion dam.

After some further mild climbing, the road enters a magnificent grove of live oak trees and sidles up against the high banks of the river. At 1.9 miles, the fire road turns east toward Highway 79, while two other trails continue north toward Green Valley Falls and Green Valley Campground. This is the turnaround point for the simple, 3.8-mile, round-trip hike just described.

Those on foot or horseback may continue on the narrow trails ahead; they connect to the more than 100 miles of footpaths and fire roads in the central part of Cuyamaca Rancho State Park. Mountain bikers going farther must stick to the fire road bending east; they are not allowed on most of the "single-track" trails within the park.

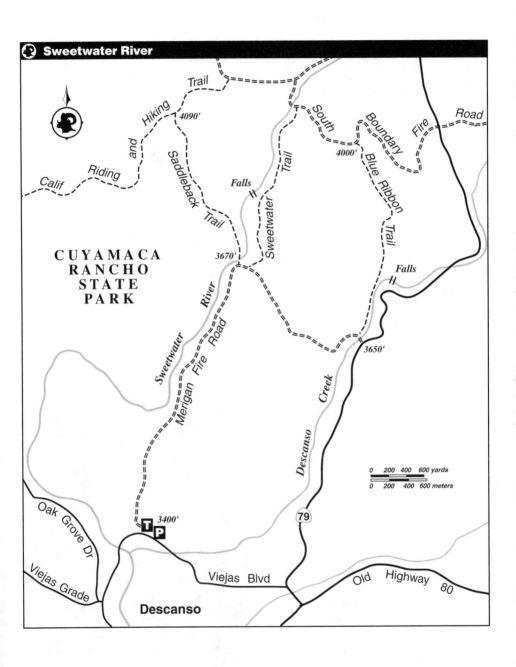

Sweetwater River

CUYAMACA
RANCHO
STATE
PARK

Calif

Riding

and

Hiking

Trail

4090'

Saddleback

Trail

Falls

3670'

Sweetwater

Trail

South

4000'

Boundary

Blue Ribbon

Fire

Road

Trail

Falls

3650'

Sweetwater

River

Merigan Fire Road

Descanso Creek

79

Oak Grove Dr

3400'

T P

Viejas Grade

Viejas Blvd

Old Highway 80

Descanso

| 0 | 200 | 400 | 600 yards |
| 0 | 200 | 400 | 600 meters |

HIKE 84

Horsethief Canyon

Location	Pine Creek Wilderness
Highlights	Cascades and shallow pools
Distance	3.2 miles round trip (to Pine Valley Creek)
Total Elevation Gain/Loss	500'/500'
Hiking Time	2 hours (round trip)
Optional Maps	USGS 7.5-min *Barrett Lake, Viejas Mountain*
Best Times	November through June
Agency	CNF/DD
Difficulty	★★

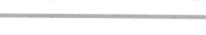

The croak of a soaring raven cracks the stillness as my companions and I saunter down the green-fringed path. A groggy dragonfly flits through a beam of morning sunlight. Cool air, slinking down the night-chilled slopes, caresses our faces and sets aflutter the papery sycamore leaves overhead. Approaching the pools and cascades of Pine Valley Creek, we smell the moist exudations of mule-fat and willow trees. We cup the clear, cold water in our palms and dash it across our heads.

If you want this kind of escape from the city—and you want it relatively quickly—Pine Creek Wilderness, east of San Diego, is one great place to find it. The 13,000-acre wilderness, in the Cleveland National Forest, was created by an act of Congress in 1984, and now includes about 25 miles of hiking trails within its borders. Dayhiking the wilderness requires no permit, though you must obtain a wilderness permit for overnight backpacking.

Average or better winter rains followed by spring sunshine transform the place into a foothill garden, with water dancing down the larger ravines and careening off boulders in Pine Valley Creek—the large drainage bisecting the wilderness. The tough chaparral vegetation coating the slopes gets to looking temporarily soft, the green of emerging

annual grasses turns positively lurid, and the live oaks, sycamores, and cottonwoods send out new leaves and branches in a burst of growth.

To Reach the Trailhead: The quickest and most impressive route into the wilderness is by way of Horsethief Canyon. The trailhead, at mile 16.4 on Lyons Valley Road, is similarly quick and

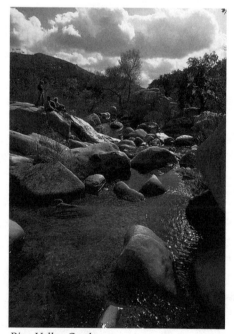

Pine Valley Creek

easy for San Diegans to reach. From I-8 at Alpine, follow Tavern Road 2.7 miles south, Japatul Road 5.8 miles east, and Lyons Valley Road 1.5 miles south to the trailhead. From Jamul, in south San Diego County, drive east and north, using Skyline Truck Trail and Lyons Valley Road, to get to the same point.

Description: From the trailhead parking lot, a sign directs you north along a gated dirt road for about 300 yards. You then veer right down a ravine on the signed Espinosa Trail. After a fast 400-foot elevation loss, the path bends right (east) to follow oak- and sycamore-lined Horsethief Canyon. True to its name, this corral-like canyon was used in the late 1800s by horse thieves to stash stolen horses in preparation for their passage across the international border. The canyon bottom is dry most of the year, but agreeably shaded throughout. After another mile and not much more descent, you reach Pine Valley Creek, which in winter and early spring brims with runoff from the creek's headwaters in the Laguna Mountains.

Upstream from the pool, you can make your way alongside or over a jumble of car-sized boulders and past several small cascades. Tangled willows and mule-fat (a willow look-alike) impede your progress. Watch your step on slippery slabs of rock, and be aware of poison-oak thickets, possible rattlesnakes, and fast water if your visit comes immediately on the heels of a big storm. You can continue in this manner—straight up the canyon bottom—for 3 picturesque miles or more.

If you're hooked on loop hikes, you can try the following, less-scenic return route: Proceed downstream from Horsethief Canyon along the west bank of Pine Valley Creek for 0.7 mile. At a point opposite the Espinosa Creek confluence, turn right (west) on an old roadbed paralleling a ravine. Follow its steep course upward through chaparral and over a summit to the trailhead parking lot.

Operation Gatekeeper, the federal government's attempt to stave off illegal immigration from Mexico into the United States, resulted in an eastward shift in migration patterns, and a huge increase in migrant foot traffic through the canyons of the Pine Creek Wilderness during the 1990s. By now, however, much of this continued migration has shifted far east into Imperial County and Arizona. Possibly you will see some travelers making their way north during your visit.

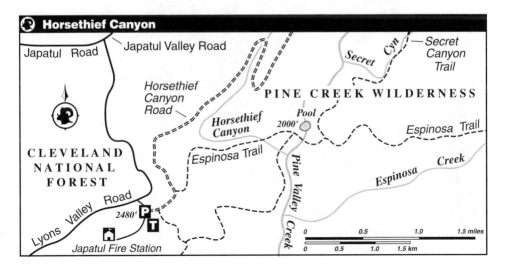

HIKE 85

Corte Madera Mountain

Location	South of Pine Valley
Highlights	Panoramic views
Distance	6.5 miles round trip
Total Elevation Gain/Loss	1750'/1750'
Hiking Time	4 hours (round trip)
Optional Maps	USGS 7.5-min *Morena Reservoir, Descanso*
Best Times	November through May
Agency	CNF/DD
Difficulty	★★★

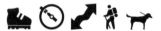

On a clear day atop Corte Madera Mountain, you can see forever—or at least as far as Santa Catalina and San Clemente islands to the west, and the mile-high Sierra Juarez plateau in Baja California to the south. From many parts of San Diego, Corte Madera Mountain's sheer south face appears as an abrupt drop in the profile of the eastern horizon. On the summit, you stand near the edge of that 300-foot-high precipice.

To Reach the Trailhead: To reach the hike's starting point, exit I-8 at Buckman Springs Road and proceed 3 miles south to Corral Canyon Road. Turn right (west), and proceed 4.8 miles on narrow pavement to a sharp hairpin turn. Unsigned, gated Kernan Road goes northwest from the hairpin. Park nearby off the road.

Description: First, squeeze around the gate and walk 0.5 mile uphill on Kernan Road. Where the road bends right in a

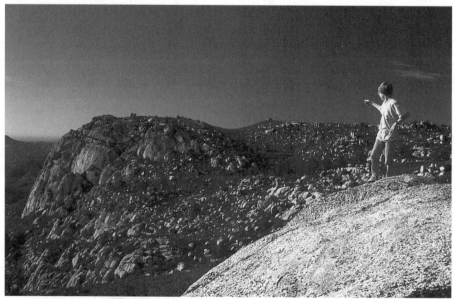

On the left, Corte Madera Mountain

horseshoe curve, go left on the Espinosa Trail and continue northwest. After one more mile of climbing, you top a saddle and intersect Los Pinos Road. Turn right and continue 0.3 mile to another saddle, this one a half mile southeast of boulder-studded, Coulter-pine-dotted peak 4588. Leave the road there and find and follow a path that works its way up past peak 4588 and across another saddle just northwest of the peak.

Continue following the path northwest, then finally southwest along a crest to the summit plateau of Corte Madera Mountain. The view north includes a fabulous vista, available nowhere else on public land, of privately owned Corte Madera Valley. A beautiful lake and oak-studded meadows fill the valley. The name Corte Madera ("woodyard") apparently refers to the use of this area as a source of timber during the building of the San Diego area missions.

Corte Madera Mountain's summit plateau is covered by large sheets of granitic rock supporting patches of chaparral. From the southernmost point on the plateau you can peer over the abrupt face into the canyon drained by Espinosa Creek. To the southeast is Los Pinos Mountain, topped by a fire lookout, one of the few remaining in Southern California that is used on a regular basis.

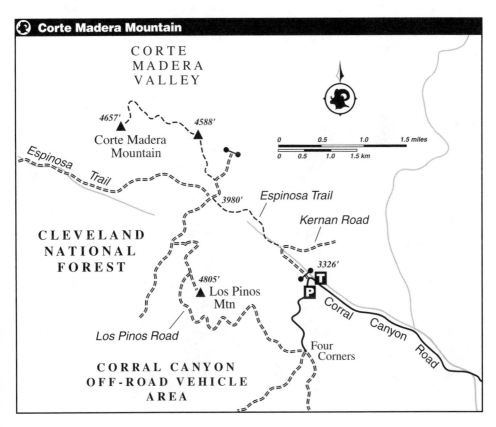

HIKE 86

Cottonwood Creek Falls

Location	Laguna Mountains
Highlights	Cascades and shallow pools
Distance	1.8 miles round trip
Total Elevation Gain/Loss	500'/500'
Hiking Time	1 hour (round trip)
Optional Map	USGS 7.5-min *Mount Laguna*
Best Times	December through June
Agency	CNF/DD
Difficulty	★★

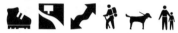

Hidden in the apex of a narrow valley in the Laguna Mountains near the town of Pine Valley, a small stream has worn its way down to metamorphic bedrock. Engorged on occasion by spates of heavy rain or melting snow, the stream comes alive, alternately dancing over ledges or inclined slabs, and pausing in placid pools. This is no Yosemite Falls, to be sure, but merely one of many secret beauty spots tucked away in the Southern California's mountainous folds. Known as Cottonwood Creek Falls, it remains attractive through spring and early summer. By July or August, summer's heat sucks it dry.

To Reach the Trailhead: From I-8 just east of Pine Valley, exit at Sunrise High-

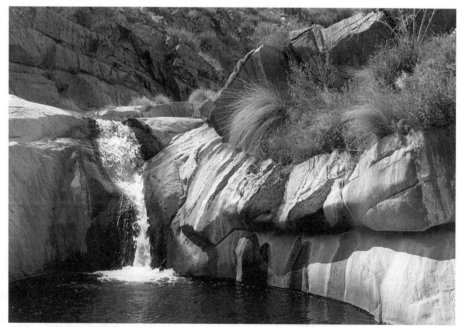

Cottonwood Creek Falls

way and proceed 2 miles north (uphill all the way) to two large turnouts on opposite sides of Sunrise Highway (near mile marker 15.0). Park a the north end of either turnout, and don't forget to display your National Forest Adventure Pass.

Description: From your parked car, walk over to the start of the unmarked trail, which is directly beneath a small powerline at the north end of the east-side turnout. The trail descends quickly at first. In the late spring white-blossoming ceanothus, beard tongue, and woolly blue curls, and blooming yuccas brighten the trailside all the way down, suffusing the air with a heady fragrance.

As you approach Cottonwood Creek, 0.7 mile down, turn sharply left and go upstream past some large oaks toward the cascades. After a bit of rock scrambling, and two easy crossings of the stream,

you'll reach the uppermost fall, where the stream drops 10 feet into a crystalline pool at least head-high deep. By May or June, the water warms to a temperature suitable for comfortable bathing, though by that time the flow in the creek may be sluggish and the water unappealingly tainted by algae.

The broad banks of the creek just below the falls area provide some nice camping space—if you don't mind packing overnight gear and hauling it on such a short journey.

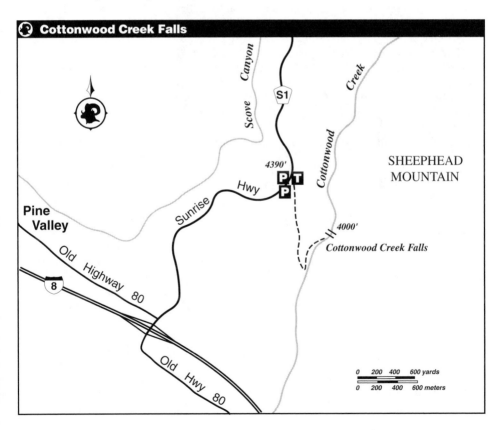

HIKE 87

Noble Canyon Trail

Location	Laguna Mountains
Highlights	Sparkling mountain stream; wildflowers
Distance	10.0 miles
Total Elevation Gain/Loss	650'/2400'
Hiking Time	5 hours
Optional Maps	USGS 7.5-min *Monument Peak, Mount Laguna, Descanso*
Best Times	October through June
Agency	CNF/DD
Difficulty	★★★

The Noble Canyon National Recreation Trail is an extension and reworking of an older trail built across the Laguna Mountains in the 1930s by the Civilian Conservation Corps. Since its completion in 1982 the trail has become popular among hikers, equestrians, and mountain bikers. With transportation arrangements set up in advance, you can travel one-way along this trail in the relatively easy downhill direction.

The route is a good one for backpacking, with suitable campsites located at frequent intervals along the way—particularly on shady terraces along the mid-portion of Noble Canyon. (Remember to establish your camp no less than 100 feet from water). Water flows in the canyon bottom year-round, though it slows to a trickle before the first rains of autumn. Purification is necessary if you intend to rely on it for your drinking or cooking.

To Reach the Upper Trailhead: Just east of Pine Valley, exit I-8 at Sunrise Highway and turn north. As you drive north (uphill) on Sunrise Highway, observe the green mile markers posted at half-mile intervals. The I-8/Sunrise Highway interchange is approximately at mile 13. You'll find the top end of the trail at the Penny Pines trailhead, mile 27.3 on Sunrise Highway, where parking space is plenti-

ful along the highway shoulder. A National Forest Adventure Pass is required for parking here.

To Reach the Lower Trailhead: From the town of Pine Valley, drive west 1 mile on Old Highway 80 to Pine Creek Road, next to a bridge over Pine Creek. Turn right and proceed 1.6 miles to the Noble Canyon trailhead on the right. A National Forest Adventure Pass is required for parking here.

Description: From the Penny Pines trailhead, head west along the marked Noble Canyon Trail, along the southern border of the burn caused by the 2003 Cedar Fire. Possibly only a few of the Jeffrey pines that grew here will survive; the black oaks will likely far better during the recovery period.

As you rise a bit along the north slope of a steep hill, your view to the north extends to the distant summits of San Jacinto Peak and San Gorgonio Mountain. You descend to cross dirt roads three times, then climb and circle around the chaparral-clad north end of a north-south trending ridge. This seemingly out-of-the-way excursion avoids privately owned "in-holdings" in the national forest, and it opens up interesting vistas to the north and west. Three varieties of blooming ceanothus brighten the view in springtime.

Next, you descend into the upper reaches of Noble Canyon, where you will exit the Cedar Fire burned zone. After a wet season, the grassy hillsides show off springtime blooms of blue-purple beard tongue, scarlet bugler, woolly blue curls, yellow monkeyflower, Indian paintbrush, wallflower, white forget-me-not, wild hyacinth, yellow violet, phacelia, golden yarrow, checker, lupine, and blue flax.

The trail sidles up to the creek at about 3.0 miles, and stays beside it for the next 4 miles. Past a canopy of live oaks, black oaks, and Jeffrey pines, you emerge into a steep, sunlit section of canyon. The trail cuts through chaparral on the east wall, while on the west wall only a few hardy, drought-tolerant plants cling to outcrops of schist rock.

Back in the shade of oaks again, you soon cross a major tributary creek from the east. This drains the Laguna lakes and Laguna Meadow above. Pause for a while in this shady glen, where the water flows over somber, grayish granitic rock and gathers in languid pools bedecked by sword and bracken fern. Look for nod-

ding yellow Humboldt lilies in the late spring or early summer.

You continue through oak woodland and riparian vegetation for some distance downstream. Mixed in with the oaks, you'll discover some incense-cedar and California bay trees. The creek is screened by a typical growth of willows and sycamores. The understory vegetation includes dense thickets of poison oak, Indian-basket bush, wild rose, and wild strawberries.

You may discover some mining debris—the remains of a flume and the stones of a disassembled arrastra (a horse- or mule-drawn machine for crushing ore), dating from gold-mining activity in the late 1800s. Old cabin foundations are also in evidence.

Crossing to the west side of the creek, you break out of the trees and into an open area with sage scrub and chaparral vegetation. The trail contours to a point about 100 feet above the creek, then maintains this course as it bends around several small tributaries, open to the midday sunshine nearly the whole way. Yucca,

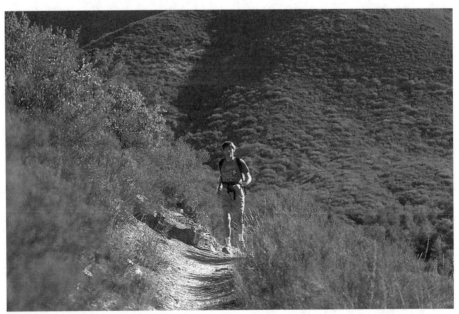

Jogging lower Noble Canyon Trail

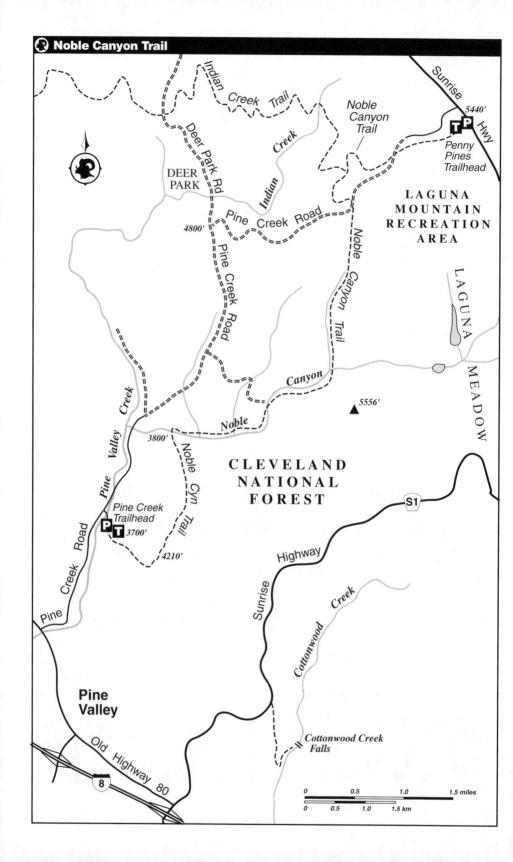

Indian Creek Trail

Noble Canyon Trail

Sunrise Hwy

5440'

T **P**

Penny Pines Trailhead

Deer Park Rd

Indian Creek

DEER PARK

LAGUNA MOUNTAIN RECREATION AREA

Pine Creek Road

4800'

Noble Canyon Trail

LAGUNA MEADOW

Pine Creek Road

Canyon

5556'

Pine Valley Creek

Noble

3800'

CLEVELAND NATIONAL FOREST

S1

Noble Cyn Trail

Pine Creek Trailhead

P **T** 3700'

4210'

Pine Creek Road

Highway

Sunrise

Cottonwood Creek

Pine

Pine Valley

Old Highway 80

8

Cottonwood Creek Falls

0	0.5	1.0	1.5 miles
0	0.5	1.0	1.5 km

prickly-pear cactus, and even hedgehog cactus—normally a denizen of the desert—make appearances here.

At about 7 miles, the trail switches back, crosses the Noble Canyon creek for the last time, and veers up a tributary canyon to the south. The trail joins the bed of an old jeep road, reaches a saddle after nearly 2 miles from Noble Canyon, then diverges from the old roadbed, going right (west) over another saddle. It then descends along a particularly rocky course (tough on mountain bikes, but not too bad for hikers) directly to the Noble Canyon trailhead near Pine Creek Road.

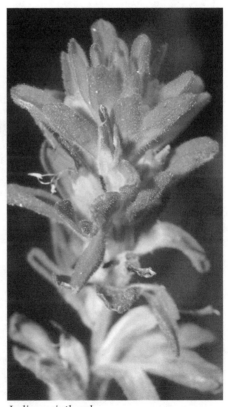

Indian paintbrush

HIKE 88

Oasis Spring

Location	Laguna Mountains
Highlight	Hidden, shady spot with a spring, overlooking the desert
Distance	2.0 miles round trip
Total Elevation Gain/Loss	300′/300′
Hiking Time	1 hour (round trip)
Optional Map	USGS 7.5-min *Monument Peak*
Best Times	All year
Agency	CNF/DD
Difficulty	★

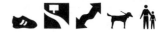

A more restful place could scarcely be imagined. A warm breeze from the desert below wafts up the narrow canyon, bringing with it the scent of sage and California bay. A bigleaf maple tree shimmers in the sunlight. A sparkling stream gushes out of the ground and begins a headlong rush toward the dry desert sands a half mile below. "Oasis" is a perfectly apt name for this idyllic spot.

To Reach the Trailhead: Just east of Pine Valley, exit I-8 at Sunrise Highway and turn north. As you ascend, observe the green mile markers posted at half-mile intervals along the Sunrise Highway shoulder. They increase from approximately mile 13 at the I-8/Sunrise Highway interchange. At mile 26.7, a gated dirt road takes off down along the slope to the right (east). Parking is very limited here;

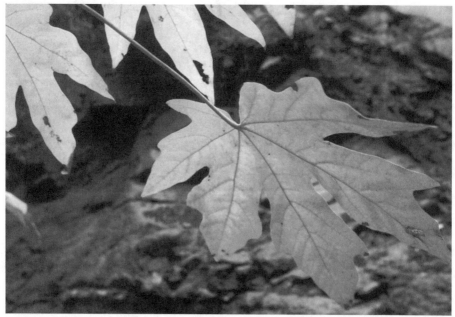

Bigleaf maple

an east-side turnout at mile 26.5 offers more room. Don't forget your National Forest Adventure Pass.

Description: From the turnout, you can pick up the Pacific Crest Trail alongside and follow it north. After about 300 yards, the PCT dips into a shallow ravine and briefly joins the dirt road to Oasis Spring. Once you're on the dirt road, stay on it and continue descending through a chaparral zone largely burned during the 2002 Pines Fire, and now showing signs of regrowth.

Curving left, the road leaves the ravine and briefly traverses the abrupt face of the Laguna escarpment. From the lip of the road there's a dramatic view of distant alluvial fans and barren peaks in the Anza-Borrego Desert far below. The road soon ends, but a narrowing trail continues, zigzagging down through growths of live oak and bay laurel to reach an old pumphouse. The bigleaf maple tree here may have been planted. The normal range of the bigleaf maple within the Pacific coast states extends no farther south than the Santa Ana and San Bernardino mountains.

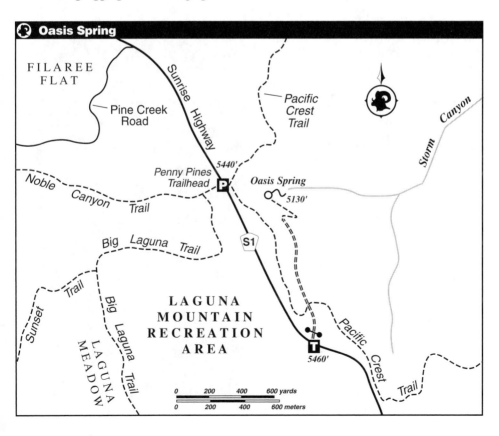

HIKE 89

Garnet Peak

Location	Laguna Mountains
Highlights	Outstanding desert views
Distance	2.4 miles round trip
Total Elevation Gain/Loss	500'/500'
Hiking Time	1 ½ hours (round trip)
Optional Map	USGS 7.5-min *Monument Peak*
Best Times	All year
Agency	CNF/DD
Difficulty	★★

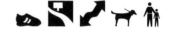

Although Garnet Peak isn't the highest peaklet along the Laguna Mountain rim, its exposed position makes it a good place to view both the pine-clad Laguna plateau and the raw desert below. Especially rewarding is a predawn pilgrimage to observe the sunrise from its summit. Around the time of the winter solstice, the sun's flattened disk peeps up over the desert wastes of northwestern Sonora, Mexico, some 150 miles away. On the clearest mornings at that time of year, you might witness the famed "green flash," an event occasionally seen on the horizon at sunset on the coast, but seldom seen at sunrise anywhere.

To Reach the Trailhead: Just east of Pine Valley, exit I-8 at Sunrise Highway and turn north. As you drive uphill, observe the green mile markers posted at half-mile intervals along the Sunrise Highway shoulder. They increase from approximately mile 13 at the I-8/Sunrise Highway interchange. Find a place to park off the pavement of Sunrise Highway near mile 27.8, and find the start of the Garnet Peak Trail on the right (east) side of the highway. Be sure to post a National Forest Adventure Pass on your parked car.

Description: Follow the Garnet Peak Trail 0.5 mile north through burned timber to where it crosses the Pacific Crest

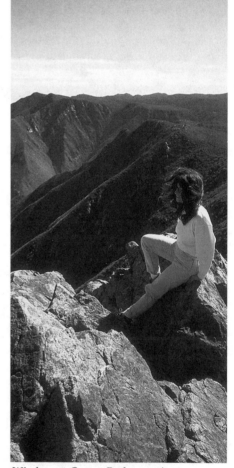

Windswept Garnet Peak summit

Trail. The area you are traversing was where the eastward-moving Cedar Fire of 2003 met the edge of the burn area of 2002's Pines Fire and essentially died due to lack of fuel.

Continue north, away from the burned timber and onto a rocky path that slants up along the shoulder of the peak. Before many years go by, these slopes will again see Lord's candle yucca stalks, heavy with white flowers in the spring and early summer poking through ceanothus and manzanita brush along the trail.

Garnet Peak'summit is crowned by a jagged cluster of layered, tan-colored metasedimentary rock, the type seen along much of the Laguna escarpment. The peak falls away abruptly to the east and south, revealing a vertiginous panorama of Storm Canyon and its distant alluvial fan. Along the horizon lie the

Salton Sea and Baja's Laguna Salada, both desert sinks. To the south and west, the Laguna crest, dusky with patches of pine and oak trees and chaparral, seems to roll like a frozen wave to the edge of the escarpment.

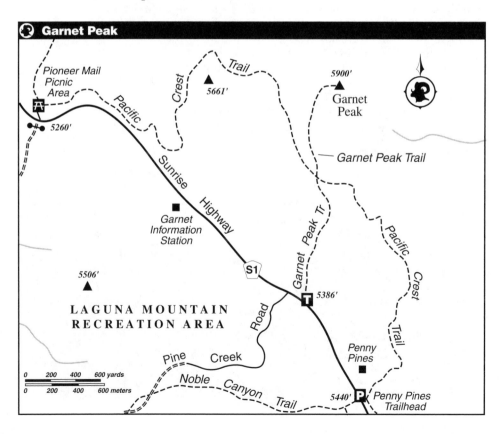

HIKE 90

Sunset Trail

Location	Laguna Mountains
Highlight	Colorful spring and autumn vegetation, views
Distance	7.2 miles
Total Elevation Gain/Loss	700'/700'
Hiking Time	4 hours
Optional Map	USGS 7.5-min *Monument Peak, Mount Laguna*
Best Times	September through June
Agency	CNF/DD
Difficulty	★★★

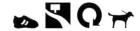

The Sunset Trail, opened in 1993, permits easy access by foot along the west rim of the high Laguna Mountain plateau. Like its analog a few miles east—the sunrise-facing Pacific Crest Trail—the Sunset Trail offers fine panoramas, but on the sunset side of the mountain. Early mornings are by far best (certainly during the warm summer season) to take advantage of cool temperatures and clear, tangy air. In the hour or two after sunrise, you can often look down upon a white and frothy ocean of stratus clouds hugging a hundred-mile strip of coastline.

To Reach the Trailhead: From I-8 just east of Pine Valley, drive about 5 miles uphill along Sunrise Highway. At or near the Meadows Information Station, mile 19.1, park along the highway shoulder, which is wide enough in this area to accommodate parking by visitors who come up by the hundreds in winter to play in the snow.

Description: From the information station itself, walk a little way uphill along the highway shoulder to reach the trailhead, marked by a wooden sign. An unmarked fork in the trail in about 100 yards

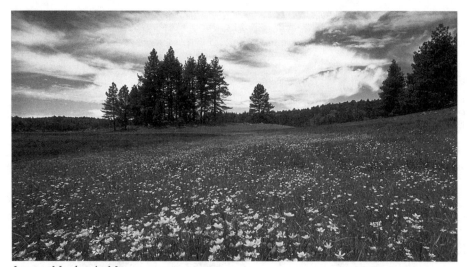

Laguna Meadow in May

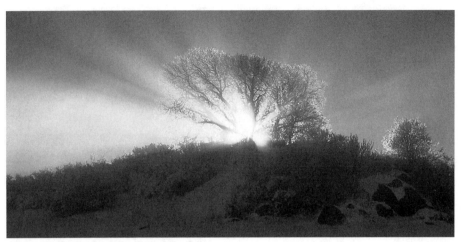

An icy morning along the Sunset Trail

may confuse you. Stay left, and gradually climb toward a gently undulating ridge crest dotted with vanilla-scented Jeffrey pines and black oaks. After nearly a mile, the trail suddenly veers left to circle a rocky outcrop. There, a view opens of velvet-smooth Crouch Valley, some 500 feet below, and much of coastal San Diego County whenever clear air prevails at lower altitudes. The view is certainly worth the trivial effort invested so far.

Onward, you descend gradually for a while, then rise again, reaching (at 1.5 miles) the lowermost edge of Laguna Meadow and a beautiful pond called "Water of the Woods." Veering left, the Sunset Trail follows the edge of the pond for a short while, then slants up the ridge to the left (northwest).

You climb back up to the viewful crest, with more opportunities to scan the broad western horizon. Farther north, you pass over a hilltop and descend to the northernmost arm of Laguna Meadow. Turning east, the trail meets, at 3.9 miles, the Big Laguna Trail. If the ground is soggy, you may want to turn around here and return the same way. Otherwise, you can loop back across Laguna Meadow as follows:

Turn right on the Big Laguna Trail and follow it south about 1.5 miles to Big La-

guna Lake, the biggest of several shallow, ephemeral lakes in the meadow. In an average rainy season, these lakes begin to fill with water or snow by December or January. By April or May, as the meadow dries, carpets of wildflowers—tidy tips, buttercups, goldfields, dandelions, wild onions, and western irises—begin to appear. Summer heat causes water levels in the lakes to decline rapidly.

Just past Big Laguna Lake the trail turns decidedly east. You can leave it at this point and head straight across the broad meadow, almost due south, toward some structures associated with the Laguna Ranch. During the wet season, snow covers the meadow on several occasions, but it quickly melts. In February or March the meadow may be too soggy to easily cross. Later in the year you may have to thread your way through cattle in the meadow. The ranch and the meadow are on public land, but ranchers retain grazing rights. As you get closer to the ranch, veer right so you can get through a gate in a barbed-wire fence some 300 yards west of the ranch house. Continue bearing southwest until you intersect the Sunset Trail near the point where you began your hike.

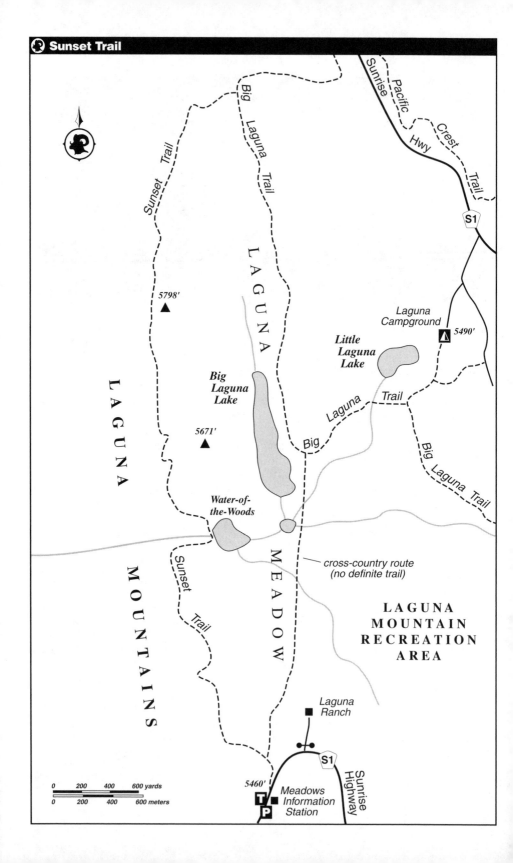

5798'

L A G U N A

Big Laguna Trail

Sunset Trail

Sunrise Hwy

Pacific Crest Trail

S1

Laguna Campground

5490'

Little Laguna Lake

Big Laguna Trail

Big Laguna Lake

5671'

Big

Laguna

Trail

Water-of-the-Woods

L A G U N A

M E A D O W

cross-country route (no definite trail)

LAGUNA MOUNTAIN RECREATION AREA

Sunset Trail

M O U N T A I N S

Laguna Ranch

S1

Sunrise Highway

5460'

T P

Meadows Information Station

0 200 400 600 yards
0 200 400 600 meters

HIKE 91

Culp Valley

Location	Northern Anza-Borrego Desert State Park
Highlights	Secluded, oasis-like spring; desert views
Distance	1.7 miles
Total Elevation Gain/Loss	300'/300'
Hiking Time	1 hour
Optional Map	USGS 7.5-min *Tubb Canyon*
Best Times	September through June
Agency	ABDSP
Difficulty	★

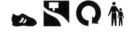

While the low desert swelters, the temperature hovers in a more moderate register at Culp Valley, 3000 feet higher. This is the only designated camping area in the Anza-Borrego Desert where the heat on the cooler days of May, June, or September is quite bearable. July and August daytime temperatures there are probably too warm for most people's tastes—typically the 90s and 100s.

Stark, gray boulders are piled up all around the floor of Culp Valley, thrusting upward into an azure sky. The west wind blows capriciously, often whistling eerily through the rocks. Nearby, out of sight from the valley, is a hillside spring surrounded by an oasis of green grass and shrubs. It's this kind of contrast that makes hiking here especially rewarding.

To Reach the Starting Point: Drive to mile 9.2 (according to the green mileage signs posted every half mile) on County Highway S22, Montezuma Highway. Turn north onto the unpaved entrance road leading into the no-frills Culp Valley Campground. This turnoff is 4 miles east of Ranchita, and about 9 miles west of Borrego Springs. The campground is free, with newer restrooms and several scattered open spaces where you can park your car or small RV, day or night.

Description: On foot from the campground head back toward the highway

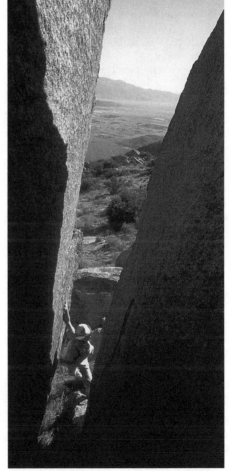

Split boulder below Culp Valley vista point

and take the road branching west toward Pena Spring. After a few minutes, the road ends on a crest. You continue north down a narrowing trail following the bottom of a shallow ravine. You quickly pass the signed California Riding and Hiking Trail. Note this intersection; you will return here after visiting the spring.

Going downhill for another 0.2 mile, you pass into the burn zone of the August 2002 Pines Fire, which managed to lick its way northeast into the remote Hellhole and Borrego Palm canyons farther northeast before dying out due to lack of anything further to burn.

On the hillside to the left look for Pena Spring, an oozing acre or so nourishing a verdant patch of green grass and fire-following vegetation. The spring is a nocturnal mecca for rabbits, coyotes, deer,

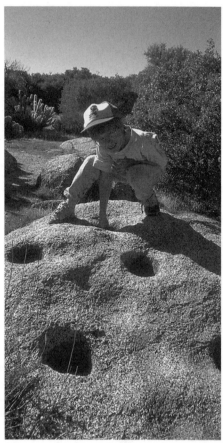

Morteros near Pena Spring

bighorn sheep, and other animals partaking of the clear, cold groundwater reaching the surface here. Nearby, you can look for a large, flat boulder pocked with several deep *morteros*, or Indian grinding holes.

After visiting the spring, backtrack up the road 0.2 mile to the intersection of the California Riding and Hiking Trail. Turn left (east) on this trail, climbing up, then along, a flattish ridge offering good views of nearby Culp Valley on the right, and tantalizing glimpses of the deep gorge on the left—Hellhole Canyon. The ridge wasn't recently burned, so you'll find juniper, catclaw, desert apricot, buckwheat, white sage, buckhorn and prickly pear cacti, and Mojave and Lord's candle yucca—collec-

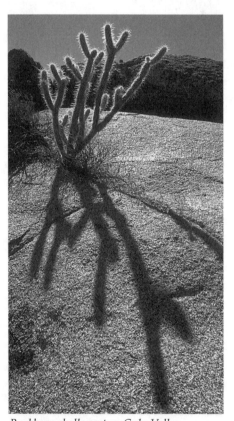

Buckhorn cholla cactus, Culp Valley

tively representing a transition zone between montane chaparral and high-desert scrub.

After 0.5 mile on the California Riding and Hiking Trail, you come to an unmarked trail junction in a saddle. To return to Culp Valley, veer right and continue 0.3 mile south into the campground. Before doing that, try climbing the low rock outcrop just north of the trail junction. There, you get a jaw-dropping view of the Hellhole Canyon gorge, Borrego Valley, and the towering Santa Rosa Mountains. About 0.2 mile farther east there's a slightly higher "vista point" on a hilltop that offers a more panoramic view.

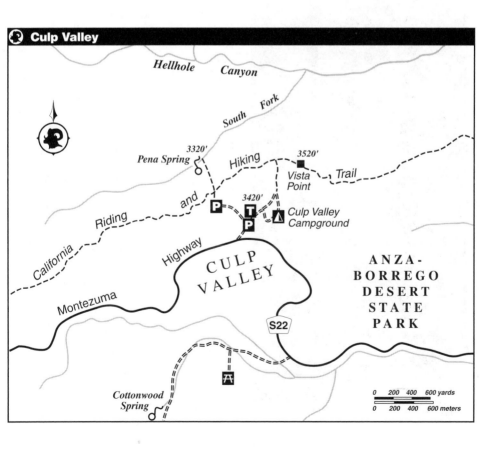

HIKE 92

Hellhole Canyon

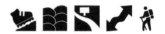

Location	Northern Anza-Borrego Desert State Park
Highlight	Hidden waterfall in desert canyon
Distance	5.0 miles round trip
Total Elevation Gain/Loss	900'/900'
Hiking Time	3 ½ hours (round trip)
Optional Map	USGS 7.5-min *Tubb Canyon*
Best Times	December through May
Agency	ABDSP
Difficulty	★★★

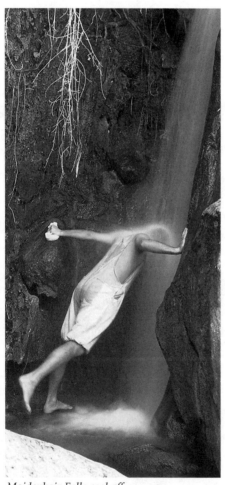

Maidenhair Falls cool-off

In the midst of one of America's hottest and driest deserts, it seems a bit surprising to find a place where mosses, ferns, sycamores, and cottonwoods flourish around a sparkling waterfall. Maidenhair Falls is such a place, and it lies not far from Borrego Springs and the popular Anza-Borrego Desert State Park visitor center.

To Reach the Trailhead: From Christmas Circle (the traffic circle in the center of Borrego Springs), drive 1.3 miles west on Palm Canyon Drive to Montezuma Highway, and go south 0.7 mile to the large trailhead parking area on the west side of Montezuma Highway.

Description: From the parking lot, head west on a wide trail (an old roadbed) straight across and up an alluvial fan toward the gaping mouth of Hellhole Canyon. The sandy surface of the fan supports a variety of vegetation, stratified according to elevation. Indigo bush, chuparosa, cheesebush, burroweed, creosote bush, desert lavender, and buckhorn cholla are the common plant species of the lower fan. They're largely replaced by jojoba, brittlebush, ocotillo, and teddy-bear cholla on the upper fan. Everywhere, jackrabbits flit among the bushes, startled by your approach.

As you approach the canyon mouth, a mile from the trailhead, you may hear (in a wet year, at least), the sound of flowing water. Usually the water doesn't get very far on the surface; it quickly sinks into porous sand as it spreads out and slows on the fan below. As the canyon walls pinch in, you soon find yourself threading a path near the flowing water. Generally, you'll want to stay away from the boulder-filled and vegetation-choked canyon bottom. Sooner or later you'll get involved in difficult scrambles over large boulders and fallen trees, and perhaps have unpleasant encounters with catclaw thorns. The remnants of trees that litter the canyon are a result of past wildfires. Fan palms—the signature tree of the Anza-Borrego Desert—begin to appear.

About 200 yards past a dense cluster of palms, the canyon walls pinch in really tight. Tucked away in a corner of the canyon bottom—hard to find—you'll discover the grotto containing Maidenhair Falls. The falls plunge about 25 feet into a shallow pool. Tiers of maidenhair fern adorn the grotto, and sopping wet mosses cover the places the ferns don't.

Further travel up-canyon from Maidenhair Falls involves much battle with the underbrush—slow going on a dayhike, and slower if you're backpacking. Ambitious hikers can explore the remote higher reaches of the canyon. Some have traveled up the canyon's South Fork tributary, which leads to Pena Spring near Culp Valley.

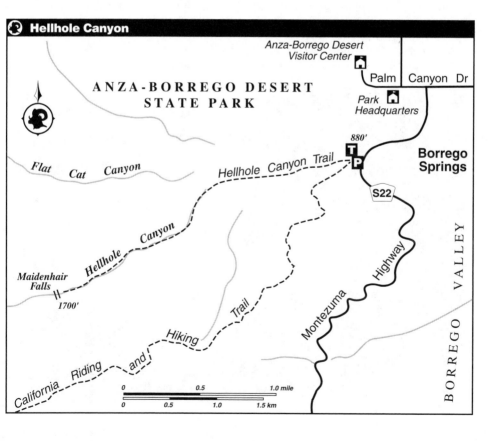

HIKE 93

Borrego Palm Canyon

Location	Northern Anza-Borrego Desert State Park
Highlights	Most dramatic display of native palms in California; spring wildflowers
Distance	3.0 miles round trip
Total Elevation Gain/Loss	450'/450'
Hiking Time	1 ½ hours (round trip)
Optional Map	USGS 7.5-min *Borrego Palm Canyon*
Best Times	October through May
Agency	ABDSP
Difficulty	★

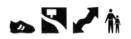

Borrego Palm Canyon has long been famous for harboring many hundreds of native palm trees in an otherwise austere setting of rock and sun-blasted vegetation. Perhaps 80 percent of these palms, which have surprised and delighted thousands of visitors over several decades, were summarily evicted from the canyon at 4:45 P.M. on September 10, 2004. On that afternoon an isolated, intense summer thunderstorm dumped buckets of rain over a relatively small area of the San Ysidro Mountains above. Sheets of water falling down the steep slopes gathered strength and speed as they joined forces in the narrow constriction of the canyon. A wall of water perhaps 30 feet high tore away nearly everything in its path.

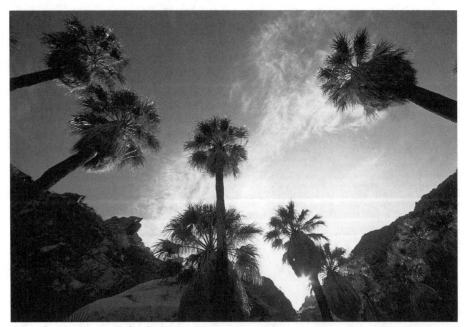

Fan palms in Borrego Palm Canyon

Borrego Palm Canyon Campground was hit soon after with a roiling mass of muddy water—carrying palm trunks and other debris—about 100 feet wide and moving at least 40 miles per hour. Witnesses ran for higher ground, or escaped down the campground's entrance road in speeding cars. Ironically, not drop of rain fell that day in Borrego Springs, just three miles away.

Dubbed a "hundred-year flash flood" by some, the event was indeed a rare occurrence for that particular location in the Anza-Borrego Desert. But it was not unusual for the geographical region as a whole. Isolated and locally intense thunderstorms commonly strike the Anza-Borrego Desert and Colorado Desert region during mid-July through mid-September's "monsoon" season.

Since the 2004 flash flood, Borrego Palm Canyon Campground's facilities have been repaired, and hikers are again making their way up the Borrego Palm Canyon Nature Trail to what remains of the "First Palm Grove" just inside the canyon's lower portal. You can learn more about the California desert flora on that trail than anywhere else around Anza-Borrego. Be sure to pick up the interpretive leaflet for the trail at the Anza-Borrego visitor center, or when you enter Borrego Palm Canyon Campground. The nature trail begins at the far end of the campground.

To Reach the Trailhead: From Christmas Circle (the traffic circle in the center of Borrego Springs), drive 1.4 miles west on Palm Canyon Drive toward the Anza-Borrego Visitor Center. Just before reach-

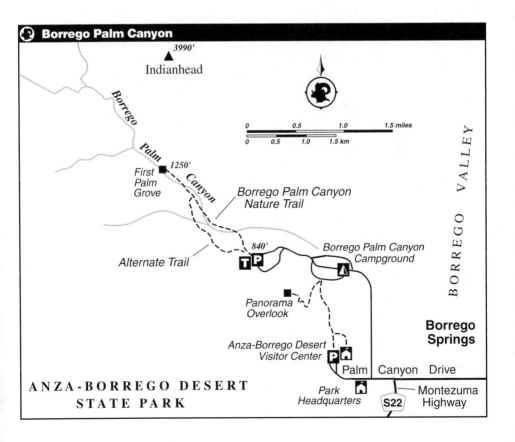

ing the visitor center, turn right on the access road leading into Borrego Palm Canyon Campground. At the gate pay the day-use or camping fee; then proceed to the Borrego Palm Canyon trailhead at far west end of the campground. Next to the trailhead are rest rooms and a pond holding transplanted desert pupfish.

Description: Interpretive markers and plaques line the main nature trail, which roughly parallels the canyon bottom and measures about 1.5 miles along its revised alignment. (It is also possible, either on the way up or on the way back, to follow a somewhat circuitous alternate trail on the left, or south, side that stays high above the canyon floor and visits a zone thick with thorny ocotillos.)

The initial crossing of canyon bottom on the main trail lets you inspect the flood-torn riverbed, which may be wet or dry, depending on recent rainfall. You then ascend moderately on the rocky alluvial fan toward the canyon's mouth. You'll be able to see and identify (using trail markers or plaques) mesquite, sage, catclaw, indigo bush, desert lavender, creosote bush, brittlebush, ocotillo, desert-willow, chuparosa, and various kinds of cactus. This vegetation looks drab most of the year, but really lights up in a rainbow of colors by March in a wet year. In the past couple of decades, the native bighorn sheep that frequent the canyon have become quite accustomed to passing hikers. Sometimes they may graze contentedly only a stone's throw from the trail.

As you approach the canyon's narrow mouth, desert-varnished rock walls soar dramatically 3000 feet upward on both sides. You follow the trail up a series of steps hewn in the rock, passing a gauging station and a small waterfall, and then enter the formerly abundantly shaded zone of the First Grove. The grove is a ghost of its former self, its stream-hugging riparian vegetation peeled away along with nearly all lower-lying palms. Higher-growing palms remain. They are of one variety, *Washingtonia filifera*, the only palm indigenous to California.

Fan palms are invasive wherever water is permanently present—if not on the surface then at least underground. The palms will likely return in force to this site over the next quarter century, as will alders, sycamores, and other lush types of vegetation.

The Borrego Palm Canyon Nature Trail ends at First Grove. Further exploration of canyon ahead is not for casual tourists. The game is to work your way upward on sketchy paths high above the canyon bed, or more often along the flood-scoured bed itself, which is paved unevenly with sand and flood-tossed rocks, and granitic or metamorphic bedrock slabs. As riparian vegetation returns to the canyon bottom in the years to come, it will increasingly slow the pace of intrepid hikers.

At 3.3 miles from the trailhead, the South Fork of Borrego Palm Canyon branches obviously to the left (southwest), its discharge of water less than that of the main fork. A spectacular double-cascade of water lies 0.4 mile ahead up this rough gorge—a worthy destination for motivated hikers willing to clamber over angular rocks.

HIKE 94

Villager Peak

Location	Northern Anza-Borrego Desert State Park
Highlights	Ever-present dramatic views
Distance	13.0 miles round trip
Total Elevation Gain/Loss	5000'/5000'
Hiking Time	11 hours (round trip)
Recommended Maps	USGS 7.5-min *Fonts Point, Rabbit Peak*
Best Times	October through May
Agency	ABDSP
Difficulty	★★★★

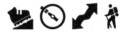

Despite its remoteness, Villager Peak is one of the more popular destinations for "serious" Southern California peak baggers. More than a hundred people every year succeed in reaching the summit, and the box containing the peak register is often overflowing with business cards and other mementos. Many people backpack the route, but others, who must start at or before sunrise, manage to complete the round trip as a dayhike. The importance of taking plenty of water on this wholly waterless route cannot be overemphasized.

The approach to Villager Peak is straightforwardly up, using a single north-trending ridge of the Santa Rosa Mountains. One or more paralleling trails follow this ridge—the result of recent use by hikers, prehistoric use by desert-dwelling Indians, and more or less continual use by bighorn sheep. On the way down, however, navigational difficulties may be encountered where watershed di-

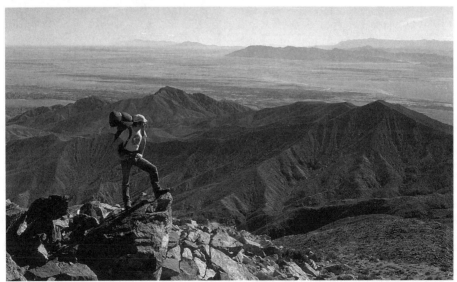

A pause at mid-elevation enroute to Villager Peak

vides split and go their separate ways. Bighorn sheep don't necessarily stick to the main route, and their trails may lure you off the main ridge onto some steeply plunging side ridge.

To Reach the Trailhead: From Borrego Springs, drive 13 miles northeast on Borrego Salton Seaway (County Highway S22). Park in the northside turnout at mile 31.8.

Description: On foot, proceed north toward the east end of a long, sandy ridge 0.5 mile away. The north face of this ridge is a huge scarp along the San Jacinto Fault—said to be one of the largest fault scarps in unconsolidated earth material in North America. North of this ridge, flash-floods exiting from Rattlesnake Canyon have cut a series of braided washes in a swath about 0.6 mile wide. A faint path marked by "ducks" (small piles of stones) takes you over this dissected terrain to the base of the long, ramplike ridge leading to Villager Peak.

The initial climb is very steep, but the route soon levels off to a rather steady gradient averaging about 1000 feet per mile. Stay on the highest part of the ridge to remain on route. Creosote bush, ocotillo, and glistening specimens of barrel cactus, hedgehog cactus, and silver, golden, and teddy-bear cholla cactus grace the slopes below 3000 feet. Dense thickets of wicked-looking agave at 3000 to 4000 feet will slow you down. At times, you feel as if you were threading a spiny gauntlet.

Along the lower part of the ridge you'll come upon several Indian "sleeping circles," which may have been used as windbreaks or to anchor shelters made from local vegetation. At about the 3000-foot level (3.0 miles) a green patch marking Rattlesnake Spring comes into view in a tributary canyon of Rattlesnake Canyon, about 1.5 miles east.

At 4100 feet (4.3 miles), you'll pass along the edge of a spectacular dropoff overlooking Clark Valley. The white band of rock prominently displayed along the

face of this escarpment is marble—metamorphosed limestone. Thought to be some of the oldest rock exposed in San Diego County, it originated from ocean-floor sediments deposited about half a billion years ago. Just beyond the 4800-foot contour (5.0 miles), the ridge descends a little to a small, exposed campsite with airy views both east and west.

In the next mile the ridgeline becomes quite jagged. Pinyon, juniper, and nolina (a relative of the yucca) now dominate. At 6.5 miles, you reach the rounded, 5756-foot summit of Villager Peak, offering good campsites amid a sparse forest of weather-beaten pinyon pines. The views are practically aerial all around the compass. A clear, calm, moonless night spent here is an unforgettable experience. Despite the horizon glows of cities from Los Angeles to Mexicali, the stars above shine fiercely in a charcoal sky. At dawn, the silvery surface of the Salton Sea mirrors the red glow spreading across the east horizon.

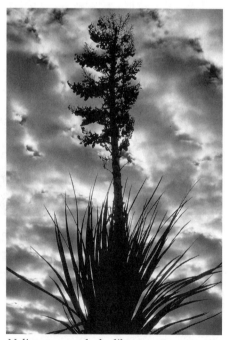

Nolina, a yucca look-alike

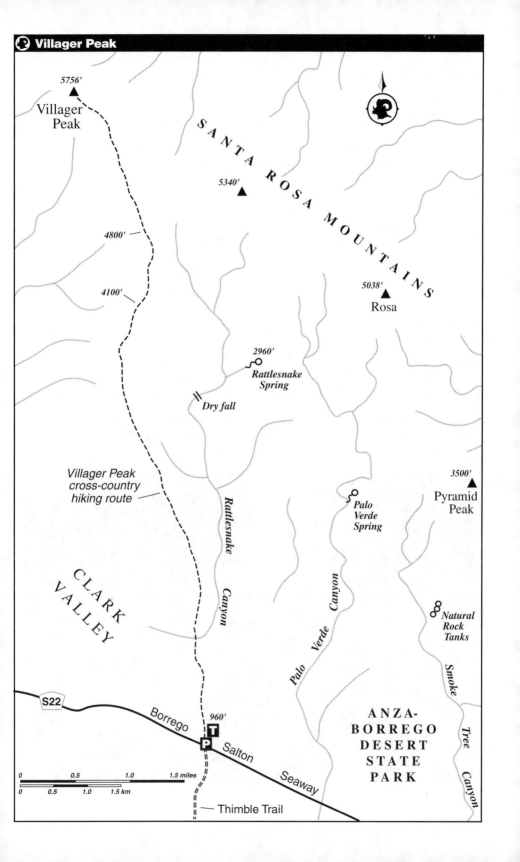

5756'
▲
Villager
Peak

S A N T A   R O S A   M O U N T A I N S

5340'
▲

4800'

4100'

5038'
▲
Rosa

2960'
○
Rattlesnake
Spring

Dry fall

3500'
▲
Pyramid
Peak

Villager Peak
cross-country
hiking route

Palo
Verde
Spring

Rattlesnake Canyon

C L A R K
V A L L E Y

Palo Verde Canyon

Natural
Rock
Tanks

S22

Borrego

960'
T
P

Salton

Seaway

A N Z A -
B O R R E G O
D E S E R T
S T A T E
P A R K

Smoke Tree Canyon

0   0.5   1.0   1.5 miles
0   0.5   1.0   1.5 km

Thimble Trail

HIKE 95

Calcite Mine

Location	Northern Anza-Borrego Desert State Park
Highlights	Eroded, slotlike gorges; historic interest
Distance	4.2 miles
Total Elevation Gain/Loss	800'/800'
Hiking Time	2 hours
Optional Map	USGS 7.5-min *Seventeen Palms*
Best Times	November through April
Agency	ABDSP
Difficulty	★★

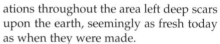

Thousands of years of cutting and polishing by water and wind erosion have produced the chaotic rock formations and slotlike ravines you'll discover in the Calcite Mine area. The highlight of this hike is, of course, the mine itself. During World War II, this was an important site—indeed the only site in the United States—for the extraction of optical-grade calcite crystals for use in gunsights. Trench-mining operations throughout the area left deep scars upon the earth, seemingly as fresh today as when they were made.

Lately the old jeep road leading to the mine has become increasingly rough and eroded, with partial washouts daunting enough to turn back only the most nimble 4-wheel-drive vehicles and dune buggies. This has made the route quieter for hikers.

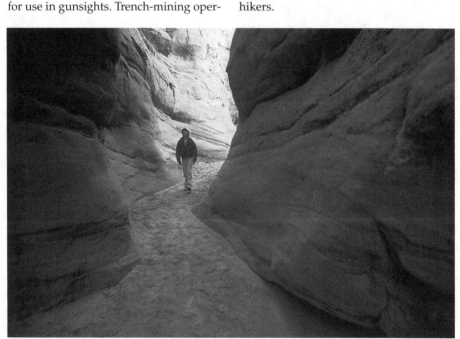

South Fork Palm Wash

To Reach the Trailhead: From Borrego Springs, drive 13 miles northeast on Borrego-Salton Seaway (County Highway S22). Park in the roadside turnout at mile 38.0.

Description: From the turnout, walk 0.1 mile east to the Calcite jeep road intersection. An interpretive panel here gives some details about the history of the mine. Follow the jeep road as it dips into and out of South Fork Palm Wash, and continues northwest toward the southern spurs of the Santa Rosa Mountains. Ahead you will see an intricately honeycombed whitish slab of sandstone, called Locomotive Rock, which lies behind (northeast of) the mine area.

About 1.4 miles from S22, the road dips sharply to cross a deep ravine. Poke into the upper (north) end of this ravine and you'll discover one of the best slot canyons in Anza-Borrego. (Skilled climbers can squeeze through the slot and go up a break on the right side to reach a point above and northwest of the mine area.)

At road's end you may find bits of calcite crystal strewn about on the ground, glittering in the sunlight. You could spend a lot of time exploring the mining trenches and the pocked slabs of sandstone nearby.

Palm Wash, a frightening gash in the earth, precludes travel to the east.

On the return, try this alternate route: Backtrack 0.5 mile to the aforementioned deep ravine. Proceed downstream along its bottom. As you pass through deeper and deeper layers of sandstone strata, the ravine narrows until it allows the passage of only one person at a time. When you reach the jumbled blocks of sandstone in Palm Wash at the bottom of the ravine, turn right, walk 0.3 mile downstream, and exit the canyon via a short link of jeep trail that leads back to the Calcite road.

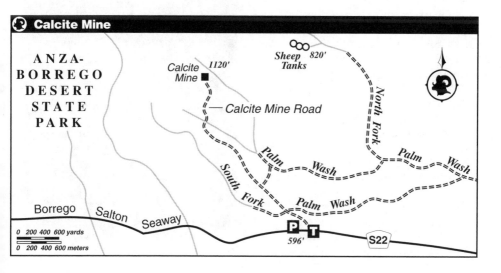

Calcite Mine

ANZA-
BORREGO
DESERT
STATE
PARK

Calcite Mine ■ 1120'

Sheep 820'
Tanks

Calcite Mine Road

North Fork

Palm Wash

Palm Wash

South Fork Palm Wash

Borrego Salton Seaway

0 200 400 600 yards
0 200 400 600 meters

596' P T

S22

HIKE 96

Oriflamme Canyon

Location	Southern Anza-Borrego Desert State Park
Highlight	Hidden waterfall
Distance	2.6 miles round trip (to waterfall)
Total Elevation Gain/Loss	500'/500'
Hiking Time	2 ½ hours (round trip)
Optional Maps	USGS 7.5-min *Earthquake Valley, Julian*
Best Times	November through April
Agency	ABDSP
Difficulty	★★★

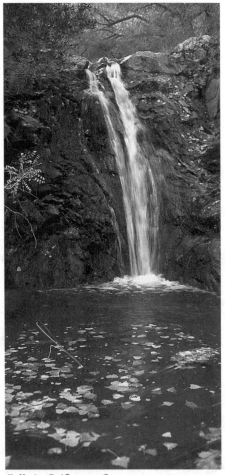

Oriflamme Canyon's gurgling waters are borne to the open air at a spring high on the east slope of the Laguna Mountains. For 5 miles or so they trickle over polished granite and schist bedrock, tumble over small waterfalls, and nourish a line of oaks, sycamores, willows and cottonwoods. At Mason Valley, down on the Anza-Borrego Desert floor, they finally sink into porous sand.

As soon as the late-fall or winter rains come, the flow of water down Oriflamme Canyon is copious. At one point the water cascades impressively over a 15-foot precipice within a hidden grotto of rock and riparian vegetation. This is the destination of the short but semi-rough hike described here. Wear long pants, or you'll be subjected to intolerable levels of flagellation meted out by the low-growing catclaw, prickly pear, and cholla cactus. Also be aware that this is prime rattlesnake habitat, so be especially alert and cautious during warm weather.

To Reach the Trailhead: From "Scissors Crossing"—the intersection of State Highway 78 and County Highway S2 on the west edge of Anza-Borrego Desert State Park—drive 9 miles south on Highway S2 to a dirt road (at mile 26.8 according to the green highway mileage markers) signed ORIFLAMME CANYON, 4-wheel drive recommended. Drive in for 2 miles, then stay left

Falls in Oriflamme Canyon

as the road forks at Rodriguez Canyon. Continue for another 0.8 mile to a rough side road on the left, leading down to a Depression-era road construction camp. Park off this road.

Description: From your parked car, find and follow an old, partly overgrown cattle trail that follows, in the upstream direction on the right bank, a sloping bench overlooking the canyon bottom. After 0.5 mile the trail dips and then crosses the stream for the first time. In the narrower canyon bottom ahead, you walk back and forth across the bubbling stream and over orange and brown leaf litter. Look for Indian *morteros* (grinding holes) worn into some of the streamside boulders.

After 1.3 miles, a major tributary comes in from the right (west). Proceed another 0.1 mile south and you'll come upon the sublime, almost hidden 15-foot cascade and a shallow pool, framed by the twisted trunks of sycamores. Watch out for poison oak growing along the stream here.

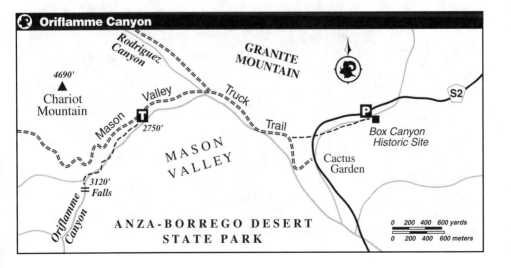

HIKE 97

Ghost Mountain

Location	Southern Anza-Borrego Desert State Park
Highlight	Historic interest
Distance	2.0 miles round trip
Total Elevation Gain/Loss	400'/400'
Hiking Time	1 ½ hours (round trip)
Optional Map	USGS 7.5-min *Earthquake Valley*
Best Times	October through May
Agency	ABDSP
Difficulty	★★

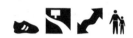

The California desert has been home to many an eccentric person, but possibly none so audacious as Marshal South. From 1931 until the mid-'40s. Marshal and his poet wife, Tanya, lived atop Ghost Mountain, a rock-strewn, remote mountaintop in the Anza-Borrego Desert, depending in large part on local resources for food, water, and shelter. There, they built an adobe cabin, "Yaquitepec"; fash-ioned an ingenious rainwater collection system; raised three children; and tried to emulate, to one degree or another, the life of the prehistoric Indians.

The ruins of Yaquitepec are today one of Anza-Borrego's noted attractions—and quite easy to reach.

To Reach the Trailhead: From "Scissors Crossing"—the intersection of State Highway 78 and County Highway S2 on the

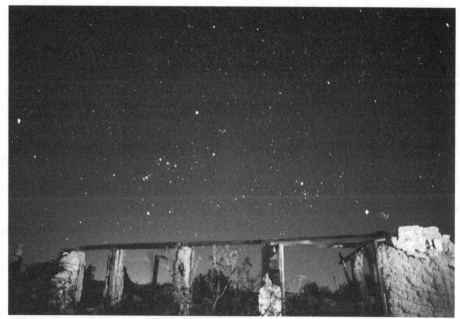

Winter constellations over Yaquitepec ruins

west edge of Anza-Borrego Desert State Park—drive 5 miles south on Highway S2 to a dirt road on the left (at mile 22.9 according to the green highway mileage markers) into Blair Valley, a large, flat expanse of land spreading east. Stay left as you enter the valley, and follow the main dirt road around the north and east sides of Blair Valley for 2.7 miles. On the right is a signed spur road going southwest, leading toward a trailhead at the base of Ghost Mountain.

Description: From the parking area at the end of the road a trail climbs in switchbacks up the rocky slope, and turns east along the ridge to the Yaquitepec site. Little remains of the dwelling except melting mud walls and the water cistern, but the view from the site is impressive.

When not consumed with the business of survival, Marshal South wrote maga-

zine articles detailing the family's experiences on what was then a nearly inaccessible mountaintop. His writings appeared frequently in *Desert Magazine* during the 1940s. These articles are well worth looking up in the library.

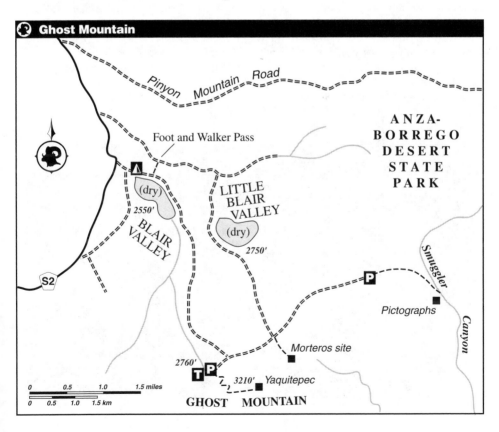

HIKE 98

Whale Peak

Location	Southern Anza-Borrego Desert State Park
Highlights	Dwarf pinyon-juniper forest; huge boulders; panoramic desert views
Distance	4.5 miles round trip
Total Elevation Gain/Loss	1500'/1500'
Hiking Time	3 ½ hours (round trip)
Recommended Map	USGS 7.5-min *Whale Peak*
Best Times	October through May
Agency	ABDSP
Difficulty	★★★

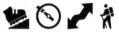

Whale Peak is probably the most visited major summit in Anza-Borrego Desert State Park. Hundreds of people every year day-hike or backpack into this serene, wooded island in the desert sky. Whale Peak yields to approaches from nearly every direction. The area around it, however, can prove distressing from a navigational point of view. The peak lies within a complex of similar-looking hogback ridges and gentle valleys, and the peak itself remains hidden from view until you are almost upon it. Count on no sources of water along the way—even storm runoff sinks immediately into the porous, decomposed granite soil.

Whale Peak's north-approach hiking route is the shortest of all, with the least elevation gain. To reach the starting point, though, you face a possibly challenging drive up a primitive dirt road, which has deteriorated in recent years. Light-duty SUVs won't make it up this road anymore.

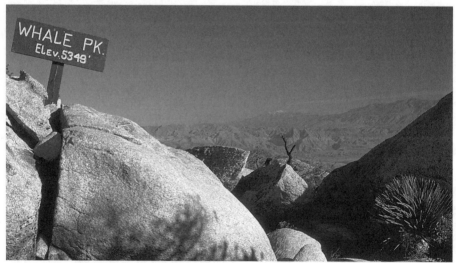

The summit of Whale Peak

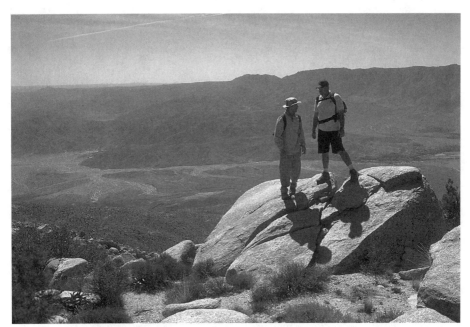

West shoulder of Whale Peak

To Reach the Trailhead: From "Scissors Crossing"—the intersection of State Highway 78 and County Highway S2 on the west edge of Anza-Borrego Desert State Park—drive 4 miles south on Highway S2 to a dirt road on the left (at mile 21.4 according to the green highway mileage markers) signed PINYON MOUNTAIN AREA. Stay right (east) at a fork in 0.1 mile, and continue up the alluvial fan toward the Vallecito Mountains and their domelike crown, Whale Peak. After 5.7 miles the road tops a watershed divide at 3980 feet elevation in the middle of a saddle called Pinyon Mountain Valley, a remote place that's terrific for car camping (assuming your vehicle will get you there). A spur road going south from the saddle ends at the foot of a ravine that will be your starting point for the hike.

Description: On foot head directly up the ravine, climbing south over and around small trees and big boulders. Near the top of the ravine you bend left and emerge onto a sandy flat just below 4400 feet. You can now find and follow the main informal trail—or just as effectively one or more alternate routes marked by hiker's ducks (small piles of stones)—trending southeast over and around several rocky summits. You might want to keep track of your position by map and compass techniques, or with the help of a GPS receiver. Flat areas for trail camping are quite abundant along the way to the top.

The assemblage of pinyon pine, juniper, scrub oak, manzanita, yucca, and nolina on these north facing slopes of Whale Peak are what botanists call the pinyon-juniper woodland plant community. Similar habitats lie on the rim of the Mojave Desert to the north, and on the Sierra Juarez plateau south of the Mexican border.

Eventually, you'll come to a small valley west-northwest of the Whale Peak summit. From this point you climb south up to the peak's west shoulder, and then scramble east over and around boulders to the flattish top of the mountain. A large boulder complex marks the peak's 5349-

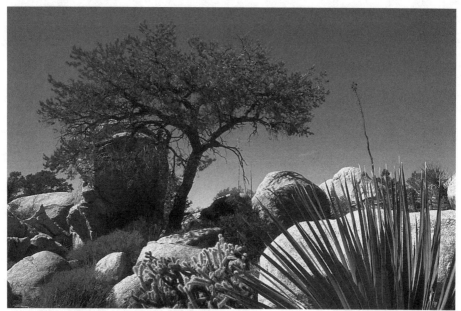

Pinyon pine, nolina, and cactus cling to life on the bouldery slopes of Whale Peak

foot maximum elevation. Nearby you can find a climbers' register where you can add your name to the long list of hikers who have enjoyed being where you are.

On a clear day atop Whale Peak, the panorama is superb: the Salton Sea in the east, Baja's mesalike Sierra Juarez in the south, and the dark wall of the Laguna Mountains to the west.

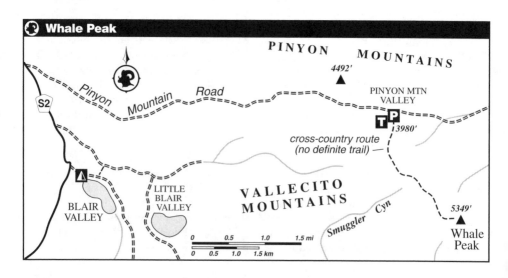

HIKE 99

Moonlight Canyon Trail

Location	Agua Caliente Regional Park (Southern Anza-Borrego)
Highlights	Desert views; geologic interest
Distance	1.5 miles
Total Elevation Gain/Loss	350'/350'
Hiking Time	1 hour
Optional Map	USGS 7.5-min *Agua Caliente Springs*
Best Times	October through May
Agency	SDCP
Difficulty	★

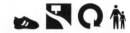

Take in a deep breath of clean, dry air. Bask in the larger-than-life brilliance of the desert sun. Sink into the womblike comfort of warm spring water. At Agua Caliente Springs you can have your cake and eat it too—hike first, then enjoy a relaxing soak in the hot springs. A San Diego County park has been established here in the midst of state park lands at the foot of the Tierra Blanca Mountains.

A splinter of the Elsinore Fault is responsible for the upwelling of warm, mineral-rich water here. The same fault passes through the Lake Elsinore area and Warner Springs, where hot springs are also found. There are two options for soaking at Agua Caliente Springs: a shallow outdoor pool with spring water flowing through at its ambient temperature of about 95°F, and a large indoor jacuzzi pool where the water's temperature is boosted to more than 100°F.

To Reach the Trailhead: You'll find Agua Caliente along County Highway S2, 27 miles northwest of I-8 at Ocotillo, and 22 miles southeast of Highway 78 at Scissors Crossing. Currently, the park is open September through May, and closed during the hot summer months.

Description: As for hiking, the Moonlight Canyon Trail—one of several short trails in the area—is a good one to start on. This well-marked but somewhat steep

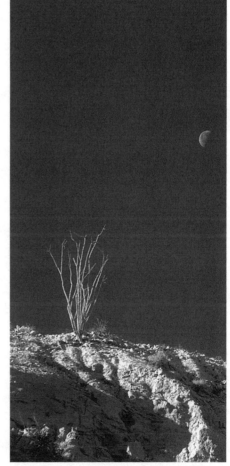

Ocotillo above Moonlight Canyon Trail

and rugged trail, starts at the south end of the campground, climbs over a rock-strewn saddle, drops into a small wash mysteriously named Moonlight Canyon, descends past some seeps and a little oasis of willows in the wash bottom, and finally circles back to campground. Although moonlight treks around this trail are possible, a good flashlight wouldn't hurt after dark.

True to their name, the Tierra Blanca ("white earth") Mountains are composed of light-colored granitic rock. In some areas this type of rock gradually acquires a patina of oxidized iron and manganese minerals called desert varnish. Right here, however, the rock has been pounded and fractured by movements along the Elsinore Fault. It easily decomposes into the light-colored mineral crystals the make up the coarse sand you will be walking on.

From the high point on the Moonlight Canyon Trail, 300 feet above the campground, you can climb off-trail an additional 250 feet to reach Peak 1882, offering a superb view of Carrizo Valley and the Vallecito Mountains, including Whale Peak. Another, longer side trip, again cross-country, can be made up-canyon (south) in Moonlight Canyon to a point overlooking the Inner Pasture, an isolated valley ringed by the boulder-punctuated Tierra Blanca and Sawtooth mountains.

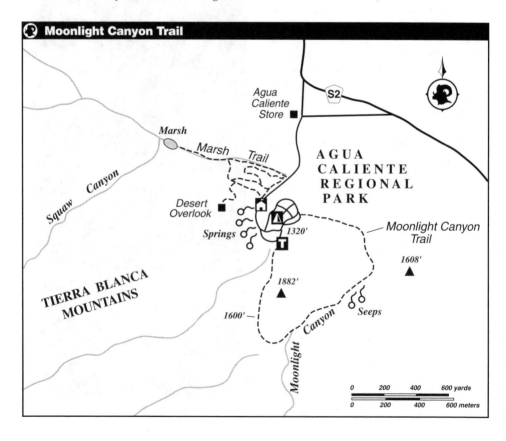

HIKE 100

Mountain Palm Springs

Location	Southern Anza-Borrego Desert State Park
Highlights	Groves of native palms
Distance	2.5 miles
Total Elevation Gain/Loss	350'/350'
Hiking Time	1 ½ hours
Optional Map	USGS 7.5-min *Sweeney Pass*
Best Times	October through May
Agency	ABDSP
Difficulty	★★

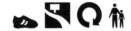

If you like the contrast between palm-tree oases and a raw landscape of sand and eroded rock, you'll love Mountain Palm Springs. The palms here are gregarious, growing in dense clusters, often with pools of water at their feet. Some have never been burned: they still hold full skirts of dead fronds around their trunks, the better to serve the local population of rodents and snakes. In late fall and early winter, the sticky, sweet fruit of the palms hangs in great swaying clusters, sought after by birds and the sleek coyotes that prowl up and down the washes. The palm groves are distributed along several small washes that drain roughly a square-mile area on the east side of the Tierra Blanca Mountains near the south end of Anza-Borrego Desert State Park.

Consider the loop hike described here as a fairly complete tour of the area; but do be enticed to extend your explorations in the form of side trips or extended loop trips if the spirit moves you.

To Reach the Trailhead: At a point 20 miles northwest of I-8 at Ocotillo, and 29 miles southeast of Highway 78 at Scissors Crossing (mile 47.1 on County Highway S2 according to the green roadside mile markers), take the dirt road going 0.7 mile west to the Mountain Palm Springs primitive camping area in a bowl-shaped area at the foot of the mountain range.

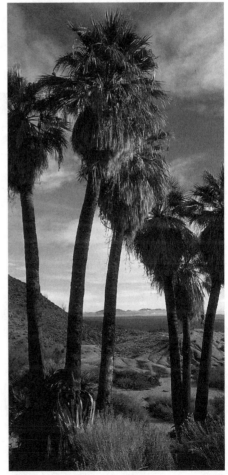

Palms at Southwest Grove

Description: From the camping area, begin by walking up the small canyon to the left (southwest). Past some small seeps you'll come upon the first groups of palms—Pygmy Grove. Some of these smaller but statuesque palms grow out of nothing more than rock piles.

A long pause is in order ahead at Southwest Grove, a restful retreat shaded by a vaulted canopy of shimmering fronds. A rock-lined catch basin fashioned for the benefit of the local wildlife mirrors the silhouettes of the palms. A couple of elephant trees cling to the slopes just above the grove, but for a better look at these curious plants, you can climb a spur trail to Torote Bowl, where a bigger group of elephant trees will be found.

From Southwest Grove, pick up the well-worn but obscure trail that leads north over a rock-strewn ridge to Surprise

Canyon Grove in Surprise Canyon. Up-canyon from this small grove lies Palm Bowl, filled with tangled patches of mesquite and fringed on its western edge by more than a hundred tall palms. On warm winter days, the molasseslike odor of ripe palm fruit wafts upon the breeze, and phainopepla hoot and flit among the palm crowns, their white wing patches flashing.

North of Palm Bowl Grove, an old Indian pathway leads over a low pass to Indian Gorge and Torote Canyon, where many more elephant trees thrive—another possible diversion. To conclude the loop hike, however, you return to Surprise Canyon Grove and continue down-canyon to the campground. On the way, you pass North Grove, hidden in a side drainage on the left.

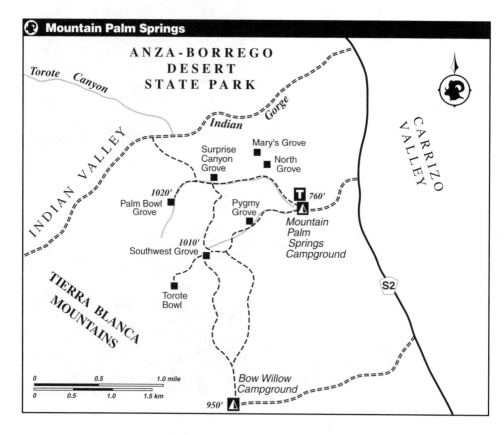

HIKE 101

Mortero Palms to Goat Canyon

Location	Southern Anza-Borrego Desert State Park
Highlights	Rugged, palm-filled canyon; view of historic railroad
Distance	5.0 miles round trip (to view of trestle)
Total Elevation Gain/Loss	2500'/2500'
Hiking Time	5 hours (round trip)
Recommended Map	USGS 7.5-min *Jacumba*
Best Times	November through April
Agency	ABDSP
Difficulty	★★★

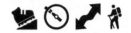

The 200-foot-high, 600-foot-long trestle over Goat Canyon on the San Diego & Arizona Eastern rail line is revered among railroad buffs everywhere. It has been called the longest curved railroad trestle and one of the highest wooden trestles in the world.

Dubbed the "impossible railroad," the San Diego & Arizona Eastern tracks were laid through southern Anza-Borrego's Carrizo Gorge in the second decade of the 20th Century. Starting in 1919, the railroad carried freight, and for a time passengers, between San Diego and the Imperial Valley. The gorge section features 11 miles of twisting track, 17 tunnels, and numerous trestles. The current Goat Canyon trestle, built over a tributary of Carrizo Gorge, was completed in 1933 as part of a re-alignment of the original route. In 1976 Hurricane Kathleen churned northward up along the Gulf of California, dropped about 10 inches of rain on southern Anza-Borrego, and severely mangled the gorge section of the railroad—rendering it impassable for almost five years. After reopening in 1981, the line was quickly severed again, this time by a fire that burned several trestles. Not until 2004 did the line open yet again, starting with limited freight service. Sightseeing passenger excursions along the Carrizo Gorge segment are being considered.

Walking the tracks is expressly forbidden. On the following, practically beeline hike over rough terrain, however, it is possible to get a fine view of the magnificent Goat Canyon trestle, which lies in the middle and most remote section of Carrizo Gorge.

To Reach the Trailhead: You'll start hiking at the Mortero Palms trailhead, close to the rock outcrop known as Dos Cabezos ("two heads"). To get there from I-8 at Ocotillo, proceed north and west on Highway S2 for 4 miles to a dirt road on the left (from this point on, high clearance or 4-wheel drive may be needed). Go south on this road and swing right after 1.1 miles. Continue west for another 4.6 miles, and turn left across the railroad tracks on a paved crossover. Go right, continue another 0.1 mile, then veer left, away from the tracks. Go another 1.6 miles, staying left at the next two junctions, and then go right to the end of the road, where you can park.

A detailed topographic map of the area is recommended, and these directions assume you have one.

Description: A wide wash lies below the roadend. The Mortero Palms grove, your first destination, is in the canyon to the west (not the narrower canyon to the south). So, head west along the south side of that west-trending canyon for a while,

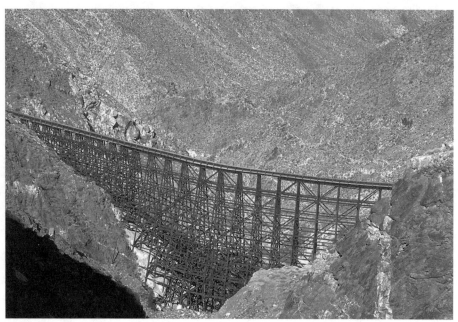

Goat Canyon trestle

avoiding the vegetation-choked streambed. After you've climbed over some boulders, look for a half-dozen *morteros* (Indian mortars), namesakes of the palm grove, in the center of the drainage 100 yards below the lower end of the grove.

Groundwater close to the surface supports the dense cluster of palms amid an otherwise dramatically desolate scene of rounded granitic boulders set against the deep blue sky. On warm days the grove is a seductively cool spot, and it takes some will power to get moving again to tackle the short but steep stretch of canyon ahead. Traverse left or right, or climb the water-polished rocks directly if you're a real daredevil. Any way you choose you'll get briefly involved in at least one difficult rock-climbing maneuver.

At the 2440-foot contour it's easier to leave the canyon bottom temporarily and go up on the slope to the north through stands of teddy-bear cholla. Don't trip here—this type of cholla cactus bristles with thousands of stiff, barbed spines. Drop back in at about 2750 feet, but leave

the canyon again at the 2840-foot contour. Proceed west and southwest across a small saddle and continue west over a divide into the Goat Canyon drainage.

Descend to a delightful, juniper-dotted bowl at about 3200 feet, a nice spot to spend the night if you are backpacking. Goat Canyon descends steeply farther west of here. Down at about 2700 feet in the canyon, there's an excellent, though somewhat distant view of the curved trestle, framed by the steep walls of canyon.

Further exploration in the area might include a visit to 4512-foot Jacumba Peak, the high point of the Jacumba Mountains, which lies some 2 miles south.

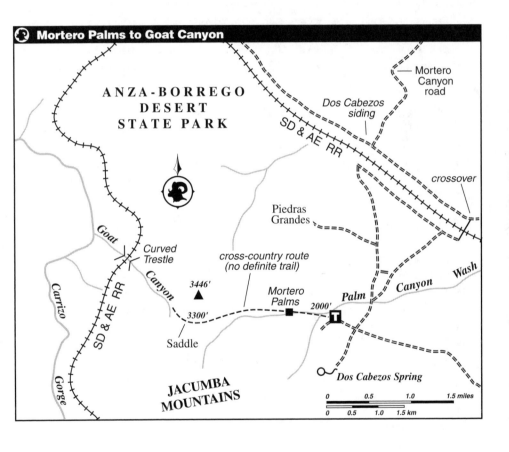

Mortero Palms to Goat Canyon

ANZA-BORREGO
DESERT
STATE PARK

Mortero
Canyon
road

Dos Cabezos
siding

SD & AE RR

crossover

Piedras
Grandes

Goat

Curved
Trestle

cross-country route
(no definite trail)

Canyon

Carrizo

SD & AE RR

3446'
▲

3300'

Mortero
Palms

2000'

Palm

Canyon

Wash

T

Saddle

Gorge

JACUMBA
MOUNTAINS

Dos Cabezos Spring

0   0.5   1.0   1.5 miles

0   0.5   1.0   1.5 km

Summary of Hikes

HIKE	DIFFICULTY*	TERRAIN	PRINCIPAL ATTRACTIONS
1 Paradise Falls	★★	Inland foothill canyon	Waterfall
2 Happy Camp Canyon	★★★	Inland foothill canyon	Oak groves; geological interest
3 La Jolla Valley Loop	★★★	Coastal foothill & canyon	Views; botanical interest
4 Sandstone Peak	★★★	Coastal peak	Views; geological formations
5 The Grotto	★★	Coastal canyon	Oak groves; geological interest
6 Charmlee Natural Area	★★	Coastal foothills	Views; wildflowers
7 Zuma Canyon	★★★★	Coastal canyon	Stream & cascades; views
8 Point Dume to Paradise Cove	★★	Beach	Intertidal exploration; views
9 Solstice Canyon	★	Coastal canyon	Sheltering oak groves
10 Temescal Canyon	★★	Coastal foothill & canyon	Views; botanical interest
11 Will Rogers Park	★	Coastal foothills	Views
12 Cheeseboro & Palo Comado Canyons	★★★	Inland foothills	Botanical interest
13 Old Stagecoach Road	★★	Inland foothills	Views; historical interest
14 Placerita Canyon	★★	Inland foothill canyon	Waterfall; historical interest
15 Verdugo Mountains	★★★	Inland foothills	Views
16 Trail Canyon Falls	★★	Mountain canyon	Waterfall
17 Mt. Lukens-Grizzly Flat Loop	★★★★	Mountain peak & canyon	Views
18 Down the Arroyo Seco	★★★	Mountain canyon	Stream & cascades
19 Mt. Lowe	★★	Mountain peak	Views
20 Millard Canyon	★★★	Mountain canyon	Stream; historical interest
21 Mt. Lowe Railway	★★★	Mountain slope	Views; historical interest
22 Eaton Canyon	★★	Inland foothill canyon	Waterfall
23 Santa Anita Canyon Loop	★★★	Mountain canyon & slope	Streams; historical interest
24 Vetter Mountain	★★	Mountain peak	Views
25 Cooper Canyon Falls	★★	Mountain canyon	Waterfall
26 Mt. Waterman Trail	★★★	Mountain slope	Views
27 Devil's Punchbowl	★	Desert canyon	Geological formations
28 Mt. Baden-Powell Traverse	★★★	Mountain peaks	Views
29 Lightning Ridge Nature Trail	★	Mountain slope	Botanical interest
30 Lewis Falls	★	Mountain canyon	Waterfalls
31 Mt. Islip	★★★	Mountain peak	Views
32 Down the East Fork	★★★★★	Mountain canyon	Cascading stream
33 Fish Canyon Falls	★★	Mountain canyon	Waterfall

HIKE	DIFFICULTY*	TERRAIN	PRINCIPAL ATTRACTIONS
34 Old Baldy	★★★	Mountain peak	Views
35 Cucamonga Peak	★★★★	Mountain peak	Cascading stream; views
36 Cougar Crest Trail	★★	Mountain slope	Botanical interest; views
37 Forsee Creek Trail	★★★★	Mountain slope & peaks	Streams; views
38 Dollar Lake	★★★★	Mountain slope	Streams; alpine lake
39 San Gorgonio Mountain	★★★★	Mountain peak	Streams; views
40 Deep Creek	★★	Mountain canyon	Hot springs
41 Big Morongo Canyon	★	Desert oasis	Streams; birding & wildlife
42 Wonderland of Rocks Traverse	★★★★	Desert canyons	Geological interest
43 Ryan Mountain	★★	Desert peak	Views
44 Ladder Canyon	★★★	Desert canyons	Slot ravine
45 Tahquitz Canyon	★★	Desert canyon	Waterfall; botanical interest
46 San Jacinto Peak (easy)	★★★	Mountain peak	Views
47 San Jacinto Peak (hard)	★★★★★	Desert to mountain peak	Views; botanical interest
48 San Jacinto Peak (middle)	★★★★	Mountain peak	Views
49 Tahquitz Peak	★★★	Mountain peak	Views
50 Toro Peak	★★	Mountain peak	Views
51 Lone Tree Point on Catalina	★★	Island peak	View; botanical interest
52 Water Canyon	★★	Inland foothill ravine	Oaks & riparian vegetation
53 Santiago Oaks Regional Park	★	Inland foothill	Stream; oaks
54 El Moro Canyon	★★	Coastal canyon	Oaks & riparian vegetation
55 Whiting Ranch	★★	Inland foothill ravine	Oak woodland; geological formations
56 Santiago Peak	★★★	Mountain peak	Views
57 Trabuco Canyon	★★★	Mountain canyon & ridge	Wildflowers; views
58 Bell Canyon Loop	★★	Inland foothill & canyon	Geologic & botanical interest
59 San Juan Loop Trail	★	Mountain canyon	Waterfall & pool
60 Sitton Peak	★★★	Mountain peak	Views
61 Tenaja Falls	★	Mountain canyon	Waterfall
62 Tenaja Canyon	★★★	Mountain canyon	Cascading stream; oaks
63 Santa Rosa Plateau Ecological Reserve	★★	Inland foothills	Wildflowers; vernal pools
64 Dripping Springs Trail	★★★★	Mountain slope	Wildflowers; views
65 La Jolla Shores to Torrey Pines Beach	★★	Beach	Unspoiled coastline
66 Torrey Pines State Reserve	up to ★★	Coastal hills	Unique pines; wildflowers; views
67 Los Penasquitos Canyon	★★	Coastal canyon	Oaks; waterfall
68 Bernardo Mountain	★★★	Inland peak	Wildflowers; views
69 Cowles Mountain	★★	Inland foothill peak	Views
70 Blue Sky Ecological Reserve	★★	Inland foothill canyon	Botanical interest; views
71 Woodson Mountain	★★	Inland foothill peak	Geological formations; views
72 Iron Mountain	★★	Inland foothill peak	Views

HIKE	DIFFICULTY*	TERRAIN	PRINCIPAL ATTRACTIONS
73 El Capitan Open Space Preserve	★★★★	Foothill slopes & peak	Views
74 Doane Valley	★★	Mountain meadow	Streams; botanical interest
75 Barker Valley	★★★	Mountain slope & canyon	Waterfalls
76 Love Valley	★	Mountain meadow	Wildflowers
77 Agua Caliente Creek	★★★	Mountain canyon	Cascading stream
78 Hot Springs Mountain	★★★	Mountain peak	Views
79 Cedar Creek Falls	★★	Mountain slope	Waterfall
80 Volcan Mountain	★★	Mountain ridge	Views
81 Cuyamaca Peak	★★★	Mountain peak	Views
82 Stonewall Peak	★★	Mountain peak	Views
83 Sweetwater River	★★	Mountain canyon	Oak woodland; canyon stream
84 Horsethief Canyon	★★	Mountain canyon	Cascades & pools
85 Corte Madera Mountain	★★★	Mountain peak	Views
86 Cottonwood Creek Falls	★★	Mountain canyon	Cascades & pools
87 Noble Canyon Trail	★★★	Mountain canyon	Wildflowers; cascading stream
88 Oasis Spring	★	Mountain ravine	Hidden spring; views
89 Garnet Spring	★★	Mountain peak	Views
90 Sunset Trail	★★★	Mountain slope & meadow	Views; botanical interest
91 Culp Valley	★	Desert slope	Views; hidden spring
92 Hellhole Canyon	★★★	Desert canyon	Waterfall
93 Borrego Palm Canyon	★	Desert canyon	Cascading stream; native palms
94 Villager Peak	★★★★	Desert ridge & peak	Views; botanical interest
95 Calcite Mine	★★	Desert slope	Geological & historical interest
96 Oriflamme Canyon	★★★	Desert canyon	Waterfall
97 Ghost Mountain	★★	Desert slope	Historical interest
98 Whale Peak	★★★	Desert peak	Botanical interest; views
99 Moonlight Canyon Trail	★	Desert slope	Geological interest; views
100 Mountain Palm Springs	★★	Desert slope & ravine	Botanical interest
101 Mortero Palms to Goat Canyon	★★★	Desert canyon & slope	Botanical & historical interest

* Difficulty ratings are as follows:

★ Easy

★★ Moderate

★★★ Moderately strenuous

★★★★ Strenuous

★★★★★ Very strenuous

Recommended Reading

Anderson, Kristi and Tavernier, Arleen (eds.), *Wilderness Basics*, 3rd edition, The Mountaineers Books, 2004.

Bakker, Elna, *An Island Called California*, 2nd edition, University of California Press, 1984.

Belzer, Thomas J., *Roadside Plants of Southern California*, Mountain Press Publishing Company, 1984.

California Coastal Commission, *California Coastal Access Guide*, 6th edition, University of California Press, 2003.

Clarke, Herbert, *An Introduction to Southern California Birds*, Mountain Press Publishing Company, 1989.

Dale, Nancy, *Flowering Plants, The Santa Monica Mountains, Coastal & Chaparral Regions of Southern California*, Consortium Book Sales and Distributing, 1986.

Ferranti, Philip, *120 Great Hikes in and near Palm Springs*, Westcliffe Publishers, 2003.

Furbush, Patty A., *On Foot in Joshua Tree National Park: A Comprehensive Hiking Guide*, 4th edition, M.I. Adventure Publications, 1995.

Lightner, James, *San Diego County Native Plants*, San Diego Flora, 2004.

Lindsay, Diana and Lowell, *The Anza-Borrego Desert Region*, 4th edition, Wilderness Press, 1998.

McAuley, Milt, *Hiking Trails of the Santa Monica Mountains*, Canyon Publishing Company, 1987.

Munz, Philip A., *Introduction to California Desert Wildflowers*, University of California Press, 2004.

Munz, Philip A., *Introduction to California Mountain Wildflowers*, University of California Press, 2003.

Munz, Philip A., *Introduction to California Spring Wildflowers of the Foothills, Valleys, and Coast*, University of California Press, 2004.

Peterson, P. Victor, *Native Trees of Southern California*, University of California Press, 1972.

Raven, Peter H., *Native Shrubs of Southern California*, University of California Press, 1966.

Robinson, John W., *San Bernardino Mountain Trails*, 5th edition, Wilderness Press, 2003.

Robinson, John W., *Trails of the Angeles*, 8th edition, Wilderness Press, 2005.

Schad, Jerry, *Afoot and Afield in Los Angeles County*, 2nd edition, Wilderness Press, 2000.

Schad, Jerry, *Afoot and Afield in Orange County*, 2nd edition, Wilderness Press, 1996.

Schad, Jerry, *Afoot and Afield in San Diego County*, 3nd edition, Wilderness Press, 1998.

Schaffer, Jeffrey P., et al. *The Pacific Crest Trail: Southern California*, 6th edition, Wilderness Press, 2003.

Schoenherr, Allan A., *A Natural History of California*, University of California Press, 1995.

Sharp, Robert P. and Glazner, Allen F., *Geology Underfoot in Southern California*, Mountain Press Publishing Company, 1993.

Tway, Linda, *Tidepools of Southern California: An Illustrated Guide to 100 Locations from Point Conception to Mexico*, Consortium Book Sales and Distributing, 1991.

Agencies & Information Sources

Agua Caliente Band, Cahuilla Indians
(**ACBCI**)
(760) 416-7044

Angeles National Forest
Los Angeles River District (**ANF/LARD**)
12371 N. Little Tujunga Road
San Fernando, CA 91341
(818) 899-1900

Angeles National Forest
Santa Clara/Mojave Rivers District
(**ANF/SCMRD**)
30800 Bouquet Canyon Road
Saugus, CA 91350
(661) 296-9710

Angeles National Forest
San Gabriel River District (**ANF/SGRD**)
110 N. Wabash Ave.
Glendora, CA 91741
(626) 335-1251

Anza-Borrego Desert State Park (**ABDSP**)
P.O. Box 299
Borrego Springs, CA 92004
(760) 767-4684 *(recording)*
(760) 767-4205 *(visitor center)*
(760) 767-5311 *(administration)*

Big Morongo Canyon Preserve (**BMCP**)
(760) 363-7190

Blue Sky Ecological Reserve (**BSER**)
(858) 467-4201

Bureau of Land Management
Palm Springs (**BLM/PS**)
(760) 251-4800

Caspers Wilderness Park (**CWP**)
(949) 923-2210

Catalina Island Conservancy (**CIC**)
(310) 510-2595

Charmlee Wilderness Park (**CW**)
(310) 457-7247

Chino Hills State Park (**CHSP**)
(909) 780-6222

Cleveland National Forest
Descanso District (**CNF/DD**)
3348 Alpine Blvd.
Alpine, CA 91901
(619) 445-6235

Cleveland National Forest
Palomar District (**CNF/PD**)
1634 Black Canyon Road
Ramona, CA 92065
(760) 788-0250

Cleveland National Forest
Trabuco District (**CNF/TD**)
1147 E. 6th St.
Corona, CA 92879
(909) 736-1811

Conejo Recreation and Park District
(**CRPD**)
(805) 495-6471

Crystal Cove State Park (**CCSP**)
(949) 494-3539

Cuyamaca Rancho State Park (**CRSP**)
(760) 765-0755

Devil's Punchbowl Natural Area (**DPNA**)
(661) 944-2743

Eaton Canyon Natural Area (**ECNA**)
(626) 398-5420

Joshua Tree National Park (**JTNP**)
74485 National Monument Drive
Twentynine Palms, CA 92277
(760) 367-5500

Lake Poway Recreation Area (**LPRA**)
(858) 668-4770

Los Coyotes Indian Reservation (**LCIR**)
P.O. Box 248
Warner Springs, CA 92086
(760) 782-0711

Los Penasquitos Canyon Preserve (**LPCP**)
(858) 538-8066

Mission Trails Regional Park (**MTRP**)
(619) 582-7800

Mt. San Jacinto State Wilderness
(**MSJSW**)
(909) 659-2607

Palomar Mountain State Park (**PSP**)
(760) 742-3462

Placerita Canyon Park (**PCP**)
(661) 259-7721

Point Mugu State Park (**PMSP**)
(818) 880-0350

San Bernardino National Forest
Arrowhead District (**SBNF/AD**)
28104 Highway 18
Skyforest, CA 92385
(909) 382-2782

San Bernardino National Forest
Big Bear District (**SBNF/BBD**)
North Shore Drive, Highway 38
Fawnskin, CA 92333
(909) 382-2790

San Bernardino National Forest
San Gorgonio District (**SBNF/SGD**)
34701 Mill Creek Rd.
Mentone, CA 92359
(909) 382-2881

San Bernardino National Forest
San Jacinto District (**SBNF/SJD**)
54270 Pinecrest
Idyllwild, CA 92549
(909) 382-2921

San Diego County Parks and Recreation
Department (**SDCP**)
(858) 694-3049

San Dieguito Regional Park (**SDRP**)
(858) 674-2270

Santa Monica Mountains Conservancy
(**SMMC**)
(310) 858-7272

Santa Monica Mountains National Recreation Area (**SMMNRA**)
401 W. Hillcrest Drive
Thousand Oaks, CA 91360
(805) 370-2301

Santa Rosa Plateau Ecological Reserve
(**SRPER**)
(909) 677-6951

Santa Susana Pass State Historic Park
(**SSPSHP**)
(310) 454-8212

Santiago Oaks Regional Park (**SORP**)
(714) 973-6620

Torrey Pines State Reserve (**TPSR**)
(858) 755-2063

Whiting Ranch Wilderness Park (**WRWP**)
(949) 923-2245

Will Rogers State Historic Park (**WRSHP**)
(310) 454-8212

Index

About the Author

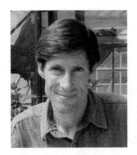

Jerry Schad's several parallel careers have encompassed interests ranging from astronomy and teaching to photography and writing. He teaches astronomy and physical science at San Diego Mesa College, and currently chairs the Physical Sciences Department there.

Schad has run or hiked many thousands of miles of distinct trails throughout California, in the Southwest, and in Mexico. He is a sub-24-hour finisher of Northern California's 100-mile Western States Endurance Run, and has served in a leadership capacity for outdoor excursions as close as San Diego County and as far away as Madagascar. More information can be found at Schad's website: www.skyphoto.com

BOOKS BY JERRY SCHAD

50 Southern California Bicycle Trips
101 Hikes in Southern California
Adventure Running
Afoot & Afield in Los Angeles County
Afoot & Afield in Orange County
Afoot & Afield in San Diego County
Back Roads and Hiking Trails, The Santa Cruz
  Mountains
Backcountry Roads and Trails, San Diego County
California Deserts
Cycling Orange County
Cycling San Diego
Physical Science: A Unified Approach
Top Trails Los Angeles
Trail Runner's Guide San Diego

Other Jerry Schad Books from Wilderness Press

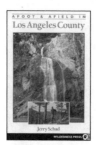

Afoot & Afield in Los Angeles County

Covering all the best L.A. adventures, from strolling along at Malibu Lagoon State Beach to trekking up a mountain on Catalina Island. Close to 200 trips explore the City of Angels' own backyard, traveling through a variety of climate zones and revealing a diverse array of plant and animal life.
ISBN 0-89997-267-5

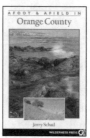

Afoot & Afield in Orange County

Whether you're up for exploring marine life at the Bolsa Chica Reserve or climbing Santiago Peak in the Santa Anas, or anything in between, this guide shows the way. Details 72 salubrious outings in every kind of natural environment, from teeming tidepools to windswept mountaintops.
ISBN 0-89997-206-3

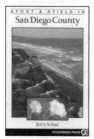

Afoot & Afield in San Diego County

San Diego's best-selling comprehensive hiking guidebook, featuring 220 detailed descriptions of every trail worth taking, from Torrey Pines to the Carrizo Badlands and beyond. Catalogs the best trips along the coast, through the foothills, up the mountains, and across the desert.
ISBN 0-89997-229-2

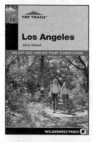

Top Trails Los Angeles

A succinct and portable guide to the 48 must-do hikes in the greater L.A. area. Get going fast with the "don't-get-lost" trail milestones, innovative trail-feature tables and more of Schad's insight and insider's knowledge of the best trails in the Southland.
ISBN 0-89997-347-7

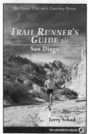

Trail Runner's Guide San Diego

A comprehensive guide to running the myriad trails of sun-soaked San Diego, from the beach at La Jolla to the summit of Palomar Mountain. Runners and hikers alike will appreciate the detailed descriptions of 50 exhilarating routes. Includes climate and topography tips, maps, photos, and more.
ISBN 0-89997-308-6

For ordering information, contact your local bookseller or Wilderness Press, www.wildernesspress.com